On the morning of January 22, 1982, Dr Charles
year-old with a world of possibilities at his feet.
was a quadriplegic facing death or at least, a life s
and mental disability. Possessing both the kno
anatomy and an indomitable will, Charles Krebs decided that whatever it took, he would walk again, and he did. He made the heroic journey back to wholeness in body, mind and spirit. An inspiration to anyone who has faced debilitating failure or the intrusion of sudden misfortune, this book also stands as the seminal text for the dawning era of energetic medicine. In seeking the scientific explanation for his own miraculous recovery, Dr Krebs synthesised the vast bounty of knowledge of the function of the human body and brain—from the 5,000 year-old texts of the East, to the very frontiers of Western neuroscience. Essentially, however, this highly readable book is about you. About why you are who you are.

Charles T. Krebs, PhD

Charles has over nine years teaching experience as an Associate Professor of Biology at St Mary's College of Maryland, part of the University of Maryland, and fifteen years research experience, including two years as Head of the Water Quality Laboratory of the Environmental Protection Authority of Victoria, and has published a number of scientific papers. Since 1984 Charles has studied Kinesiology and Eastern Energetic Sciences, and is currently Co-Director of Melbourne Applied Physiology, Instructor/Trainer for Applied Physiology in Australia, and Co-Principal of the Kinesiology College of Energetic Sciences in Melbourne. Since 1988, working with Clinical Psychologists, Speech Pathologists, Neurologists and other health professionals, Charles and his partner, Susan McCrossin, developed the Learning Enhancement Advanced Program (LEAP), a very effective program for the correction of most learning problems. LEAP is based on the neurophysiology of the brain and uses highly specific Kinesiological formatting to address stress within specific brain structures.

Charles is known for his clear and informative presentation of Kinesiology, Anatomy and Physiology. As well as conducting a busy clinical practice and teaching in the three year long Practitioner Training at the Kinesiology College of Energetic Sciences in Melbourne, he tours Australia and Europe lecturing and demonstrating Applied Physiology techniques to graduate practitioners and lay students.

Green Angel Press
7121 New Light Trail
Chapel Hill, NC 27516

Copyright 1998 CHARLES KREBS

All rights reserved. No part of this book may be reproduced in any form or by any electronic or mechanical means, including information storage and retrieval systems, without permission in writing from the copyright owner and above publisher of this book, except by a reviewer who may quote brief passages in a review.

Cover design: Concept and photograph David Verrall
Design Deborah Snibson, Modern Art Production Group
Typeset by Midland Typesetters, Maryborough, Victoria
Printed by: Axess Printing Cumming, Georgia
Reprinted with all North American rights 2007 Green Angel Press

Library of Congress Cataloguing-in-publication data

Krebs, Charles T.
A revolutionary way of thinking: from a near-fatal accident to a new science of healing / Charles T. Krebs Ph. D.
p. cm.
Includes Bibilography and index
1. Health 2. Kinesiology 3. Energy Medicine I. Brown, Jenny II Title
ISBN 978-0-9658065-3-4

Printed in The United States. First North American Edition April 2007

A Revolutionary Way of Thinking

From a near fatal accident to a new science of healing

by

DR CHARLES KREBS
and Jenny Brown

Green Angel Press
Chapel Hill, NC

Dedication

To all who have experienced learning difficulties, and to their friends and families, so that they may finally understand themselves with greater compassion.

Thank you

To Dr Stephen Sommer for creating the connection, publisher Michelle Anderson for being inspired by the idea, and to Jenny Brown, my right hand and co-writer for her stamina, for keeping me on track and for showing me when to tell another story.

To graphic artists Lynne Coleman and Elizabeth Wirt for their detailed drawings and to Louise Barrett for the computer graphics and for being my secretary extraordinaire. To photographer David Verrall for the cover photograph and the photographs in Chapter 8 of Phil Atkinson.

To James Harrison for undertaking the long haul of text editing with patience and elegance, to Pauline Sculli, Max McManus and Pollyanna Sutton for reviewing the early drafts and for their pragmatic suggestions.

To Professor Emeritus William Tiller for allowing use of his model of Positive and Negative-Space/Time and for critically reviewing Part 3 of the text. To Dr Wayne Topping for his factual suggestions, Gordon Dickson for his valuable information on the origins of kinesiology, to Dr Graeme Jackson for his expertise on hippocampal function, memory, learning and brain damage. To Dr Carla Hannaford, Dr Harry Marget and Dr Peter Bourke for their encouragement and critical reviews.

A Special Acknowledgement

To my wife, Susan McCrossin, for the ideas and for the many hours of 'our' time that were devoted to this book. Even more importantly were the four years she devoted to validating the efficacy of the Learning Enhancement Advanced Program (LEAP) for the correction of learning problems by the scientific studies she conducted in the course of obtaining her dual Bachelor of Science in Psychology and Neuroscience and her Honours Degree in Neuroscience.

AUTHOR'S NOTE

In this book I will introduce you to the new energetic healing science of kinesiology by looking particularly at what it can achieve when applied to learning difficulties.

Kinesiology and acupressure-based programs like Edu-K and Learning Enhancement Advanced Program (LEAP), can change people's lives in a way that allows their true self-confidence to flourish. The miraculous cure is nothing more or less than connecting a person more fully to their true learning potentials.

How many people do you know who have ability and potential but who never realise their promise because of a lack of self confidence in themselves and their abilities? They learn to place a lower and lower value on themselves. First they stop shooting for goals, then they stop making them.

With kinesiology, we appear to have found a way to facilitate a release from grinding cycles of frustration, anger, despair, alcoholism, substance abuse, emotional problems and often crime, just some of the fruits of learning difficulties. In most communities this list constitutes the core of serious social problems.

So what if you could be reconnected to your real innate intelligence? What if, without stress, you really were able to express yourself more fully—more easily? For one thing you could reclaim your birthright, and more importantly, reach beyond your own survival needs to make a contribution to the greater good. To society.

In some area of function in our lives we are all dyslexic. No matter how smooth the plan, there will always be blocks that brings us undone and which seem to be based in old patterns and reactions. The area of function in which we lose our brain integration then affects the choices we make and by degrees, begins to affect the expression of our spirit.

As we move into the 21st century, the world is just going to get faster and we need to be functioning with more efficient brain integration to meet these demands. Already we are changing jobs two or three times in a working life. We are also being asked to adapt to technology at a phenomenal rate.

In his lifetime (1608–1674), the poet John Milton could claim to have read every book published in the English language. Today we couldn't hope to read a fraction of what is published this year. But already, the information revolution doubles the amount of written communication published about every five years.

Until the middle decades of this century life was primarily a physical challenge. Today it is a mental one. Never before has human kind been asked to integrate so much information, so fast and while using the same evolutionary biological and neurological structure as before. The evidence is mounting that it is us human beings who are beginning to slow the pace.

We are being challenged with a critical question: What is our real speed and adaptability; what is the real capacity of the human body and mind? As the century unfolds, inevitably it will demand more. And even if we can mentally cope into the future, will our emotions, reflexes and deeply held instinctive reactions hold us up?

In this book I make the case for looking at the potential for truly smoothing the path forward for human beings by healing the body-mind-spirit. This is done through the remarkable application of a tool which combines an ancient energetic model with 5000 year old roots, and a modern western health discipline that discovered the accuracy of muscle feedback as a diagnostic tool. The analogy of the bio-computer serves to make some sense of how it operates.

As simple as the equation might seem on the surface, I sincerely believe that the advent of kinesiology, which after all only has a 30 year history, could mark the dawn of a profound era of energetic healing.

JENNIFER M. BROWN CO-AUTHOR

A freelance writer with 30 years experience in print, radio and television journalism, Jenny's abiding interest has been in presenting the stories of creative and inspiring individuals to the greater public. She has found these people in the arts, food, tourism, human and social services and latterly, in the health field. Sensing the potency of the alternative health movement, Jenny became an early advocate for their ideas and the exploration has resulted in co-authorship of two books, *Healing With Words*, with Dr Robert McNeilly, and *A Revolutionary Way of Thinking*, with Dr Charles Krebs—a labour of love that took three fascinating years to realise.

CONTENTS

Introduction	1
Part ONE	
Exploring beneath Skull Rock	3
Chapter One	
CHARLES KREBS' STORY	5
Diving to the Depths	5
A Raft on the Ocean	25
Terra Firma	30
Chapter Two	
WHAT IS KINESIOLOGY?	40
The Origins: Academic Kinesiology	40
Applied Kinesiology	43
Essential Ch'i	45
Interweaving Yin and Yang	48
Touch for Health	52
Clinical Kinesiology	54
Kinesiology: Using Muscle Response	55
The Subconscious Rules	58
Survival First	60
The Muscle-Emotion Interface	61
Emotional Stress Defusion	63
Experiencing Kinesiology	64
A Far-Reaching Healing Science	67

PART TWO
How to have a fully functional brain 71
Introduction 72

Chapter Three
MAPPING A MARVELLOUS ENTITY 73
Brain Structure and Function 73
The Neuron: Where It all begins 74
The Brain as a Three-Tiered Structure 80
The Hierarchy of the Triune Brain 82
The Small Brain 83
The Structure of the Cortex 85
THE AMAZING TERRAIN OF THE HUMAN BRAIN 87
Significant Sites of Perception and Processing 90
The Site of Mental Processing 92
The Heart of the Matter 95
White Matter: The Routes of Integration 95
Grey Matter: Where All the Decisions are Made 100
The Origins of the Subconscious 102
The Limbic System: Where Emotions Arise 111
Where Memory and Emotions Meet 116

Chapter Four
THE REMARKABLE REACH OF MEMORY 121
What Does the Brain Do? It Learns and Remembers 121
What is Known 123
The Neural Substrate of Conscious Memory 123
Reward and Punishment 128
Conscious Memory: Long-term and Short-term 131
Consolidation of Memory 134
Working Memory 136
Episodic Memory 139
Memories are Made of This: Replication or Recreation? 140
Memory Reconstruction: Can It be Trusted? 142
Rememberance of Things Unknown: Explicit/Implicit Memory 144
Dual Perception-Memory Systems: The Subconscious Control
   of Behaviour 148
Act First and Live: Think About it Later 152
Association Responses 153
Memory Triggers 156

Chapter Five
THE MIRACLE OF LEARNING 159
Learning What is Relevant 159
The Process of Learning 160
Brain Dominance: The Right and Left Hemispheres 161
Redefining the Terms 163
Concepts of Logic and Gestalt 164
Models of Learning based on Logic and Gestalt 169
Blocks in Mental Processing: Organic Blocks/Functional Blocks 171
Gestalt and Logic Lead Functions 174

Chapter Six
MAJOR PATTERNS OF DYSFUNCTION 176
Learning Difficulties 176
Major Types of Logic and Gestalt Function 176
Patterns of Dysfunction: 181
Gestalt Dominance in Mental Processing 182
Logic Dominance in Mental Processing 184
Limited Access to Gestalt and Logic in Mental Processing 185
Poor Integration of Gestalt and Logic in Mental Processing 186
The Stress Loop 188

Chapter Seven
THE NATURE OF BRAIN INTEGRATION 192
Brain Integration and Performance 192
The Choreography of Thought 193
The Stress Factor 195
The Corpus Callosum: The Routes of Integration 197
The Terrible Twos: a Crucial Age in the Loss of Integration 198
Other Integrative Pathways 202
The Role of Subconscious Processing Centres in Brain Integration 204
The Loss of Brain Integration 205

Chapter Eight
LOSS OF BRAIN INTEGRATION: WHAT YOU CAN DO ABOUT IT 207
Factors Causing a Loss of Brain Integration 207
Acupressure Techniques that affect the Brain 209
Movement and the Brain 211
I Move, Therefore I Think 214
Movement and Sensory Experience 216
Movement and the Vestibular System: Paying Attention 218

Self Help for a Disintegrated Brain	221
Further Acupressure Techniques	222
Physical Movement Techniques	231
The Whole is Worth More than the Sum of its Parts	240
Emotional Stress Defusion Techniques	240
A Daily Stress Defusion Technique	243

Chapter Nine
BRAIN INTEGRATION IN ACTION

BRAIN INTEGRATION IN ACTION	246
Deep Interventions	246
The Evolution of a New Kinesiological Paradigm	246
Damaged Hardware: Organic Brain Damage	248
Software Problems: Functional Shutdown	250
The Learning Enhancement Advanced Program: LEAP	253
LEAP in Application	254
Brain Integration under the Microscope	261
Hyperactivity and LEAP	266
LEAP into the Future	269
The Success Loop	271

Chapter Ten
ENVIRONMENTAL FACTORS THAT CAN AFFECT THE BRAIN

ENVIRONMENTAL FACTORS THAT CAN AFFECT THE BRAIN	274
The Delicate Balance of Brain Integration	274
Internal Environmental Factors:	274
Hydration/Diet/Sugar	274
Supplementation	281
Allergies or Sensitivities: Food Dyes/Food Additives	286
Candidiasis	293
External Environmental Factors: Electromagnetic Radiation	299
Mobile Telephones	301
TV and Computer Screens	302
Fluorescent Lights	303
Devices for Neutralising Electromagnetic Radiation	305
Structural and Physiological Factors Affecting Brain Integration	306
Eye Muscle Balance	306
Deformed Palate	309
Crowded Teeth	310

PART THREE
The big picture — 313

Chapter Eleven
AN ALL ENCOMPASSING REALITY — 315
The Nature of Reality — 315
Two Divergent Models of Reality — 316
The Western Physical Model — 316
The Eastern Energetic Model — 318
An Integrated Model of Reality — 319
Aspects of Positive and Negative-Space/Time — 319
Positive Space/Time, Physical Reality — 320
Negative Space/Time, Metaphysical Reality — 322
The Paradox of Life — 325
The Multi-Dimensional Being: — 327
  The Physical Body — 327
  The Etheric Body — 328
  The Astral Body — 329
  The Mental Body — 329
  The Causal or Spiritual Body — 330
Chakras—Spinning Wheels of Light — 330
Chakras and Physiology — 333
The Chakras and the Nadi System — 336
Chakras and the Subtle Bodies — 338

Chapter Twelve
REALMS OF CONSCIOUSNESS — 342
Defining the Mind — 342
Mind: Subtle Structure and Function — 343
Mind: The Neurological Substrate — 345
What is Consciousness? — 346
Near-Death Experiences — 347
Out-of-Body Experiences — 350
Lessons from Near-Death and Out-of-Body Experiences — 354
Mind: The Instrument of Consciousness — 355
Focusing the Mind — 357
The Power of Will — 359
Mind to Mind — 359

The Heart and Mind in Healing	361
Beyond Mind. Higher Consciousness	363
References	365
Source of Illustrations	394
Appendices	396
Index	408

INTRODUCTION

By Dr John F Thie DC
Author Touch for Health.
Founding Chairman International
College of Applied Kinesiology.
Founding President Touch for Health
Foundation and Association, USA
Research Director International
Kinesiology College, Switzerland

Why is it, I have often wondered, that some people find learning easy and others don't?

I've been a student and a teacher. I'm a parent and a grandparent and still find it hard to justify why some individuals manage to breeze through life without seeming effort while others struggle so hard to make the distance. We can accept differences but some are so great it just doesn't seem fair.

Charles Krebs understands. He has lived both and gained some powerful insights in the process.

Through a dramatic sequence of events, Charles learned the difference between success that could be taken for granted and the bitter blows of continual failure; the daily shattering of self esteem that comes from not ever being good enough. Almost overnight he plunged from athletic and academic excellence into an abyss of physical and mental disability.

Reading the account of his diving accident, his struggle for survival, and his return to meaningful life as an international teacher of the new healing science of kinesiology, can give hope to anyone. It shows that whatever the obstacles, it is possible to repair the essentially intelligent design of the human body and mind to regain an equal place in life.

Charles has done more. In his research into the miracle of his own healing, which led him to explore the function and dysfunction of the human brain and how it can be affected by the techniques of kinesiology, he has begun to make a real contribution to both learning and health sciences.

This book contains some of the clearest presentations of methods that can enable almost anybody to learn more easily. It also leaps beyond the bounds of structure and functional physiology to consider the interplay of mind and consciousness in all of our experiences.

With Dr Krebs, I believe that life is about learning, doing and being. And further, that when we are able to express ourselves to the highest possible degree, we are in a position to fulfill the divine purpose of our life with more ease, compassion and joy.

Charles found his purpose the hard way but like so many others in the Touch for Health/Kinesiology field, he has a passionate humanitarian determination to share his knowledge and skills to smooth the way forward for others.

Touch for Health/Kinesiology originated in the groundbreaking work of Dr George Goodheart who only 30 years ago discovered the nexus between western physical science and eastern energetic medicine. Since that time it has profoundly and positively affected the lives of millions of people around the globe.

Practitioners are constantly finding new techniques, swapping discoveries and adding into an ever-expanding paradigm of healing through touch. At international meetings these days there is need for simultaneous translation into five languages. It is a very exciting time to be involved in the exploration.

The model of brain integration that Charles and his wife Susan McCrossin have constructed represents another major step forward and this book is a brilliantly realised presentation of that work.

I know it will fascinate not only those in the healing and learning fields, but is the book for anyone with a true desire to become a fully-functioning, mindful human being.

PART ONE

Exploring beneath skull rock

Who is this whose ignorant words
Cloud my design in darkness?
Brace yourself and stand up like a man;
I will ask the questions and you will answer.
Have you descended to the springs of the sea,
or walked the unfathomable deep?
Have the gates of death been revealed to you?
Have you ever seen the doorkeepers of the
gates of darkness?
Have you comprehended the vast expanse
of the world?
Come, tell me all of this, if you know?

God's question to Job
from *Ego and Archetype*
Edward S. Edinger

Chapter One

CHARLES KREBS' STORY

DIVING TO THE DEPTHS

In German, my name means crab which is coincidental because professionally I trained and worked as a marine biologist, studying crabs. In the early 1970s I had completed my PhD at the Marine Biological Laboratory in Wood's Hole on Cape Cod, Massachusetts, and later had collaborated on some research projects with a gifted scientist named Kathy Burns. Kathy and I had hoped to do a lot more work together but these plans were shelved when she accepted an appointment to work in Australia.

The great island continent in the Southern Hemisphere had always fascinated me. When I was a small boy I had a desk in my room that had a map of the world across its surface. For some reason, I would find myself staring at this island and imagining the adventures I might have there. That fascination never waned.

So in 1980 when Kathy and her husband Robert invited my wife and me to visit them, we jumped at the chance. They had just finished building a 14-metre yacht and wanted us to join them on its maiden voyage from Melbourne on the Australian mainland, south to the little island state of Tasmania.

It was a wonderful trip, and after it Ansley and I had enough time to return to Melbourne to explore the city and some of the surrounding countryside. We loved it. We loved the openness of the people and of the land. I loved the trees.

There is something incredibly emotional for me about gum trees that I can't explain because in upstate New York, where I had grown up, there were lots of oaks and maples but no gum trees. Yet somehow the sight of a gum tree, silhouetted at dusk against a big gloaming Australian sky really affected my heart. It was an uncanny feeling of being wholly connected to a place in which I was, to all intents and purposes, a stranger.

Ansley and I very much wanted to spend more time in Australia, so towards the end of our holiday I met with the director of the Victorian Marine Science Laboratory and was interviewed for a job that was due to come up in about a year.

We returned to the States and, sure enough, when the position of research scientist was advertised internationally, I applied and was duly appointed to develop a marine pollution monitoring program for the Victorian Government.

In July 1981 we returned to Australia and took up residence in the small, charming and historic coastal town of Queenscliff, where the marine laboratory is based.

I'd been working for only about six months when another couple we had met through Bob and Kathy, Alison and Peter Barker, invited the four of us to join them on their 12-metre dive boat, *The Orca*, for a week's diving off a beautiful national park called Wilson's Promontory. This is one of Victoria's oldest national parks, a huge triangle of land with a granite core that has defied the fury of Bass Strait storms to remain the southernmost tip of mainland Australia.

Alison and Peter had a hunch that on a previous trip they may have spotted the wreck of an old ship that had foundered off the 'Prom' last century. They were hoping to locate it this time.

I was 35, at the peak of my fitness and keen to try anything. All through my life I'd been one of the lucky ones who had found most physical and academic endeavors easy. I had my doctorate. I was a good downhill skier. I was running three to six kilometres every day and playing A-grade basketball and volleyball. I practised karate two to three times a week and had played golf for only a week before I was shooting under 100.

A week of diving in the height of the summer sounded like heaven to me.

Off Wilson's Promontory the waters vary in depth from 15 to more than 90 metres. They are cold and very, very clear. In one place, we explored enormous underwater rock sculptures made up of huge granite boulders, some up to 30 metres high, piled one on the other. In between were crevices and caves that we could swim in and out of. The caves were full of fascinating marine organisms; hydroids with their frilly plankton-catching feet, spectacularly colored sea stars and gardens of iridescent algae, all of which I knew so it was like visiting old friends.

It was, however, the first time that I had ever swum with seals. Seals are amazing. They are so awkward on land yet are unbelievably graceful in the water and have great big, flirtatious brown eyes. The females are very inquisitive. Some would swim right up to me and poke their faces into my mask as if to ask: 'What are you doing here?' Fortunately, the 250-kilogram males aren't so curious.

I remember one wonderful moment when I was peering into a cave and found two seals looking in with me. One had tucked herself under my arm and another was leaning over my shoulder. I wished I'd brought a camera.

During that week, we had been progressively building up to do the dive to search the bottom for *The Conowara*. Alison and Peter presumed it would be about 60 metres down, about the limit of scuba diving using compressed air.

For a very deep dive you don't just plunge in. At the surface, the air is 78 percent nitrogen, a substance that is normally not very soluble in the blood, but which at greater pressure begins to dissolve in the blood. As you go deeper in water, which is 800 times the density of air, the scuba works by pushing both oxygen and the nitrogen into your lungs and bloodstream at increasing pressure.

At the surface there is one atmosphere of pressure. Ten metres under water the pressure is two atmospheres. At 20 metres you are at three atmospheres; at 30 metres, four atmospheres, and so on. As the pressure builds, so the air needs to be forced into your lungs at greater pressure, which means increasingly higher levels of nitrogen are accumulating in your blood.

Beyond 30 metres, you actually start getting enough nitrogen to affect your brain function. In diving, this can lead to a syndrome known as 'intoxication' or 'rapture of the deep'. In medicine it is called 'nitrogen narcosis'. The common wisdom has it that at 30 metres you feel as though you've consumed one martini; at 46 metres it feels like you've had two and at 60 metres you might as well have drunk three.

I'd been to 60 metres a number of times—always in warm tropical waters—and had only ever been narced once. That happened when I was doing research off the Marshall Islands, a US Protectorate in the western Pacific which boasts some of the most unspoilt coral reefs in the world. There I'd been doing research on marine organisms and diving every day—a wonderful job to be paid for.

One day I'd gone to 55 metres and was trying to place some soft coral into an equally soft plastic bag. I would open the bag and then lift the coral to put it in and the bag would collapse. I'd put the coral down, wrestle the bag open, pick up the coral and the bag would collapse again. After trying this about half a dozen times I realised I wasn't being too mentally acute and when I was tempted to pat a couple of sharks that were swimming nearby, I realised it was time to get back to the surface.

At Wilson's Prom, we were diving off a landmark called Skull Rock, a single piece of granite about 60 metres high and a half a kilometre long. On one side, this rock has a huge cleft and in certain lights it can indeed look like a gigantic human skull. As it turned out, it was a propitious place to be diving.

We had planned to take our last dive to look for the wreck. The whole week leading up to it had been about progressively acclimatising ourselves to deeper and deeper levels to progressively activate cavitation points in the body that can release nitrogen bubbles into the tissues. This is the process that can lead to a condition known as the bends.

On that last day, January 22, 1982, Alison, Peter and I suited up, strapped on our tanks and dropped a buoy line over the side. It stopped at 60 metres. We plunged in and as we went down the line, pulling ourselves hand over hand, we entered the ethereal world of the deep sea, a mysterious, silent realm with eerie lighting. As you go down, the clear blue of the surface water melts into a darker, deeper green.

We swam down for several minutes and at about 53 metres, found ourselves swimming through an extraordinary thermocline—the demarcation between a warm layer of water resting on a cold layer of water. The difference in temperature between the layers was about 10 or 12 degrees Celsius, so sharp that it was like crossing some invisible marine border. I could reach my hand down into the cold water below while my body was still in the warm water above.

Once we got through the thermocline, we were beyond any trace of plankton and the water underneath was incredibly clear, some of the clearest water I had ever seen. We could see 30 metres ahead. We could now see the bottom and here again were these boulders and caves, a few bottom-dwelling Port Jackson sharks and myriad brightly colored marine creatures encrusting every surface. At the bottom we all stopped for a few moments, staring in awe at the underwater world.

We synchronised watches and went off in different directions to search for the wreck.

I spent my time inspecting in and around some of the bigger boulder formations. Swimming over the shoulder of one rock, I must have plunged down about four metres, which meant I was at about 65 metres: deeper than I had ever been before.

Suddenly, I started to feel incredibly anxious. This is an aspect of nitrogen narcosis that is not often mentioned because divers are supposed to be tough, adventurous types.

But I found myself panicking for no reason that I could rationalise, and of course when you're panicking you breathe more quickly and deeply. It probably lasted only about 20 seconds and fortunately, I saw Alison was quite close by. To gain some comfort from the gripping state of panic, I swam towards her and as soon as I touched her shoulder, the anxiety passed as inexplicably as it had come on. Feeling pretty stupid, I tapped my watch to indicate that we only had about 10 minutes left before we were due to surface.

We didn't find the wreck so we regathered and started swimming slowly back up the line, stopping on the way to breathe and rest. The purpose of decompression stops is to allow that excess nitrogen to be degassed from the blood, out across the lung membrane and into the breath. We spent 15 minutes at 18 metres and half an hour at 10 metres, so by the time we got to the surface we had, theoretically, expiated all the nitrogen.

By the time we got to the last decompression stop there was a lot of movement on the line. It was getting turbulent at the surface and holding the line made us sway around quite a bit. I began to run out of air. I must have used a lot of air up in the panic attack, but it presented no real problem because Peter had an extra breathing device on his tank so I was able to breathe off his rig.

We got to the surface, clambered back on the boat and were talking excitedly about what a spectacular dive it had been, even though we hadn't found the wreck.

I went to pull my wetsuit top over my head and 'Wow! Jesus!' A sharp pain in my right elbow. A type one bend—a joint bend. Even though it was the first time I'd ever experienced one, I knew what it was.

Consider how bubbles form in carbonated soft drink when you take the cap off and release pressure suddenly. A similar thing happens in the body to cause the bends. If, after you've pushed all that nitrogen into your blood but haven't degassed it properly from your blood, it can be released inside your body.

When you extend your arm or leg, the excess nitrogen pops into a bubble inside synovial fluid of the joints. It puts pressure on the surrounding tissues and because that pressure hurts, you tend to bend your limbs in close to your body to contain the pain—thus they are fittingly named. I had the bends.

Realising this, Peter and I made a decision to do what is called a wet recompression. We put our wetsuits back on, grabbed two new tanks of air and jumped back into the water. We went down again to 10 metres and the second we got there, my elbow joint stopped hurting. We stayed at this depth for another 30 minutes, just breathing and looking at each other. It was pretty boring and it was getting cold so after we'd done the requisite time, we followed the stream of ever-expanding bubbles back up to the surface.

Apart from the fact that I had been in the water now for a couple of hours, I felt great. I went into the cabin to make a cup of tea and noticed on the shelf a medical book on diving. As I had just experienced a bend, I took the book down and started reading. The book said type one bends are by far the most common, and although they are painful this should disappear within eight to 10 days as the nitrogen is slowly absorbed out of the synovial fluids, back into the blood and then breathed out. They weren't life threatening.

Then I started reading about type two bends—cerebro-spinal bends. These are less common but much more dangerous, the result of nitrogen bubbles forming inside the spine. Because the spine is a bony cage, nitrogen bubbles that form in it can only expand by crushing the surrounding tissue. If a bubble gets big enough it can also block the blood flow, which leads to hypoxia, or oxygen starvation, and the neurons begin to die. The same thing can happen in the brain. According to the book, type two bends were potentially lethal.

I was reading this technical detail with some interest when I realised I needed to take a pee. One of the other details mentioned in the book about cerebro-spinal bends was that when it is starting to happen, you can get the staggers. Because motor co-ordination is affected, you start to stagger about like a drunk. But the clincher is that you cannot pass urine, which indicates that some of the function of the spinal column is beginning to shut down.

As I started to walk to the boat's toilet I was surprised to find I was terribly unco-ordinated. When I attempted to pee, I couldn't. Oh no! Type two bends. I had both symptoms. I came out, staggered over to Peter and said: 'I think I'm in a bit of trouble here.'

As it happened, we had already weighed anchor and were heading in to Tidal River, the only settlement on Wilson's Promontory. There we were due to meet up with a doctor friend, David Iser. We radioed him to get to the rendezvous point as quickly as he could; I suspected I was coming down with type two bends.

David immediately told us to contact two other doctors, Geoff Macfarlane and Paul McCallum, who run a medical clinic at the nearby regional centre of Bairnsdale. Because they take care of the deep sea and abalone divers who work on the oil rigs and fishing boats off the far eastern coast of Victoria, they know quite a bit about decompression sickness. Geoff Macfarlane suggested that I be taken straight to the little medical centre near the Ranger's station at Tidal River and there be put straight onto pure oxygen and five percent Dextrose, an intravenous sugar solution.

'Great', I thought. 'Once I get there I'll be fine. This is all very interesting but it'll be over in a little while.'

Geoff Macfarlane said he would arrange for a helicopter to fly me out to the big Esso barge, *The Polaris*, that was anchored about 45 kilometres away. He would meet me there. *The Polaris* had a big decompression chamber on board.

After motoring through rolling seas for an hour and a half, we finally got into Tidal River and by that stage I had the staggers pretty badly. Getting me off *The Orca* and into a dinghy was quite a challenge with the see-sawing of the two vessels in the two-metre seas.

On land I was shaking violently with every step but I still had to feel sorry for the doctor who was temporarily resident in Tidal River to look after the summer campers. He knew very little about the bends and when he saw me coming towards him he could only wonder if he was looking at an emotional basket case. He asked me if I was hysterical. 'No,' I said, 'I always walk like this.'

We got into the surgery and this doctor was in such a flap that he couldn't get the oxygen tank organised. Fortunately my friend David arrived and took over.

He was just in time. I was in agony. I'd been in cold water for hours, had been drinking copious amounts of tea and couldn't pee. I tell you, if ever you want to torture anyone, all you have to do is to pinch off their urethra and make them drink a couple of litres of water. A bursting bladder with no outlet causes the most excruciating pain imaginable.

There was nothing like a catheter in this out-back surgery but I was begging for somebody to do something—anything. David offered to give me an abdominal puncture to relieve the pressure. He took a big bore needle and stuck it through my abdominal wall into my bladder, without an anaesthetic. A stream of urine exploded across the room. It was the kindest cut of all. A tube was taped to the needle and my bladder could drain. At last I was beginning to feel a bit more comfortable.

An hour passed. Slowly, I could feel my feet were becoming paralysed. I could rock them a little bit from side to side but couldn't lift them. Then I found I couldn't bend my knees very much.

A helicopter arrived on the beach. I could hear the rotor blades cutting the air. I waited. Then about half an hour later I heard it fly away again. The radio call to get me a helicopter had been intercepted by two operators: the Esso rig helicopter and the Melbourne-based air ambulance service, the Angel of Mercy. The Esso helicopter, half-way out to the rig with an exchange crew and a full load of supplies on board, was about to turn back for me when the Angel of Mercy offered to take over the emergency lift.

The Angel had landed on the beach at Tidal River expecting to take me back to a small decompression chamber at the Prince Henry's Hospital in Melbourne. When Geoff Macfarlane was contacted about this he said: 'Don't let them take him. They'll kill him.' The hospital's chamber wouldn't be able to do the deep decompression that I needed.

The Angel had no pontoons, it couldn't fly over the water to land me on the barge. So the Angel flew away.

Meanwhile, the rig helicopter had made it out to the platform, unloaded one crew and all their gear and picked up another crew to bring back to shore. They had to fly back to their base, unload, refuel and then return to get me at Tidal River.

I had now been lying in the Tidal River surgery for three hours. It was five hours since the dive, and during that time my legs had become paralysed, my abdomen had become paralysed, my arms had become paralysed and my chest had stopped moving.

I had taught anatomy at St Mary's College at the University of Maryland and I knew that the paralysis was up around vertebrae C6 or C5 in my neck. I couldn't remember where the phrenic nerve came off the spine but I was desperately trying to recall the fact because this was the nerve that was now keeping me alive. This was the nerve that was running my diaphragm. Where did it come off the spine? C5? C4?

Until this moment I had been making subjective observations of my state. Once my chest stopped moving and I realised I was only breathing diaphragmatically, I knew I was within centimetres of death. Now I was frightened. If it went any further I was going to die. When the phrenic nerve stops, that's it!

I heard helicopter rotors again. Praise the Lord!

But even as the noise of the helicopter faded into the distance, Kathy Burns and Dr David Iser were walking along the beach. David said to Kathy, 'I don't think he's going to make it'.

I have to hand it to the helicopter pilot who flew me out to the rig because one of the things that happens as you gain altitude is that the nitrogen bubbles will keep expanding and I was already in lots of trouble. He didn't have to go very high to kill me. I was lying on the floor of the helicopter and it was flying so low over the water I could see the white caps on the waves virtually at eye line. The chopper actually had to fly up to get onto the barge's platform.

The enormous diving barge we landed on was a fairly unique vessel to be where it was at that time. Measuring about 300 metres long and about 100 metres wide, *The Polaris* carried a 3200-ton crane, used to lift oil platforms and position them on the ocean floor. It also had a saturation chamber, one of only two in the world. The other was in the North Sea, off the coast of Scotland. The saturation chambers on these barges operate in a way that streamlines the otherwise very expensive and dangerous business of building deep-sea oil rigs. It is used by the divers who weld and bolt steel deep underwater.

The danger in decompression isn't so much the fact of having nitrogen in the blood, it is when those levels change suddenly and produce the bubbles. When the original oil rigs were being set up to drill in the off-shore oil fields, stables of divers would be housed on the barges because they could only dive to the deep and work for a couple of hours before they had to resurface and undergo a long decompression. After each dive, the divers would rest for a day and a half and then go down again to work for another few hours. These guys had to be decompressed every time they came up and the danger point in the process is always the decompression.

To economise on the costs and the energy, and to minimise the decompression risks as much as possible, a system known as saturation diving had been introduced. On *The Polaris* there was the one big decompression chamber measuring about nine metres by three metres and it could house four divers who would work in rotation for periods of up to 28 days.

If the divers were working at 80 metres, the chamber and the diving bell (their commuter vehicle) would be pressurised to the same level on helium-oxygen, which is less dangerous than the nitrogen-oxygen in air. Two divers would work underwater from the bell and after shifts of four to eight hours, would come up into the saturation chamber and the two fresh divers would replace them and go down to work. This system meant the divers only had to be decompressed at the end of every 28-day shift, and they were slow, conservative decompressions.

Even so, keeping divers in these situations is similar to keeping someone alive on Mars. If you are living at seven atmospheres of pressure inside the chamber, all the helium-oxygen has to be regulated, so does the carbon dioxide and the moisture content. All the food and provisions come in and go out via air locks. All systems have to be monitored by a crew of four around the clock because if anything goes awry, the divers inside can die very quickly.

When I was landed on the rig, Geoff Macfarlane put me straight into the diving bell and it was pressurised steadily to a standard decompression depth of about 50 metres. After a few minutes at this depth I began to get some feeling back into my fingers and toes. I began to be able to move my arms, just a little. It was looking promising and I was thinking, 'That's good. I'll just get decompressed and my body will come back on line.'

The theory was that having been recompressed I would slowly be bought back up to surface pressure in stages to make sure all the nitrogen was out of my blood. I was going to be fine. But by the time we'd got back up to 30 metres of pressure, all of a sudden all my body movement went again. In an instant I was quadriplegic. I couldn't feel or move anything below my neck.

Because I had been so long with the nitrogen bubble in the neck, the blood clotting mechanism had done its work. The blood responds to a bubble in much the same way that it responds to a wound, and a clot had formed around the bubble that had lodged high in my spine. When I first went into decompression, the bubble had collapsed, but soon after, the solid clot had moved forward and was now plugging a major spinal artery. My spine was getting no oxygen at all. It was the worst of all possible situations.

Geoff Macfarlane directed that I should be immediately moved into the decompression chamber proper and here was another moment of synchronicity: that chamber is usually occupied by divers around-the-clock but now, through sheer coincidence, it was free. The crane operators, who belonged to different unions, were on strike over a demarcation issue. The divers were out chipping paint.

So I was moved in and with me came Geoff Macfarlane and a rig diver called Johnny Sullivan who had volunteered to help handle me; move me, wash me and feed me, the quadriplegic. Geoff directed that we should go to pressure of relief. So down we went again, slowly descending through two atmospheres, four atmospheres, five, six . . . seven.

Sometimes, when you go to a much greater pressure, you can get relief from symptoms because suddenly the blood can start flowing again, but by the time we'd reached 92 metres, or 10 atmospheres, Geoff said there was no reason to go any deeper; it was not going to make any difference. I could talk. I could move my head but I couldn't move anything else.

I didn't know this at the time, but even more synchronous events were colluding. Before we'd gone into the chamber, Macfarlane had called Dundee, Scotland, and talked to a colleague, Dr Phillip James, who took care of the North Sea divers and was an authority on decompression sickness. The two had met in England only a few weeks before my accident and had been tossing around a few ideas about possible alternative treatments for cerebro-spinal bends and other spinal conditions. One of their theories was that it might be possible to keep spinal tissue alive by using very high oxygen levels in a hyperbaric chamber such as the one we were in.

During this night's call they had decided that for me, maybe it represented a chance. Maybe they could give it a go. Macfarlane said to me: 'You're quadriplegic.' I said: 'You don't have to tell me that. I recognise that if I can't move my arms or my legs it usually means I'm quadriplegic.' He said: 'It is my feeling, based on hundreds of decompressions like this, that if we go back to surface pressure now, you'll be quadriplegic for the rest of your life. There is a possible treatment that we can try but it has never been tried before. If it works, you may regain a lot of function. If it doesn't, you'll die. I'll give you a couple of minutes to think about it.'

He left me there and all of a sudden the shock hit me. I turned my head to the wall. Hot tears were running down my face.

Here it is. What are you going to do? My mind was thinking, 'My God. I'm a quadriplegic. I can't move anything. What am I going to do?' I tried my best to take a positive view. I thought about all those incredible people who can do amazing things despite their physical disabilities. People who can paint wonderful pictures holding paintbrushes in their teeth. Disabled academics like Cambridge physicist Stephen Hawking who can still communicate his amazing ideas to the world via computers.

My mind was still working. I still had all my scientific knowledge. What kind of things might I be able to achieve if I had to go on as a quadriplegic? But the bottom line was, for me to have any life at all, someone—be it my wife, or a nurse—would have to give up a large part of theirs. I wouldn't be able to do anything for myself. Nothing. As positive as I was trying to be, I couldn't get away from the depressing fact that compared to what I had been before, it wasn't going to be much of a life.

I had no sensation in my chest but the heaviness in my heart was unbearable. Why do I deserve this? What have I done to deserve this?

I called Geoff back. 'Look,' I said, 'one of the most depressing things about being a quadriplegic is that you have no choice or control over your life. You can't even end your life, even if you want to. All you can do is hold your breath until you turn blue and even then, you'll start breathing automatically.

'Go for it. We'll roll the dice and see what we get because I'd much rather have more than I have now, or nothing. I'm willing to take the chance. I would rather be dead than half-alive.'

It sounds amazing now, but at that point I still had a choice, something most people in similar situations never get. I had another chance. What was equally hard was that because I was sealed inside the decompression chamber 45 kilometres offshore, I couldn't even talk to Ansley back on land. Whatever decision I made would affect her profoundly: If I chose to live as a quadriplegic, it would totally change her life and if I died, that would affect her too. I couldn't talk to her. I couldn't talk to anyone.

Macfarlane said it had to be now. I was right on the edge and if they were going to be able to save anything, we had to start immediately. We were at 10 atmospheres of pressure on 10 percent oxygen and 90 percent helium. Effectively every breath we took had 20 to 30 times as much oxygen as we would normally breathe at the surface. What was required now was to increase that level even more to diffuse oxygen across and into the starving spinal tissues to try to keep the neurons alive until the clot could be dissolved by medication. It was going to take up to three days to dissolve the clot and I didn't have three days to gamble with. By that time my spine would be dead.

The theory had never been tested. We were flying by the seat of our pants.

An oxygen mask was put over my mouth and nose and I started to breathe a mixture that contained about 200 to 300 times the level of oxygen that human beings normally breathe. It was so much oxygen that every time I took a breath it seared my lung tissue and hurt like hell. For 40 minutes every hour I had to breathe air that burned like fire. Then I'd have 20 minutes off the mask. It went on day and night. Every time the mask was presented to me, I recoiled. Could I handle another 40 minutes of agonising pain?

Macfarlane said: 'Charles, I know we're pushing oxygen toxicity. I know we're burning the surface of your lungs but we have to have the maximum oxygen we can get in there to save as much of your spine as we can. You're just going to have to bear it because if you live, your lungs will repair themselves. If you don't . . . it won't make any difference.' He didn't mince words.

I lost track of time. I didn't have a watch and couldn't have lifted my wrist to look at one anyway. Maybe it was 24 hours, maybe it was 48, I don't know. What I do know is that at the end of the treatment I began to get movement back into my shoulders and arms. Movement, but no sensation or feeling.

Gradually, so gradually, I was beginning to move again. I could hardly believe it. At first it was gross motor movement. When I first attempted to move my arm I found I had no control. Once I got it going I couldn't stop it. In fact, if I lifted my hand toward my face, I would strike myself quite hard on the forehead.

I was flailing about as though I had cerebral palsy but at least it was an indication that some of the tissue in my spine was still alive. It meant that perhaps I might only be paraplegic. The clot had dissolved and the blood flow in my spine had returned. The damage that had been done was done. At least no more was being caused.

The first day I came off the oxygen mask I was moving my arms uncontrollably. The following day I could at least stop my hand from striking my face, even though I wasn't too good at direction. By the next day, I had gained enough control to bring food to my mouth. I could pick up a bread roll and bring it up to my head where it would strike my cheek or my ear. Butter would smear all over my face as I moved the roll clumsily towards my mouth. It was messy but I could feed myself. The first time I managed to do it I cried like a baby because it represented such an incredible breakthrough. It meant that I wasn't going to be utterly dependent on somebody else for the rest of my life.

Every day I found I could move a little bit better and every movement was fantastic. By day five I could take a drink by myself. But because I'd damaged the nerves that controlled the sense of touch in my hands, senses that I haven't fully recovered to this day, I had no idea how much pressure I was applying to an object. And if I looked away for a second I couldn't tell whether my wrist was tilting. I would crush styrene cups, or drop them, and if I wasn't concentrating, would tip the liquid all over myself.

Each day Macfarlane would test me neurologically for the return of sensation and function. He would take a pin and prick the skin down my body, starting from my neck until I ceased to feel the prick. Every day he would progress further down my body before sensation was lost. At first the sensation travelled down my arms to my elbows and down my chest to my pectorals. Then it went down my forearms to the back of my hands. Sensation has never returned to my palms.

By day six, the sensation of feeling had progressed to my waist, then down my right leg. My left buttock and left leg still do not have normal touch sensation. At this point the chamber, which I had only half-jokingly been calling 'my tomb' had served its purpose. We began the slow decompression. It was going to take another four days, a long time to be lying in one place. Macfarlane, Sullivan and I had been together in that small space day and night for nearly a week and had pretty well run out of stories.

Sullivan had gone into the chamber expecting to be in there for a day. He'd planned to go out surfing the next. Little did this young, blond man know that he was going to score the role of nursemaid—bathing me daily and attending to my every need. He did whatever he could to make me comfortable. And it was his daily job to wash the entire chamber, from top to bottom with an anti-biotic solution to prevent extensive bacterial and fungal growth that was encouraged by the warm temperature, high oxygen and moisture in our otherworldly environment. He was a big, affable Aussie bloke with a heart of gold. I was deeply touched by his warmth and openness.

Macfarlane was a complete contrast in character. With his neat, jaw-rimming beard and craggy features, he showed the strain more than Sullivan. He was a man in control. I sensed he knew what he was doing and I trusted him totally. I sensed he was intense, as I can be at times, but he was unflagging in his support. Macfarlane and I had many extensive discussions about what was happening to me physiologically and neurologically. He would highlight every milestone I reached, telling me quite factually, exactly what was happening in my body.

When we ran out of conversation, I made an attempt to read a book. To understand my condition more fully, I grabbed for a book on the medical physiology of decompression sickness. I couldn't feel the pages and had great difficulty with co-ordination, so I couldn't turn them very easily. It would take me so long to turn a page that by the time I managed it, I had forgotten the sense of the last paragraph. I didn't want to turn back again because that would take me just as long, so I gave up reading and instead did some very gentle shoulder exercises on a trapeze the riggers had built for me. It was put up above my bed so I could at least lift myself.

I also started to practise writing again. I found that despite the loss of touch sensation, I could hold a pen. But all my motor patterning had been disrupted so I had to learn all over again how to write, how to even make the letters: For hours I sat there with a pen and a notepad, scribbling the letters of the alphabet: *a,a,a,a, b,b,b,b, c,c,c,c.*

The exhilaration of each tiny moment of progress was great but it was just as rapidly offset by the distraction of the physical discomfort that was arising. I hadn't been able to use my bowels for all that time. I was paralysed from the waist down and unable to push. Macfarlane and Sullivan could use the toilet in the chamber, but I couldn't and they weren't able to give me an enema because it would have been too dangerous to risk exposing bowel bacteria to such an oxygen-rich atmosphere. I was increasingly uncomfortable but at least I knew I was on my way back to the surface.

No one had ever undergone such a long, deep decompression and on the last day—day 10—I remember watching this huge dial in the chamber as it moved incrementally from 30 feet to the surface. I also remember how arresting it was to suddenly realise that Sullivan and Macfarlane didn't sound like Donald Duck after all. As the helium content had come down, so had our voices dropped, from castrati to baritone.

It was a bizarre transition that didn't completely mask the fact that those two guys had taken an incredible risk for me. In undergoing such a long compression and decompression they had taken the gamble of becoming bent themselves. They had willingly risked their lives to save mine.

I also owe my life to Esso (Exxon) for providing the manpower, facilities and funds to run this incredible rescue operation which I found out later was estimated to have cost $3 million. Helium is quite an expensive gas and every time dirty towels or food went in or out of the chamber $100 of helium was released. The only trouble with being a $3 million man is that you don't get any bionic parts.

Finally, after the longest day I had ever known, we got back to surface pressure. The doors of the chamber were opened and I was carried out on a stretcher into the midst of a bunch of burly divers who had been outside all the time, rooting for me. When I emerged they all started clapping spontaneously and at that point I experienced the most profound moment of love I had ever known. All I could see coming from the faces of these men was pure love. It was my first point of recontact with the outside world.

During all those long days *The Polaris* had been slowly moving towards the shore and when I came out of the chamber Ansley was able to come aboard to see me. Although she was trying to keep a brave face, she couldn't contain the shock or her tears. Her husband had been delivered back to her as a cripple.

I was transferred to Bairnsdale Base Hospital to stabilise for a couple of days before being moved down to the Royal Melbourne Hospital where, on February 7, I spent my 36th birthday. Some good friends came in to share it with me. One of the presents I received was a T-shirt with the word 'Jogging' printed on the front. It was a generous gesture but what could I say? I was a paraplegic. The most I could do at that stage was to stand up with support and by locking my legs until they collapsed on me again.

After a couple of weeks under observation at the Royal Melbourne, I was transferred to the Royal Talbot Rehabilitation Centre, where I shared a ward with eight other people, all of whom had suffered major spinal or head injuries. The centre was a long commute for Ansley, so she was only able to visit a couple of times a week. Apart from trying to support me, she was undergoing her own traumas. She had experienced a tough childhood; she had only recently buried her mother and was a new resident in a strange town in a strange country. She wasn't by nature as self-sustaining and outgoing as me. She was lonely, bereft and having great difficulty coping.

Even in the best of circumstances it is difficult for the mate of a profoundly injured person to cope: not only is their partner physically injured but they too are psychologically affected to an enormous degree. I was angry, depressed, self-absorbed and traumatised and it took me a long time to see she was having a terrible time, too. She would come and see me and be as supportive as she could but I was so self-focused, so obsessed with a determination that I was going to walk again, that I couldn't see the stress she was under.

My parents, too, on the other side of the world, were having their own understandable reactions to suddenly finding they had a crippled son. I remember the first time I managed to get myself out of bed and into a wheelchair without aid, I was so elated that I rang my mother in the United States. It was another major breakthrough for me, another major marker that indicated I was reducing my dependence on other people.

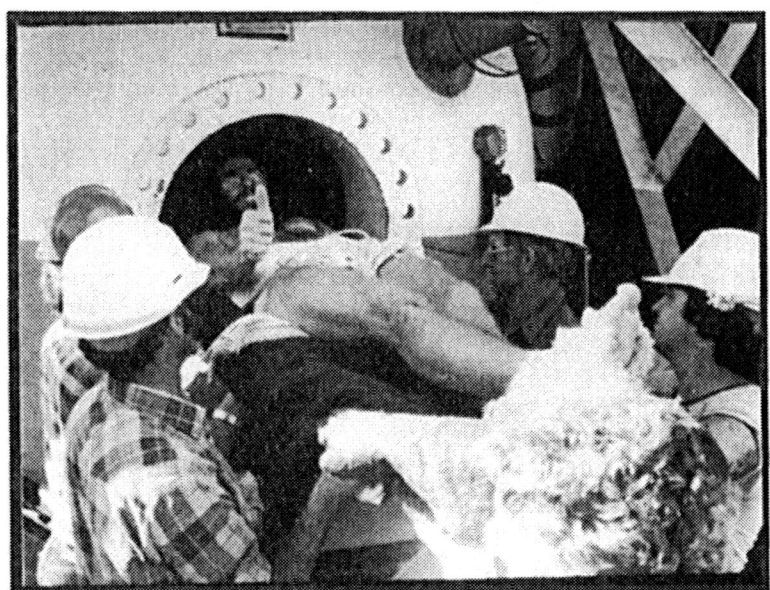

Figure 1.1. After a record 10 days in decompression Charles Krebs emerges from the chamber. PHOTOGRAPH COURTESY OF THE HERALD AND WEEKLY TIMES.

'Guess what, Mum? Today I got myself from my bed to my wheelchair without any help at all!' There was no reply. On the other end of the line all I could hear was my mother crying.

The doctors had told me I would never walk again because the nerves running into my legs had been too badly damaged. But I made a conscious decision that I was going to give it one hell of a shot. If the only other choice I had was to spend the rest of my life in a wheelchair feeling hard done by, I was going to try. I remember the day, lying in my bed looking around the ward, and saying to myself: 'Move legs'. They didn't move.

Why me? Why me? Why me? I had two choices: I could lie in my bed and piss and moan about why me and how unfair it all was. That's what most of the other people in my ward were doing. Or, I could give it my all.

For the first few weeks of my rehabilitation I would spend an hour in physiotherapy and then be put back into my bed. 'There's got to be something else I can do because at this rate I'm not going to make any progress.'

I had studied karate for a number of years and when you get to the higher levels of martial arts you begin to work with an energy known as *Ch'i*. I knew that when I broke boards and tiles with my hand, I wasn't using sheer physical force, I was using Ch'i, projected from my mind through my hand. I also knew my anatomy and physiology from teaching at university for nine years, so I knew all the muscles and nerve pathways in my body. While I was lying in my hospital bed, I started doing something that I didn't know had a name, but which I now know is called 'creative visualisation.'

I would pick a muscle in my leg that didn't work, which was pretty easy because none of them did, then I would visualise Ch'i in my mind as an electric charge and mentally project it down the visualised nerve pathways to a specific muscle. When I got to the damaged area in my neck, I would visualise the Ch'i smashing through the blockage. I focused everything I had on this process and pretty soon I was able to make the selected muscle flicker. Once I could make it flicker, just a little bit, I could then use physiotherapy exercises to make it stronger.

It had already been a month since my accident so my muscles were fairly atrophied. Yet I had a lot going for me. First, I was incredibly strong-willed. Second, I knew about Ch'i and how to direct it with my mind. Third, I knew my anatomy and physiology inside out and fourth, before my accident, I had been in phenomenal physical shape. I had been so fit that even after weeks of paralysis I had muscle tone that allowed me to detect the merest flicker in a muscle.

Every day after that I would go down to the physiotherapy gym and work out for seven hours a day. I remember one Sunday wheeling myself into the gym and one of the nurses asking me, 'What are you doing here?' I told her,

'I'm here because I don't want to be in this hospital for a minute longer than I have to be.' I wanted out. I wanted out of there real bad.

Working out took all the willpower I could summon. If I was working on my hamstring, the muscle running down the back of the thigh that lifts the heel towards the butt, I would lie on my stomach and visualise the Ch'i coursing down towards the muscle. Then I would attempt to activate the muscle and lift the leg slightly. The effort of raising my leg just a few centimetres off the table would make me sweat and shake. I'd collapse until I could recover my energy sufficiently to try again. I'd lift my leg, maybe a centimetre or two more, then collapse in a sweat. I'd try again, lift a little higher and collapse.

The next day I'd start the whole set again and keep doing it until I finally managed to get my leg all the way off the table. As soon as I could do that, I'd put a half kilogram weight on my ankle and I'd be right back to sweating and shaking and progressing by a few centimetres at a time. Once I could lift half a kilogram, I would double the load. Lift, sweat, shake, collapse. Then two kilograms, then three. Every time I increased the load I'd be right back at the start; sweating, straining and collapsing. When finally I could manage to lift my leg 10 times in a row under a five-kilogram weight, I'd start the process all over again on another muscle.

I worked out in this manner all day, every day and as I began to get more strength in my legs so I began to regain some of my dignity. I was able to get myself in and out of the shower chair. I could go to the toilet without help. I began to look around at the other people who were sharing the ward. There was Ben in the bed next to me. After undergoing surgery for tumors on his spine this young man was in a total body cast—in plaster from his neck to his knees. He'd talk to me about how he was going to take up karate once he got out of hospital. I knew that his prognosis was far worse than he was letting on.

There was Tom who had been riding his motorcycle on a very hot day. When he was within a few kilometres of his home, he removed his helmet to cool off a bit and had an accident which had left him severely brain damaged.

There was another young man, a dentist and champion distance bicycle rider who had suffered a massive stroke which had affected his mind so that he could no longer remember anything. He was in beautiful physical shape but mentally he was totally disabled.

I remember watching these young men and thinking whatever the new challenges my own situation presented, I was far better off to have a spinal problem and still have an intact mind, than to have a healthy body and a damaged brain. 'Thank you Lord. I would rather be in a wheelchair and able to think than to be able to run and not think.' I began to get some perspective on my life. I began to recognise that I had a lot to be grateful for. It could have been a whole lot worse.

I was making slow but tangible progress. After four months in the rehabilitation hospital I was getting enough strength in my leg muscles to be able to stand and shuffle. I progressed from a wheelchair to a walking frame and being upright was a real triumph. The first time the physiotherapist saw me standing up she said, 'Gosh, I didn't realise you were so tall.'

I had to practise balancing again and had to try to remember how, exactly, I used to walk. When I first tried it, I walked, or shuffled, homolaterally. That is, when I moved my right leg I would move my right arm and when I moved my left leg I would move my left arm. That's how scrambled my nervous system was. But, God, I was up and going again. I set a new goal. I was going to walk out of the hospital without a walking frame.

By the fifth month of rehabilitation I had progressed to two arm crutches and all the time was getting better at balancing. By the sixth month I was on two walking canes. I was able to walk out of the hospital—not very fast, not very steady. I walked out to pick up the pieces of my shattered life.

During all of those months Ansley had been going though her own trauma, yet I was still so self-focused that I wasn't able to give her the support she needed. Within a few weeks of arriving home I dared to realise that she was so stressed by everything that had been happening to her, and to us, that she could no longer cope.

When a situation exceeds your ability to cope mentally or emotionally there are only three courses of action open: You can leave and get yourself away from the stressful situation; you can go crazy (another way of coping); or you can kill yourself. Of those three options, leaving was by far the best thing to do. She knew it and I knew it.

It was going to be hard on me but we knew that if she stayed we would only end up hating each other. It was a horrible option for her because there were so many implications of guilt that she would carry away with her but there was no other choice. At least, if we severed the relationship here, we might be able to preserve our friendship and the memory of the love we had shared during our seven-year marriage.

Ansley left and moved to Melbourne. I stayed on in the house in Queenscliff. I was still pushing my progress like a person possessed. I made it to moving about on one cane and I started to be able to drive a car again. Yet, because I had a syndrome known as 'foot drop', and because I couldn't react physically very quickly, any little irregularity on a walking surface would cause me to catch my toe and fall. I would fall down maybe 15 to 20 times a week. I got really good at falling and would rarely hurt myself thanks to all those years of karate training.

Still, it would take me at least half a day to get going. Everything was so hard. To get out of bed was a major effort. To get into the shower and dry myself was a major effort. How do you dry your feet when you can't bend over to them? Getting dressed was a major effort and I was having to catheterize myself about four or five times a day. Everything I did took such an unbelievable amount of time that it would be 11am before I was organised.

It was so frustrating but at least I was able to go back to work for half of each day and that put me back with people again, back to some feeling of being useful. At the laboratory, I picked up a desk job, organising a major literature review looking into biomonitoring.

As I started to get further and further into this task, I began to realise that something was very wrong with the way my brain was working. The residue of the cerebro-spinal bends was showing up a new aspect. Where at first all my overt problems had been generated by the spinal damage, the cerebral or brain damage I had also suffered was beginning to show up. It hadn't been apparent until then because the damage was fairly subtle, affecting my frontal lobes. But I needed to use abstract thinking on the literature review project and this was exactly where the new problems were manifesting.

As I moved on into the project it became increasingly difficult, so I applied for time off. Time that I would use to go home to visit my family in America and time, I hoped that I could use to redress the mental scramble. I was going to be fine in just a little while. I flew home to Glens Falls in northern New York State and though it was obviously very difficult for my parents to see me as crippled as I had become, they were happy to see me and I was very, very happy to be able to spend some time with them.

To this day, I find it hard to comprehend why I didn't stay in the US. I had no wife, I wasn't sure about the job I was doing, yet I had a compulsion to return to Australia. Maybe it was Ansley. Maybe she needed me after all. Maybe I wanted to pick up my life. Maybe, if I'd stayed with my parents in that very supportive environment, I wouldn't fight so hard. Maybe I would slide into dependence. I just had a sense that for my own survival I had to go back. My mother knew it too. As hard as it must have been for her to hold back, she didn't ask me to stay.

So I went back to Queenscliff, back to work and back to the project. Within a very short time, however, it became clear I wasn't going to be able to do it. Before my accident, whenever I had needed to write anything up, I had simply reviewed all the literature, lodged the data in my brain and then selected the major themes to argue my case. It had all been very easy. Now, I was gathering the information all right but I couldn't organise it. I was left floundering in a sea of facts and I was having to negotiate longer and longer deadlines.

One day my boss, Alan Bremner, called me into his office and said, 'Charles, you're going to have to accept that there is something wrong. I'd like you to have a neuropyschological assessment. I think it's important that we're realistic about what is going on because there is clearly a difference between your performance now and the way you were working before your accident. You're going to have to face it.' The test showed, that as well as spinal damage, I had indeed suffered damage to my frontal lobes. Brain damage.

Deceiving yourself can help you marshall the will to go on, determination you may not have been able to summon had you really faced the cold, hard facts straight up. For all those months in the hospital, for all those months out of the hospital, for the entire year that has passed since the accident, I had been lying to myself that all my problems were the result of spinal bruising and that when it went away, I would be fine again. I had repeated a mantra to myself: 'I'll be back to myself soon. I'll be back to myself soon. I'll be back to myself soon.'

Now, being confronted with the results of the neurological test, my feet had been kicked out from under me again. I was devastated. I was virtually being told that I was going to be like this for the rest of my life. I couldn't kid myself any longer.

According to neuropsychological theory, six months after major damage you have seen 90 to 95 percent of all the improvement you are ever going to see. I was a hell of a long way from walking normally and now I was being told that in some sense, I was also a mental cripple.

I had never failed at anything—ever—and here I was failing one test after another. Failing again and again and again. It was the greatest lesson in humility I had ever faced. For the first time in my life I began to have compassion for other people, who like me, were trying as hard as they possibly could and were failing. It was recommended to my employers that I be placed on extended sickness benefits for six months or a year, and then be reassessed. Instead of that I was retired permanently. My job, which would be held for me had I been granted extended sick leave, was now gone. It had been reclassified into another area.

My career was taken from me. My wife had left and I now had no job. I even had to get rid of my dog because he was young, strong and boisterous and I couldn't walk him. My mental and physical abilities had been compromised. My dreams were gone. I was crushed. I had no vision about where I could go in life. I could envisage no future for myself.

All the mechanisms I had previously employed to cope with stress involved physical explosions of energy. If I ever got frustrated or angry I used to run farther or play basketball or volleyball harder. But now I had 10,000 times more stress in my life and no way to ventilate it. I had to work out some new way of dealing with incredible levels of frustration and emotional pain. I started to cry. Day after day I would wake up in the morning and cry until lunchtime.

I plunged into such a deep depression that I couldn't even make a list of things to do, much less do anything. I'd wake up and cry every day until there were no more tears left. After I'd exhausted myself I would attempt to get going again, try to keep my house in some semblance of order or go out shopping to get some food and provisions. That was just as bad.

I still walked so poorly and fell over in the street so often that I would attract attention to myself. People would either come over to try to help me, which was a caring gesture, I knew, but it simply compounded the fact that I was a cripple. Otherwise, they would watch me stagger and fall and presume I was drunk which called forth other reactions, mostly of condemnation.

I had other physical problems. My bladder was a problem as was my bowel. I had to pee all the time and if I couldn't make it to a toilet I would wet my pants. Sometimes, I'd have insensate urination, when I had no idea I had wet myself. I'd just suddenly find my trousers and my shoes were soaked.

I also had a spastic colon which meant I either couldn't open my bowels, which would put even more pressure on my bladder or, I would get about 30 seconds notice that it was about to happen involuntarily. If I didn't make it to a toilet, which I couldn't often manage because I moved so slowly, I would shit my pants.

What could I do? Isolate myself or shit myself in public? It happened about twice a month. I had never felt so hopeless. The sinkhole of depression that I was in seemed bottomless.

Then I met Sharon.

A RAFT ON THE OCEAN

Sharon was a local girl. She was 19, very attractive and very strong in her intrinsic character. She fell in love with me and I fell very much in love with her. She knew nothing about the old me, before I was crippled—she was loving me for who I was now.

Before she came into my life, I'd been wondering who could ever accept me: who would want to be with me when I couldn't walk properly, when I was shitting and pissing myself—when I only felt like half a man? The fact that she could love me as I was became a great turning point in terms of my self esteem and the reinstatement of my masculinity. She moved into my house and, by refusing to let me sit around feeling sorry for myself, she helped me regain a feeling of self-worth, of being a Man again.

She said: 'Charles, I don't care what you do but I love you too much to let you sit there and do nothing with your life. You have to get up and do something. I don't care what it is, but you have to do something.' So I started doing one thing, like gardening; and then another, like tinkering with the car or cleaning the kitchen. Action provided the first rungs on the ladder that freed me from my emotional pit. Sharon also taught me a lot about dealing with my anger.

Apart from the frustration of my new life, I was in constant pain because all the major muscles in my back were in spasm 24 hours a day. I was given pain killers but they had side-effects and even though they brought some temporary relief, the pain always returned, and worse than before. The muscle relaxants I tried were no better. They made me feel nauseous, yet I had to keep increasing the dose, and that relaxed the already weakened muscles in my legs so much I would fall even more.

In desperation I learned self-hypnosis, through which I was able to turn down the pain a little. But still, I wasn't aware of the rage I was trying to hold inside until Sharon pointed out to me how distressing she found the way I exploded over slightest incidents. My yelling and screaming helped me but made her incredibly fearful for hours. I knew I had to find some other way of dealing with the anger. Almost as soon as I came to that realisation, another woman friend, a regular meditator, came around to see me and suggested that I should go to see a Swami near Sydney called Akanandana, who ran the Satyanada Ashram at Mangrove Mountain.

Sharon and I packed the car and left for Sydney the next day. We were driving out of Melbourne, through peak-hour traffic that was going at snail's pace when I found I desperately needed to pee—again. There were no service stations, no public toilets in sight, so I blew my top.

'Look Charles,' Sharon said. 'I know it's uncomfortable for you but I really don't want to hear about it and going on and on about it isn't going to help.'

'Well,' I screamed back, 'I'd like to see how well you would cope with this!'

Her retort was gentle: 'Not nearly as well as you Charles. But in truth, it's your problem.' She was right. It was *my* problem.

I spent a week at the Ashram, talking with Akanandana, learning some yogic breathing exercises and interacting with the other residents. In such environments, people tend to be more open with each other than they are on the streets and a number of them pointed out to me that I had a tremendous amount of repressed anger. More and more I was getting the message that in spite of all my efforts I wasn't dealing with it at all well.

On my final day at the Ashram, I went for a walk with Akanandana and the last thing he said to me was: 'Charles, you really have to put more joy back into your life.' I knew what he said was true. I had no idea how to do it.

When Sharon and I got back home to Queenscliff we found ourselves deep in the full flush of early love. We were very sexually active and although my sexual pleasures had been compromised by the accident, she got so much enjoyment out of our sex life that I was able, for the first time, to derive my own sexual pleasure from the joy of another . . . Joy. There it was.

Six months passed in this domestic hiatus but as time went on, it became apparent to both of us that as good as it was, this was not going to be a long-term relationship. Sharon was very kind but very young and I was 38. All the love in the world was not going to bridge the gap in our relative life experiences.

We parted knowing it was what we had to do. But knowing that didn't make it any less painful. But now I had meditation to help me deal with the loss. Alone in the house I was meditating seriously for an hour and a half a day and doing the breathing exercises Akanandana had given me. It was changing my energy structure and my outlook. The depression was definitely lifting. I was beginning to feel better about myself.

The old Charles had died. The grieving process for the loss of the man I had been had been protracted and difficult but I was beginning to recognise that there was a new person arising. A person who still had some value, who still had potential. The old tree had withered. A new shoot was growing and I knew I was ready to do something in the world again.

I started to look beyond what I used to do. I liked to teach and in a more positive mood came across an advertisement in the local newspaper seeking instructors for an improved reading course to be taught in the local provincial centre of Geelong. I was accepted for the training course.

The literature made sense to me in terms of neurolinguistic theory about how people read efficiently and why some read inefficiently. If we read efficiently, we read quickly and with high comprehension. It wasn't about speed reading, it was about improving reading strategies, a process most people don't reassess after about the age of eight when they are told to read to themselves.

Some lucky individuals, who have good mental integration, automatically move to a process called chunking, which means they take words in as chunks of information. Techniques to achieve this were among the processes I began to teach on a part-time basis. Ever the scientist, I couldn't help but notice that most people would at least double the speed of their reading, but there were others who didn't show much improvement at all. I made note of the differences.

I was recalled for the second neurological assessment and this time it went very well. My IQ had gone up about 15 points which indicated that the damage to my frontal lobe had either been repaired or that in the interim period, I had worked out efficient strategies to get around the damage. Maybe it was the meditation—whatever had happened in the year between assessments, my mental function had returned and my IQ was back up to 160. Now I had it in writing that I was fit to return to my job at the marine laboratory.

I found the door shut. My job had been reclassified and there was no longer a position there for me. I was pensioned off, effectively retired until the public service could find the first position that came up in my field. The catch was that my field was a limited specialty. My qualifications and experience did not make me the practical choice for most of the other jobs on offer. I sent off one application after another and became used to receiving very thin letters in reply: 'We regret to inform you.'

So I continued on with the teaching, spending most of my class time with children in schools and local colleges. I would walk into the schools, still dragging my feet in a reasonably crippled way and still having to be careful because I could fall so easily. I had steel caps on my shoes to prevent wearing the tips off at a 45 degree angle. Even so, the steel would wear through every month. The kids accommodated me with good humor and as the meditation softened my inner self I came to accept that yes, I was crippled, but I was not without worth.

I decided to go even more deeply into meditation and went up to a country retreat centre to do a week-long course called Antar mona, or 'awareness of silence' which required the participants not to talk for five days while they pursued a number of different meditation strategies. Deep in my own thoughts and witnessing my own experience of reality, I reached a new consensus. I really was OK.

On the sixth day, we could all speak to each other and one of the people I started talking to was Satyamurti, a woman in her early forties whose spiritual name meant 'essence of truth'. We discovered an instant and mutual attraction. I was a lonely guy and it wasn't long before I took the chance to drop into her home whenever I came up to Melbourne. Very quickly it became an intense physical and spiritual relationship. I was spending as much time as I could spare from my teaching schedule in Melbourne and whenever she could, Satya and her three children would come to stay with me in Queenscliff.

My ardor was bridled to some degree when a chance to go back into my field presented itself with the offer of a temporary teaching position, replacing a professor of marine science at Deakin University, which was quite near to Queenscliff. During his six-month sabbatical, I became an adjunct professor, able to get back into doing what I knew and loved and back again in the questioning intellectual atmosphere of the university.

At the end of the six months, I moved up to Melbourne permanently, to be with Satya. Soon after I did so, I received a call from my brother, Don, in the States to say that my mother was dying of cancer. She was going to be operated on the next day and was given only a 50 percent chance of surviving. Don told me there was no sense in my rushing home as we would know the result so soon.

My mother survived the operation but was given, at most, two months to live. I wanted to go home and be with her and I wanted to take Satya and the kids. I wanted my mother to know my new family, Jon, 19, Peta, 15, and Andrew, 13.

Before going home Satya and I made the decision to be married. The day after our wedding we flew to the US to spend our honeymoon with my family. Within days of my arrival, my mother was showing improvement. When I had arrived I had seen no life in her eyes. By the end of the first week the spark had returned. She lived for another two years.

Satya was a sensitive, intuitive person who was very interested in subjects that I had once considered wacko and, to be quite honest, still found quite bizarre. New-age pursuits like astrology, numerology, tarot and alternative healing therapies were among ideas I was more open to now, because they represented a chance that I might still improve. I had made amazing progress but still wanted to be much better. I started visiting naturopaths, faith healers and massage therapists, even Chinese doctors and acupuncturists. Although not a lot changed in terms of my physical condition, I was stimulated to keep looking.

One of the people I saw for the pain in my back was an acupuncturist named Rob Crickett, who had spent seven years as a monk in Buddhist monasteries in Asia. After our sessions, Rob and I would have a cup of tea and a conversation. On one occasion, quite out of the blue, he said to me, 'Charles. One day you are going to be a very powerful healer.' I wondered what on earth he was talking about. I was a scientist.

Another of the people who regularly dropped in was a guy called Hugh Simmons, who was into everything alternative. He would try every healer coming down the road and report back to us about all the new ones he had found. He romped into the house one morning announcing that he had found yet another new healing therapy. He had made an appointment for me to see the practitioner at 2 pm that day.

With nothing else on my agenda, I went along to see Dr Bruce Dewe, a medical doctor who had moved into an alternative acupressure therapy called kinesiology. I had a treatment with Dewe and two other kinesiologists that lasted for an hour and a half and they were doing the weirdest stuff I had ever seen.

I was lying on the table with one of my arms extended and they would push on my arm, ask my body questions and twiddle different points on my anatomy, concentrating particularly on my throat. I was lying there thinking;

'What on earth has this got to do with my legs and the pain in my back?'

Dewe appeared to be using a coherent system, yet in my knowledge of neurophysiology, it made absolutely no sense at all. Had nothing happened, I would have walked away thinking they were all very peculiar. At the conclusion of the treatment, Dewe told me to get up off the table and walk.

When I first stood up I could hardly balance. I certainly couldn't walk. So much change had occurred in my neurology that I couldn't walk for about 15 minutes. Then, suddenly, I was walking in a totally new way. Instead of arching my hips and dragging my feet, I was walking with my feet aligned under my hips.

It was a massive functional change. Something profound had happened. I was walking in a much more efficient way than I had been able to in the more than two years that had passed since the accident. Dewe was working from a model that said something could change. And it had. My model said that what had happened was impossible. But it had happened.

I walked away exhilarated but incredibly perplexed. Suddenly my model of how the body worked was incomplete. It was no longer valid. It couldn't explain what had happened to me.

Dewe's model, which was based on an energetic system, had worked. But how had it worked? How had the pushing of particular points on my body caused such amazing change in such a short time?

TERRA FIRMA

The treatment had taken place on a Wednesday. Two days later, I was a participant in a class Dewe was leading called 'One Brain Kinesiology.' I was that desperate to find out what had happened to me.

The method Dewe taught purported to deal with emotional stress issues as well as dyslexia and other learning problems. At the workshops we learned various methods of assessing the different problems that can interfere in the learning process, and I watched with great interest as other people went through similar profound changes of function that had occurred within me.

There was one man of about 50 who had problems with reading. When he read out loud, he would read slowly, faltering painfully over every word. Dewe ran him through a stress diffusion technique called age recession which allowed this man to go back through events that had happened in his early life.

Using muscle monitoring, Dewe could locate particular stresses and he found this man had a major issue that related to an event which had occurred when he was six. At that time, he was a school beginner and because his family was relatively poor, he always wore hand-me-down clothing. The first time he was asked to get up and read to the class he happened to be wearing a pair of shoes that had belonged to an older brother. The shoes were big and sloppy and as he clomped to the front of the room the class started laughing at him. From that day, he had been overcome by anxiety whenever he had been asked to read out loud.

After applying an acupressure technique specifically to diffuse this long-held stress, Dewe had the man read in front of the kinesiology class again. He read fluently. Tears streamed down his face. For the first time in his life, he was able to read out loud without stumbling and without being terrified.

This change had taken place before my eyes. He was amazed and so was I. I could see that the techniques worked. But how? How did they work? No one in the class could explain how such a complex function like reading could be changed with such apparent ease and speed. How had Dewe, who had never met this man before, been able to access such intimate information about a specific emotional block just by pushing on the man's arm? How had this man gone from being a manifestly poor reader to an excellent reader in the space of about 10 minutes?

In that weekend workshop, I learned some rudimentary muscle monitoring techniques, which allowed me to effect changes for some of my classmates. One of the techniques was very simple. It involved drawing a big X on a piece of paper and holding it in front of a subject while testing a muscle in their arm for its ability to lock when manual pressure was applied.

We learned that if the person being tested had good visual integration, the arm muscle would hold strong and firm. If they didn't, the muscle would give and the arm could easily be pushed down.

We used the same technique to test subjects while they were looking at two parallel lines. Generally, the theory said, people who tested strong on the Xs would be weak on the parallel lines and vice versa. This was an observable way of testing visual integration which is so essential for reading.

I tried it with a few people and found if I asked someone who was strong on the Xs if they had difficulty reading, they would say 'No'.

Do you comprehend well? 'Yes.'

Do you get tired when you read? 'No.'

But when I asked people who tested weak on the Xs, Do you have difficulty reading? They would say 'Yes.'

Do you comprehend well? 'No'. Do you get tired reading? 'Yes.'

I had the perfect opportunity to test the hypothesis in a broader sphere. I had classes full of people who were attempting to read more efficiently. So for a lark, during class breaks, I would test a few volunteers using the X and the parallel lines.

The correlations proved to be so sound that quite soon, before almost every new class, I would test people and be able to predict who would improve and who would not. Those who tested strong on Xs could be predicted to improve their reading speed and efficiency. Those who tested weak on Xs could almost never improve.

At the end of the courses, the hypothesis was generally proven. I never once found a student who tested strong on Xs who did not improve significantly. Over 90 percent of those who tested weak, showed no improvement. A small percentage of this latter group would improve to some degree through the application of sheer will. If you have enough willpower you can overcome virtually any disability and some of the students with poor integration did indeed manage to improve their reading proficiency.

At first I reasoned that because I was working mainly with school students, they might have had varying degrees of motivation. Some were trying hard, others were not. But as I was also teaching lawyers and telecommunications executives, I had access to another group who, by definition, were highly motivated. They were paying big money and taking time out of their busy schedules. With the professional group, the hypothesis didn't change. Those weak on Xs still didn't improve significantly in spite of the fact that I could observe they were trying very hard.

To my mind, these results gave great validity to the techniques that kinesiology was presenting. It was predictable and reproducible and the tests supported the hypothesis. The outcomes had scientific validity. Inspired, I began to take every kinesiology workshop I could find.

In 1985, kinesiology was just being introduced into Australia so along with many other early practitioners I did more of the One Brain series and various courses in Educational Kinesiology, which dealt more directly with learning problems. But through all of these courses I remained constantly frustrated because there was no explanation that I could really get my teeth into. No model that had any real substance for me.

Kinesiology students who were very intuitive, could feel and see the results and so could I. But whereas they weren't too concerned with finding out why, coming from a more logical bias, I desperately wanted to know why it happened. I had to find out how this stuff worked.

In kinesiology you are pushing on a physical arm that is neurologically connected to the nervous system and the reason the arm muscle locks and stays locked, or gives and is weak, is because of something that occurs at a neurological level.

But, I had observed mental events—such as just thinking of a stressful issue—to also cause this response. Could the mind also affect what was happening neurologically? If it could, this meant the muscle could indicate both neurological and mental events with equal clarity. Somehow I was beginning to sense that the mind must interface with the physical body in some real, yet indeterminable way.

It was at this junction of awe and frustration that I met Richard Utt, an American who was the founder of a powerful form of kinesiology. Utt came to Australia to teach the course he had developed called Applied Physiology. I took the first workshop in the series, called Advanced Muscle Testing, and for the first time, I was being offered an explanation that I understood. Utt was able to talk about neurological pathways that I knew to exist and he hypothesised their role in muscle testing.

In muscle testing, when you ask someone to hold their arm out, and apply pressure to push it down, there are sensors in the muscle that send messages to the central nervous system. In a sense these messages say 'I am being pushed down.'

Now the central nervous system had asked the arm to resist the pressure. Automatically, the incoming message of pressure activates an outflow of messages that say 'Equal the pressure. Contract harder! Do what the brain asks!' If there is no interference in this conversation between the muscle sensors and the central nervous system, the arm will easily do as it is asked and resist the pressure. In kinesiology it is said that the muscle *locked* or remained strong.

If, on the other hand, something interferes with this conversation between the muscle and the central nervous system it is as if you are having a conversation and someone interjects and talks over you. Because of this interference, you may miss information and because you didn't hear the instructions, you will not be able to perform the task requested. Where such interference occurs in the neurological flow that maintains coherent muscle function, the arm may give, or in kinesiology terminology, unlock or be weak. With kinesiology or muscle monitoring, what you are really looking at is the ability to monitor biofeedback in the truest sense of the word. Biofeedback is feedback from a biological system that is used to guide that system.

What Richard Utt had perceived was that a muscle circuit is like an electrical circuit. From the feedback of the muscle sensors, the central nervous system, which is the central processing unit, then acts upon that information to guide the next response.

When a pilot is flying a plane he is, in effect, the central processing unit. He is making the decisions but to do so he needs feedback from the plane's sensors and instruments. The sensor indicates that the plane is tipping to the left. The pilot receives this feedback from the dial in front of him and, based on this feedback, he then guides the plane back to horizontal. This is a classic feedback situation: information in; assessment; then, action in response to that information to restore balance. As with aircraft, so it is with human bodies.

I then found out that Utt's background was indeed in feedback systems. He was a computer expert who had specialised in aircraft guidance systems, which he hypothesised were analogous to the wiring of the human body. One of his great fortunes in life was that when he first entered kinesiology, he had no anatomical or physiological understanding, but had clocked up many years of training in analysing feedback circuits. Like many other great discoverers or inventors, he came to the field of kinesiology with no preconceived ideas of how things worked. He was free to look at the connections within the human body from an entirely new standpoint.

What he presented to me was a cohesive model of the nature of neurological circuits. A muscle does not operate in isolation. Every muscle in the body is wired not only to itself, in a feedback loop, but also to those muscles that cooperate with it to perform a task. These helper muscles are called synergists because they assist the main muscle or prime mover, perform its action. There is more to it. Because muscles can only pull, every muscle is arranged with another muscle that opposes its action or, can pull the bone in the opposite direction. For instance, the biceps muscles lift the lower arm up. Its antagonist, the triceps muscle, pulls the arm down.

For integrated muscle function it is clear that these two muscles must be synchronised in their action. If I ask my biceps to contract and simultaneously, my triceps contract, clearly my arm cannot move. In fact, if you tighten both your triceps and biceps at the same time your lower arm cannot move at all. If you want to raise your hand to scratch your nose, you tell your biceps to contract. The sensors in the biceps automatically tell the triceps to relax to exactly the degree to which the biceps are being contracted. It is an incredible arrangement, which allows a single command from the brain telling only one muscle to perform an action, which then automatically synchronises all the other muscles involved in that action.

And here I was, this research scientist, sitting in a classroom enthralled by the explanation of this fantastic thing called kinesiology which was being given by a former computer expert, who like me, had survived a life threatening circumstance and whose recovery had similarly been facilitated by this pioneering science.

After kinesiology had saved Richard Utt's life he, like me, became obsessed with trying to understand how it had happened. He knew that meant learning about anatomy and physiology so over the next few years he read extensively and his reading encompassed an in-depth investigation of eastern energetic sciences. He made a mental connection: between the nature of the energetic systems on which eastern medicine is based, and his understanding of electricity—the flow of energy that we recognise in the West. Immediately, his computer knowledge had a new application.

Using his knowledge of electrical feedback systems to understand the muscular systems he saw in the anatomy and physiology textbooks, Utt realised that there must also be a connection between the energy flows of the East, which apparently controlled the physiology of the body, and the physiology of the body as it was seen in the West. He then sought this interface and found it in the acupuncture meridian system of Chinese medicine.

In the Chinese system, 'dis-ease' and physiological dysfunction are seen to be nothing but blocked energy flow. When energy flow is harmonious there is physiological balance. When energy flow is distorted by a block or some kind of interference somewhere in the energy circuit, there is disharmony, which is reflected in disturbed physiology. These interferences or blocks do not show up under x-rays or other physical examination. The Chinese had recognised that we are more than a physical being. We are, in their terms Body-Mind-Spirit—one integrated unit. In their model an emotion or a negative thought could be as powerful a block to energy flow as a physical problem. Emotions of course, cannot be seen, touched or x-rayed.

Finally, I had an explanation for the observations I had made of a muscle going weak because of a mere thought or by someone remembering an emotional issue. Utt provided many dynamic illustrations of how some sort of energetic, or as he termed it electromagnetic resistance, had caused a failure in the system, and how, when that resistance was released there was a return to function.

Having found Utt so inspiring as a teacher I took every course he taught in Australia over the next two years. The other thing Utt did, and something that really convinced me of the effectiveness of kinesiology, was a treatment for my chronic back pain, pain that was a constant background of distraction. In just two hours, by the application of acupressure and Applied Physiology techniques, he eliminated 80 percent of this pain and it has been gone to this day.

I was still teaching the reading course, when I finally landed a permanent science job running the analytical chemical laboratory for the Victorian Government's Environment Protection Authority. I was still taking kinesiology workshops on the weekends and as I was beginning to attract a few clients who wanted me to work on them as a kinesiologist, I was fitting a few treatments into my evenings and free weekends.

It was becoming a 90-hour a week schedule, which was starting to affect my marriage. In fact I was being torn three ways: to Satya, to science (my past) and kinesiology (my future).

The man who employed me for the reading courses was fascinated by the results I was achieving and asked one day whether I would explain my methodology to him and a couple of invited visitors, one of them a clinical psychologist. I made a presentation of my work to this group and at the conclusion, the clinical psychologist said that although she didn't fully understand what I was doing, she was keen to challenge me by sending along some of her more difficult clients, young children with significant learning problems who were showing no progress at all with traditional remediation.

I worked on several of her clients and when she reviewed them she congratulated me on how manifestly they had changed. Their school performance, self-confidence and self-esteem had risen so markedly she asked whether she could send more children along to see me. Throughout 1987 she sent more clients to me and the results were gratifying for all of us.

In the other area of my life, however, the stresses and strains from needs that couldn't be met or satisfied were causing the relationship to buckle after only three years. Neither Satya nor I felt we were growing. Neither of us was really happy. I was facing another relationship that had to be ended. I desperately wanted to begin teaching kinesiology but Satya was against it. The frustration was enormous and mutual. We stuck it out for the sake of the children for as long as we could.

During this time my friend Rob Cricket, the former monk, said to me, 'It is so difficult to watch you going through this Charles because it is like watching a B52 only gliding. You have all this tremendous power and you are only gliding—you are going down.'

I had been so desperately trying to rein in my instincts to move forward that I had progressively been turning myself off rather than confront the issues in the relationship. In the context of that relationship I couldn't turn my power back on. After Rob had made me realise what I was doing to myself, I knew I had to go.

As soon as I left, I immediately started to teach kinesiology and really enjoyed it. I also perused more of Richard Utt's work in the courses he came out to teach because I was learning something new every time.

Utt decided that because his program was so content-rich, and required such intense study in anatomy and physiology, it was impractical to do it on flying visits. He would start a new five-month program at his institute, the International Institute of Applied Physiology, to begin in 1988 in Tucson, Arizona.

I had left my wife. We had decided on a property settlement which meant I was selling my house and would have money in the bank. I had paid off my car and had decided that my former career in mainstream science was now over for me. I resigned from the Environment Protection Authority and all the signs were pointing me towards America. I had found my path with heart, the path that Carlos Castananda had described in the *Teachings of Don Juan* as the choice that makes the distinction between the ordinary man and the warrior.

I really felt a calling to work in healing and to pursue the new path of working with people with emotional, physical and learning problems. I had seen such tremendous change in myself and in so many other people that I wanted to be able to do it for more people. I wanted to help people to succeed in their lives. I went to Tucson and did the course and then stayed on for another six months working with Utt doing research. I came to regard him as a creative genius when it comes to working with energy and using acupressure in a new way. I was able to synthesise many of his methods into those I was already using.

At last too, I was beginning to piece together a model of what had happened to me that day I went to see Dr Bruce Dewe and encountered kinesiology for the first time. What I couldn't understand then, was how dysfunctional neurology, which in the western terms indicates damaged nerves, could so quickly be undone by stimulating a few acupoints?

When there is nerve dysfunction, it can be based on two factors, only one of which is currently recognised in the West. This factor is overt nerve damage. From this point of view, if you are instructed to move a muscle that has been shown by electrical stimulation to work, and you cannot move it, the usual prognosis is: 'the nerve must be cut or damaged beyond repair.' This is analogous to entering a room, turning on the light switch and finding that the light does not go on, and immediately concluding that 'the wires have been cut.' Most thinking people would not leap to this conclusion—'the wires have been cut' but more sensibly would conclude (assuming they knew the bulb was okay) that 'the circuit breaker has switched off.' All modern circuit breakers switch off the instant there is too much current in the circuit, and then, as the circuit-breaker cools, they should automatically switch back on again.

What appears to have happened in my case and in many other cases of paralysis that both Richard and I have worked on, was that the muscles didn't work because a circuit breaker had switched off in my nervous system. The result was that nerves running to certain muscles had stopped conducting neurological flow and hence appeared to be 'cut' or 'damaged'.

On closer examination, the circuit breakers of the nervous system do not appear to be in the physical body, rather, they are located in the energetic body. When the energetic circuit breaker switches off, the nerves remain intact but conducts no impulses. This is similar to the modern circuit breaker above, that switches off to prevent damage but then gets stuck in the 'off' position. The appropriate acupressure treatment appears to miraculously 'switch on' this energetic circuit breaker returning neurological flow and thus function, to the nerve. This is how some of my muscles had remained effectively paralysed for years and then following only minutes of treatment had been turned on again. It wasn't a miracle, it was merely an energetic reality.

From these observations we might conclude that neurons are more 'intelligent' than had been presumed. Their first response to hypoxia, as in my case, or traumatic damage, is not to die but to switch off or to go on stand-by until

the energetic system is reactivated. This could explain many miraculous cases in which people have recovered from serious neurological injuries, including brain damage to regain full function.
I feel very humbled to be able to count myself among this number.

I returned to Australia at the end of 1988 and decided to establish a business working out of a room in a suburban doctor's surgery with the steady stream of clients the psychologist continued to send to me—mostly children with learning problems.

I often found myself musing about why I was focusing so much of my time and energy on children with learning problems. The answer was simple and circumstantial. Since my accident when I had found myself so often unable to succeed, even with my best effort, I had developed a new level of compassion and understanding of what it was like to fail . . . to lose and to constantly feel less able than others.

I knew exactly what that felt like. I knew what it did to my self-esteem and I could see what it was doing to these children. With what I had recently discovered I also knew that I could help them.

The new techniques meant that I was getting even better results, so I was rapidly getting many more clients than I could possibly deal with. I was booked up months in advance. I needed a partner.

The person I figured I would feel most comfortable working with was a Melbourne-based woman, Susan McCrossin, who had been on the course in America with me. She had originally come to me as a client and had become so excited about what kinesiology could achieve that she wound up her career in computer software and gave away a six-figure income to pursue her own path with heart, learning about and applying the techniques of kinesiology and applied physiology. She struck me as a very independent person, the type of woman I now knew would work best with me.

The two marriages and the relationship with Sharon had all failed and I had been forced to review why my partnerships with women had been so problematic—so costly, in an emotional sense, to all of us. When I really got honest with myself I had to admit that my need to be needed was so overpowering that I was consistently attracted to needy women. The relationships would work for a short time but eventually, one, or both of us would become exhausted by needs that could never be fulfilled. Finally, I became conscious that I was creating the need situation and the reason for the failure. I resolved that I wanted to become self-sufficient and look for someone who was equally independent. Then maybe a relationship could be interdependent and mutually supportive. Right then however, I wasn't actively looking for anyone.

Sue was more than happy to come into the business because, she said she had enormous respect for me. From then on we worked together and started to develop our own program of procedures which we called the Learning Enhancement Advanced Program, or LEAP. While we were getting great results for most clients there were always some who eluded our methods. To understand why we had to undertake some intensive research into brain function, looking at it from the perspective of our kinesiological and applied physiological models. That work constitutes the second part of this book.

Suffice to say that we had been working with each other for some time before we began looking up from our notes to realise our friendship and working partnership was blossoming into something more meaningful. We found ourselves in a much more romantic frame. We dated after work and by 1989 began living together as a couple.

We have now been married eight years. I also have a dog in my life again, a gentle, soulful friend called Darius.

My journey to find my path with heart, my purpose and my life's partner had consumed almost a decade. It had begun with a near-fatal accident that could have taken me out of mainstream life, yet looking back, I realised the day I took the dive beneath Skull Rock was the day I passed through a portal into a life that was far more meaningful and enriching than anything I could ever have dreamed of had I remained an able-bodied research scientist.

I still limp but I have found spiritual, emotional and professional dimensions of myself that I can share with the world. Susan and I truly believe that we have found an application to a new science that can change people's futures. And when you can change the future for one person, as the masters promise, you can effectively change the world.

I no longer see what happened beneath Skull Rock as an accident. It was an event that redirected my life and put me in touch with my soul. My path has changed from that of a seeker of scientific truth to an emissary of truth in healing.

Chapter Two

WHAT IS KINESIOLOGY?

THE ORIGINS: ACADEMIC KINESIOLOGY.

What was this wonderful thing, kinesiology, that had such a profound effect on me and that I was beginning to see could have an equally profound effect on other people?

As I investigated its origins, I began to see it was both a science and an art. Although it had method, rules, principles and logical techniques, it also involved direct interaction between practitioner and client, which meant intuition and feel, the characteristics of an art form, were a major component of its application.

Kinesiology has an interesting lineage: The science of manual muscle testing was first developed in the early 20th century by a Boston orthopaedic surgeon, R.W. Lovett, who also invented the first turnbuckle brace for treating scoliosis. Lovett used his muscle testing to analyse disabilities resulting from polio and nerve damage. He applied muscle testing to trace spinal nerve damage because muscles that tested 'weak' often had a common spinal nerve.

The system of muscle grading that Lovett developed was first published in 1932, and it introduced the five levels of testing muscles that remain the basic formula used in today's physical therapies. At first he had only used three levels of testing muscles against gravity, but later added the more subjective levels four and five to include pressure from the therapist in addition to gravity.[1]

Henry and Florence Kendall, also working with people recovering from paralytic polio myelitis, modified and systematised Lovett's ideas and in 1949 published their pioneering book, *Muscle Testing and Function*.[2] Muscle testing became a new science in the field of Academic Kinesiology, the in-depth analysis of the exact motion of muscles and the way they move joints.

Each muscle has a unique job, described as its position of greatest mechanical advantage. Basically, muscles, joints and bones are lever systems that use the mechanical advantage of a fulcrum to magnify the mechanical force of muscle contraction. This allows a short muscle contraction to be both powerful and to produce a large range of motion. When the muscle is in the position of its maximum mechanical advantage it is called the prime mover or the agonist.

When a muscle is isolated by testing position as the prime mover, and then manually monitored and it can develop its full integrity of function and lock firmly, it is rated a Plus Five response. If however, firm pressure is applied and the muscle gives in the direction of the pressure, then it is a Plus Four response. If only medium pressure is applied and the muscle gives way, then it is rated Plus Three.

If the person can move the muscle into the test position against gravity, but only slight pressure results in the muscle giving way, then it is rated Plus Two. If there is difficulty just getting the muscle into the monitoring position against gravity and any pressure causes it to give, it is rated Plus One. Zero on the scale is when the muscle will not move at all against gravity, a condition known as Flaccid Paralysis. Because the strength of individual muscles varies in different people, the scale is not an absolute measure of strength but rather of the relative integrity of muscle function.

One who took an interest in the work of Kendall and Kendall was a Detroit-based chiropractor, Dr George Goodheart. A very keen observer he was one of those rare people who are able to make fantastic discoveries by looking at research from a different perspective and synthesising the information in a different way. It is often not just seeing new things, but rather, seeing known things in new ways that leads to discovery.

Goodheart had a client who had a problem with his scapula, or shoulder blade. When this man pushed against a wall, his scapula would lift off his back and poke out at almost a 90 degree angle. Goodheart remembered reading in Kendall and Kendall's book, that a lifted scapula related to a muscle called the anterior serratus, which connects the middle border of the scapula to the ribs under the arm. When the anterior serratus contracts, it holds the scapula close to the back. The protruding shoulder blade suggested the anterior serratus muscle was weakened.

After a busy day in his clinic, Goodheart set aside time to work on this client and as predicted found the anterior serratus weak. He then began to palpate, or firmly massage the beginnings (origins) and ends (insertions) of this muscle and in so doing found a series of hard little beads or muscle knots. As he palpated more firmly, the knots disappeared. Goodheart went along the muscle and pressed all the knots until they disappeared. Then he again had the man push against the wall. This time the scapula sat correctly. Further, when the muscle was manually retested it could develop a Plus Five lock.[3]

As Goodheart began to increasingly use muscle testing in his practice, he found some clients had specific muscles that would test weak when they had certain types of disease conditions. For instance, he found the clavicular division of the pectoralis major muscle or PMC, the chest muscle that connects to the collarbone, would generally test weak in clients who complained of stomach ulcers. He would apply certain chiropractic manipulations for the treatment of ulcers and reassess the strength of the PMC muscles. After treatment these muscles suddenly showed strength. This both confirmed the relationship between ulcers and the muscle response, and the efficacy of the chiropractic treatment. The change in muscle response was immediate and visible.

When Goodheart now found a patient with a stomach ulcer he would always assess the strength of the PMC. He would sometimes apply his newly discovered origin/insertion technique to the PMC, and to his surprise, quite often the muscle would strengthen with a concurrent improvement in the condition. He now had chiropractic manipulations to work with as well as a brand new technique that was also capable of alleviating symptoms.

In short, muscle testing was proving not only to be a diagnostic tool, but also to have therapeutic value.

An eclectic reader, Goodheart was interested in all sorts of different areas of knowledge and while he found his origin/insertion technique worked to strengthen the muscles of some individuals, many others were not helped at all. He started looking for other answers. His quest led him to the work of an early American osteopath, Frank Chapman, who had observed that many types of pathologies, or the symptoms of diseases, had their origins in sluggish lymph flow. Lymph is the bodily fluid that carries nutrients to tissues and organs and carries toxins away. Sluggish lymph flow meant that over time, tissues became more toxic and less functional.[4]

Chapman worked out that there were many points on the bodies of individuals who were showing various symptoms of disease, which, when palpated or massaged, would be tender. After a while, with continuous massage, they would become less tender and this was associated with improvement in the disease condition. He called these Chapman Reflex Points and published his findings in the 1930s.[5]

Goodheart recognised that many of the disease conditions described by Chapman as being associated with a specific Chapman reflex point, he had found were similarly associated with a specific muscle weakness. He now began to systematically investigate the relationship between Chapman Reflex Points and the muscle weaknesses he had found to be associated with the same disease conditions. He established that rubbing the reflex point Chapman had assigned to a disease would often strengthen the muscle associated with the same pathology.

The master synthesiser was at work.

In spite of the great success of his newly discovered origin/insertion technique and the application of Chapman Reflex Points, some conditions and their associated weakened muscles failed to respond. Goodheart kept looking.

In the 1930s another American chiropractor, Terence Bennett, had come up with his own model for restoring health based on proper blood flow. Like the lymph system, when blood flow becomes congested, tissues don't get the right amount of oxygen and nutrition. He reasoned that this set up the prime conditions for diseases to take hold. Like Chapman, Bennett had worked out his own set of reflex points. Most were on the head and upper body with a few points below the waist and on the legs.

Bennett found that applying light pressure to these points would stimulate increased blood flow to the associated tissues and organs. As with Chapman's work, stimulation of these Bennett Reflex Points would often result in major improvement in the conditions being treated (see Fig. 2.1). In the 1930s he formed the Neurological Research Foundation to teach his technique.

The dangers of radiation were little known in Bennett's day, so some of his experiments involved procedures that would not be considered safe today. One was to inject volunteers with radio-opaque dyes that make the blood visible to X-rays. Volunteers then lay down beneath a full length fluoroscope and by holding different reflex points he could observe change in blood flow. Unfortunately, Bennett died of cancer caused by such regular exposure to radiation, but not before he left a legacy of valuable knowledge that became known as the Bennett Reflex Points.[6]

As he had done with the Chapman Reflex Points, Goodheart began to systematically investigate the relationships between Bennett Reflex Points and those muscles that would not strengthen with his other techniques.[7] He was delighted to note that in most cases it constituted the missing link. Working primarily with the Bennett Reflex Points on the head and upper chest, he was able to assign specific Bennett Reflex Points to specific muscle weaknesses.

By synthesising his discoveries, Goodheart pioneered a system that brought together work done by his predecessors: Chapman's Points (for lymphatic function), Bennett's Points (for vascular function), the origin/insertion technique (for muscular problems), and muscle testing for feedback in both diagnosis and therapeutic efficacy. This marked the beginning of the new science of Applied Kinesiology.

APPLIED KINESIOLOGY

George Goodheart gathered together a group of other chiropractors interested in the developing field of Applied Kinesiology, who became known as the Dirty Dozen. They used his techniques in their clinics and daily began to share knowledge. But it was Goodheart who made the seminal breakthrough that remains the centrepiece of kinesiology. In the late 1960s, when the West was just beginning to explore the ideas filtering through from Asia, he began to read the Chinese medical literature that detailed the ancient knowledge of the Acupuncture Meridian System—the system the Chinese claimed mapped the flow of energy through the body.[8]

Goodheart found that when muscles did not respond either to origin/insertion stimulation, Chapman's or Bennett's Reflex Points, that sometimes, by running his hand just above a specific meridian pathway in the direction of flow that the Chinese had outlined, the weakened muscles would often strengthen. Again there was a relationship between a specific muscle response and a specific meridian. In 1966 he wrote a research manual on strengthening muscles by holding acupuncture points called Tonification Points.[9]

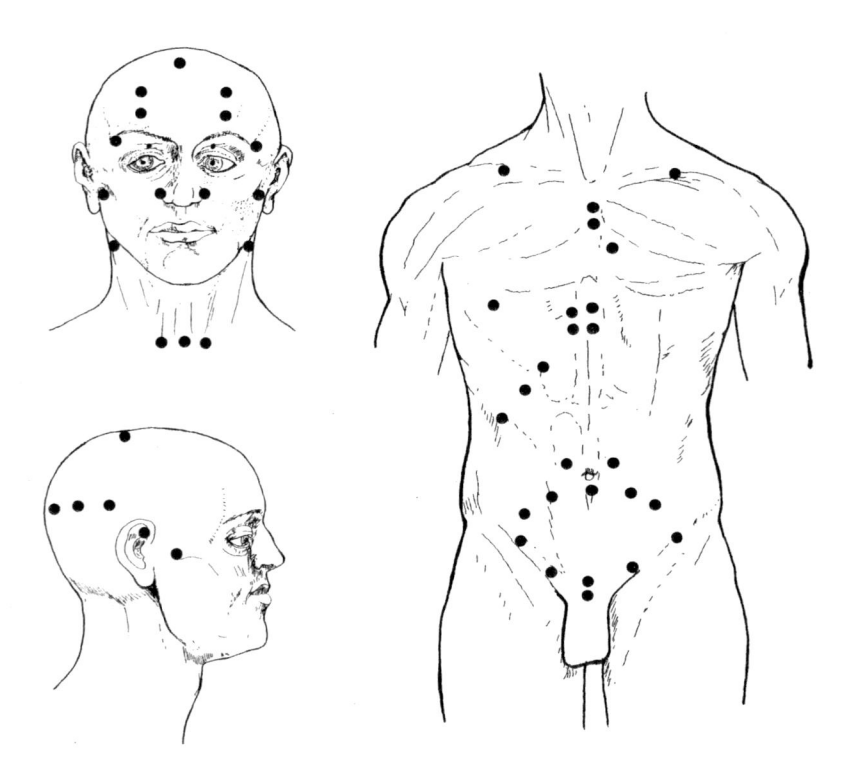

Figure 2.1. Bennett's Original Reflex Points. Goodheart used the points predominantly on the head and neck and only a few of the points on the body.

He began to recognise there was an extraordinary complex of inter-relationships linking muscle response with imbalances in the muscular system, the lymphatic system, the vascular system, and even the more esoteric energy systems of Chinese medicine. Because each muscle and reflex point reflected the state of balance of a particular organ system (such as the PMC relating to the stomach), and because the Chinese had named their meridians after the organ to which they were associated, Goodheart, in a flash of insight, realised the organ was the key in this relationship.

When the organ system was stressed (diseased); the muscle may develop an imbalance (weakness); the Chapman Reflex Point may become tender; the Bennett Reflex Point may become active, and the associated meridian flow may be disturbed.

The brilliant melding of all these observations became the Muscle-Organ/Gland-Meridian Complex, the core concept of Applied Kinesiology.

Essentially, Goodheart had started at the most physical level of knotted muscles and tender reflex points and moved to more subtle responses of reflex points that needed only light touch. Then he had entered the more esoteric domain of energy. Here, change could be effected merely by passing the hand close to the body and tracing the path of a meridian.

The Chinese system had given him a layout of thousands of years of empirical observations about the energetic system and the principles by which it works. To this body of knowledge Goodheart added the muscle response correlation, which meant the energy balance of these meridians and their associated organs, could be quickly and consistently ascertained by direct muscle feedback. According to Goodheart it remains one of the West's few contributions to the East in terms of the application of energetic techniques.

The Chinese method of accessing energy imbalances in the body was written down in the *Huang Di Nei Ching* or *Yellow Emperor's Inner Classic of Medicine* between the first century BC and the early first century AD based on a thousand years of accumulated knowledge.[10] Yet as the system was based on reading subtle energetic states of the wrist pulse, it was very intuitive and took many years to master as a diagnostic art. Goodheart had tapped into the same energy systems but now could access these systems very quickly through the instant biofeedback afforded by using muscle testing as the diagnostic tool.

But what is this energy the Chinese were tracing?

ESSENTIAL CH'I

Western science does not yet have the instruments to measure what the Chinese call Ch'i or Qi, for which the best western translation is energy.[11] But even this word does not directly equate to the western concept of energy as being a force something like electricity. Ch'i has a different quality from the coarser physical energy and is aligned more with the early Greek and Roman concepts of the elan vital or, vital energy. The notion of subtle invisible forces running through the body had been totally eclipsed in the western hemisphere by the end of the medieval era.

Western science does, however, have the instrumentation to measure the existence of acupressure points, which I call acupoints, of the Chinese meridian system. These are the points of least electrical resistance on the surface of the skin and the cells directly beneath them have a slightly different structure to their neighbors.[12] Most acupoints are situated in small surface depressions, identifiable by palpation, and are often hypersensitive. Beneath these surface depressions the epidermis is thinner and has a characteristic structure with modified collagen fibres.[13] Senelar claims that more than 80 percent of the known acupoints examined have this unique structure.[14]

Remarkably, they are in exactly the places on the body that the Chinese had mapped thousands of years ago.[15] Classical theory recognised about 365 acupoints on the surface meridians, 309 of which are bilateral or on both sides of the body, giving a total of 670 meridian acupoints.[16]

How did those ancients plot all 670 acupoints that make up the integrated acupuncture meridian system?

The short, if unscientific answer, is that some of the monks and medical practitioners who had spent many years in meditation developing extremely subtle levels of perception, were able to actually 'see' or 'sense' these acupoints and the movement of energy through the body. It was as clear to them as if they were looking at a pattern on a piece of cloth. Because these masters could see the patterns of energy, they could perceive which patterns were harmonious and balanced—indicating wellness, and which indicated imbalance or disease. From this knowledge came the Law of Five Elements, one of the central tenets of acupuncture.

The Law of Five Elements says there are certain directions of energy flow and certain points on the body which, when activated, cause the movement of energy from one point to another.[17] Bodies have only a specific amount of energy, so an *over-energy* in one place by definition, means that there has to be an *under-energy* in another place. Because the Chinese diagnosticians were using inductive reasoning (looking at the whole), they did not name diseases as such. Rather, they were interested in a complex of patterns that made up the whole and it was from these patterns that they were able to diagnose imbalances.[18]

Chinese Medicine is not less logical than the western system, just less analytical.[19]

All they needed to know to re-establish balance was where the over-energy and under-energy existed. With that knowledge, they could employ the Law of Five Elements to locate the correct acupoints. Stimulation of these acupoints would remove the block to energy flow. Once unblocked the excess energy would naturally flow to where it was deficient. When energy was in balance, theoretically health was restored.

One of the reasons why the West found the Chinese view of the body so confusing for so long, had a lot to do with the ancient language in which their medical information was couched. The Chinese explanations related to the cosmology of a Taoist and then Confucian agrarian society of over 2000 years ago. An inductive, lyrical language written in allegory and metaphor, it evokes the experience of a largely rural world. Energy flows were thus compared to

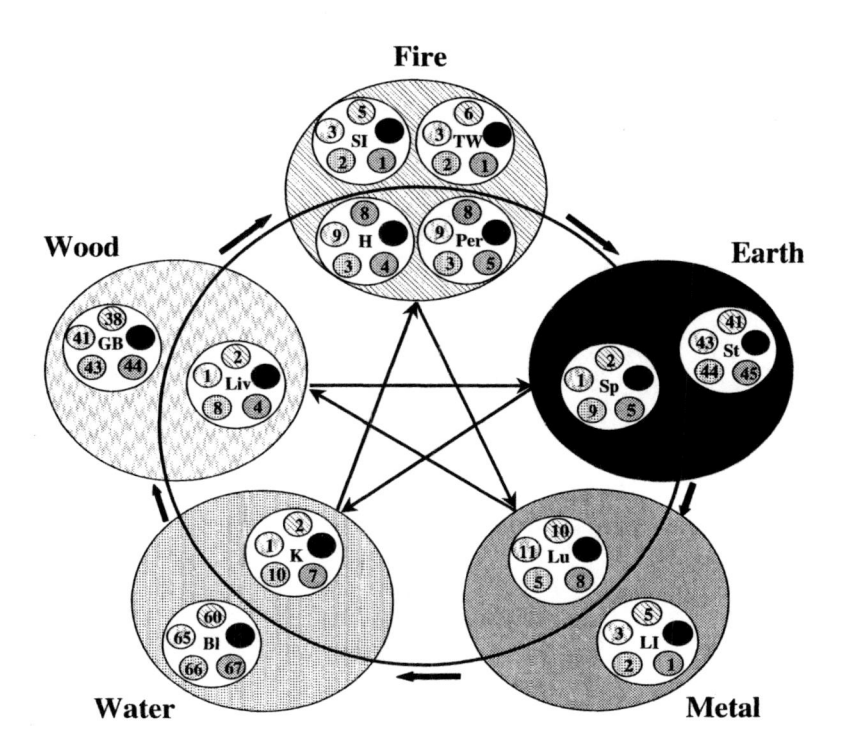

Figure 2.2. The Law of Five Elements. The arrows indicate the direction of energy flow in two cycles. The Sheng or Promotion cycle is a clockwise flow around the circle. The Ko or Control cycle is a clockwise flow around the star in the centre. Each meridian circle in each element has five numbers relating to the Command Points, specific acupoints directing energy flow.

rivers; flooded rice paddies and overflow channels. Organs were called Emperors or Ministers and the laws were called Grandmother-Son or Mother-Son Laws. The Five Elements are described as having qualities of earth, fire, metal, wood or water. Was it any wonder that when the West first came across these ideas the metaphors made the information so inaccessible?

Despite our confusion with their system and the lack of attention paid by the Chinese to internal anatomy, they were well aware of organ function. They called the meridian flows by organ names, not because they referred to the organs themselves, but because part of the energy flow of each meridian sustained the function of a specified organ.[20] Thus they talked of lung energy, heart energy and kidney energy and what they meant was the complex energy structure of which the physical organ was but one part.

To the western mind such a description immediately designates only a physical organ with a specific function. But the Chinese descriptions did not mean a heart as a muscular organ pumping blood. Rather it talked about a concept of heart: the Emperor, as the source of power in the system that drove not only the blood, but was also the power behind the emotions of love, hatred and anger.

And when the Chinese describe a meridian they were not describing a static, physical unit, but a dynamic interaction that affects all planes of the being. The Chinese do not see a physical body and a mind as being separate structures. They see a Body-Mind-Spirit that creates an integrated being.[21]

To quote the great chronicler of Chinese history, Joseph Needham, 'In accord with the character of all Chinese thought, the human was an organism, neither purely spiritual nor purely material in nature'.[22] Mind and emotions are no less influential in their view of health than the state of the physical body, that part of us which can be touched and felt'.

What ties the body to the mind and the spirit is the etheric energy of Ch'i, which is the interface between the physical body and the subtle energy bodies of mind and spirit.[23] These subtle bodies have been recognised for millennia in the esoteric traditions of China, India and Tibet. An ancient Chinese adage held that, 'There is nothing between Heaven and Earth except Ch'i and the Laws that govern it'.[24]

INTERWEAVING YIN AND YANG

Early Chinese thought developed the concept that there were two fundamental properties of the universe, Yin and Yang. These polar opposites are perceived to be present in all things and interconnected by Ch'i. As the Nei Ching states 'the entire universe is an oscillation of the forces of Yin and Yang'. Although Yin and Yang are complementary opposites, they are neither specific forms of energy nor material things, rather they are labels used to describe how things function in relation to each other and the universe.[25]

Yin and Yang really represent a way of thinking in which all things are but a part of a whole. No thing can exist in and of itself, but can only be defined by its opposite. For instance, 'hot' is the absence of 'cold'; 'dark' is the absence of 'light'; 'wet' is the absence of 'dry', and so on. Yin and Yang are thus opposite properties that define each other.

In the original metaphor, Yin was 'the shady side of the mountain', and Yang was 'the sunny side of the mountain'. Yin is associated with the qualities of cold, dark, matter, passivity and rest, and considered feminine. Yang is associated with the qualities of heat, light, energy, activity and movement, and considered masculine.[26]

In Yin-Yang theory, these two properties are in constant interaction and relation. All things have two aspects, a Yin aspect and a Yang aspect, and Yin and Yang mutually create each other and control or balance each other.

Boiling water exemplifies these abstractions: As water heats it becomes more Yang (hot), but as each water molecule escapes into the air as vapour, it cools or becomes Yin, due to water's latent heat of evaporation. This is why sweating, Yang, makes you cool, Yin.

The famous Tai Qi or Yin-Yang symbol represents the relation and interdependence between Yin and Yang (see Fig. 2.3). The white dot in the black and the black dot in the white signify that in Yin (black) there is always the seed of Yang (the white dot), and visa versa. No thing is, or can be, all Yin or all Yang. Yin and Yang are complementary properties that compose the whole, and the curved line between them expresses the movement of Yin transforming into Yang and Yang transforming into Yin. The fact that the black and white sides are equal demonstrates the 'balance of Yin and Yang' when there is harmony.

It could be said that the whole of Chinese medicine, its physiology, its

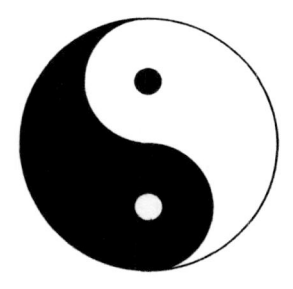

Figure 2.3. The Tai Qi or Yin-Yang Symbol.

pathology, its diagnosis and its treatment, can all be reduced to the fundamental theory of Yin and Yang. This theory serves to explain the organic structure, physical function and pathological changes in the human body, and in addition, guides the clinical diagnoses and treatment.[27] Ch'i flowing through the meridians and following the Law of Five Elements is only the mechanism by which Yin and Yang are expressed within the body.

When the Chinese talk about a meridian or vessel, they are describing conduits made of subtle matter through which Ch'i flows. Ch'i has various properties or qualities that connect the Body-Mind-Spirit into a dynamic integrated organism, an idea that western medicine is only now beginning to entertain.

The Chinese say there are 14 major meridians in the body, each of which has its own acupoints.

Two of these vessels, the Governing and Central vessels, flow up from the region of the crotch. Central Vessel runs up the mid-line of the front of the body to a point, CV24, just below the bottom lip. It carries Yin energy. Governing Vessel runs from the tip of the tailbone, up the spine, over the top of the skull to a point, GV26, just below the nose on the upper lip. It carries Yang energy. The other 12 vessels are bilateral. Some vessels run up and some vessels run down each side of the body. Of these bilateral meridians or vessels, six are Yin and six are Yang.[28]

In the Chinese anatomical position, the arms are raised above the head. All Yang meridians run from Heaven toward Earth (except Governing), and all Yin meridians run from Earth toward Heaven. Via the Law of Five Elements the Yin flowing from the Earth is thus integrated with the Yang flowing from Heaven. The old adage may therefore be restated as 'there is nothing between Yang and Yin except Ch'i and the Law of Five Elements that governs it'.

To make this simpler, the 14 major meridians can be visualised as a series of 14 tall cylinders which are arranged in a circle and filled to a certain level with fluid (Ch'i). Each of the fourteen cylinders is directly connected to the next cylinder in the circle by big pipes, and to every other cylinder by pipes beginning and ending with a command point of the Law of Five Elements (the numbered circles in Fig. 2.2). These are called 'command points' because they act as the valves on these secondary channels or meridians controlling the flow of Ch'i between meridians.

These cylinders (meridians) are in turn connected by a myriad of pipes of varying diameters (primary, secondary, tertiary, etc.) through which the fluid circulates. Some of these pipes only connect to other pipes but every time a pipe joins a cylinder or another pipe, there is a valve. The acupoint. (see Fig. 2.4).

A force impels the fluid to circulate constantly in a certain direction. Provided all the valves are adjusted correctly, the fluid in all the cylinders will remain at the same height, containing the same amount of energy, or a balance of Yin and Yang.

But what happens if a valve is turned down, restricting or blocking the flow of fluid? The level will rise in the cylinder upstream because fluid is flowing in faster than it can now flow out. This cylinder will gain an excess of fluid (Ch'i) relative to other cylinders. Since each meridian is either Yin or Yang, one part of the system will now have an excess of Yin or Yang (see Fig. 2.5).

The level in the downstream cylinder will fall compared to the others, as fluid is being lost faster than it is being replenished. This part of the system will become deficient in either Yin or Yang. In the Chinese medical system, the proper thing to do is to find the valve that is blocked and adjust it. Once the blockage is removed the fluid will seek its own level automatically to reestablish a balance of Yin and Yang. This is presented graphically in the figure below.

In the body, once the energy block is removed and the balance restored, the physiology that was affected by the previous energy or Ch'i disturbance suddenly disappears. In the Chinese system, pain is only a sign of over-energy

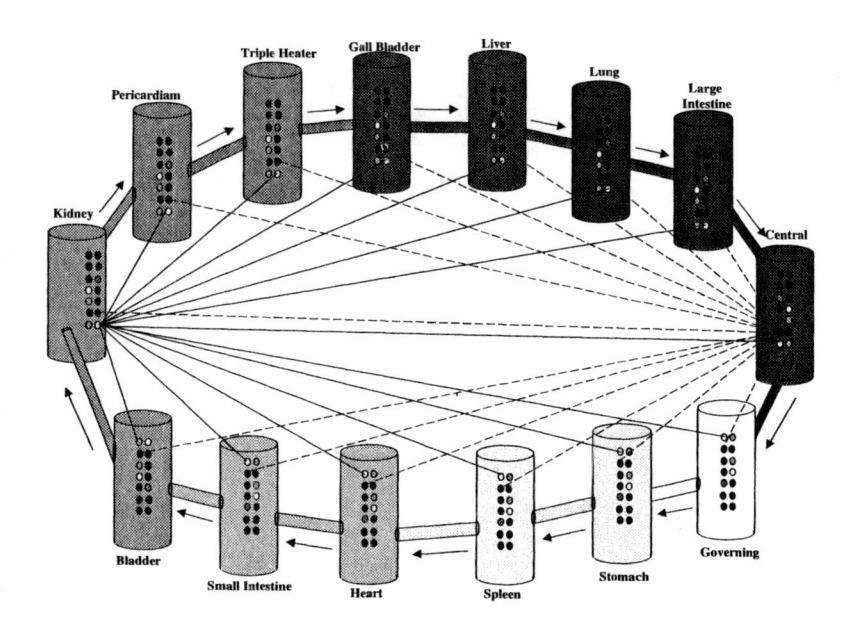

Figure 2.4. The Meridian-cylinder analogy. Note: *the connections between the meridians are only shown for two meridians. In reality there is a matrix where all 14 meridians are similarly connected.*

in a particular place and if you drain the excess energy away, the pain will also drain away. It is an effective, eloquent system whose principles are simple but whose applications are immense. It was the application of this ancient knowledge that really allowed kinesiology to take off.

TOUCH FOR HEALTH

Another member of the Dirty Dozen was chiropractor Dr John Thie, who saw the synthesis of western and eastern knowledge as very exciting. It strengthened his belief that people should be able to take care of their own health, and that the West should change the foundation of its health system from crisis management to prevention. He also versed himself in the Chinese system and realised that if everyone could balance their own energy on a regular basis

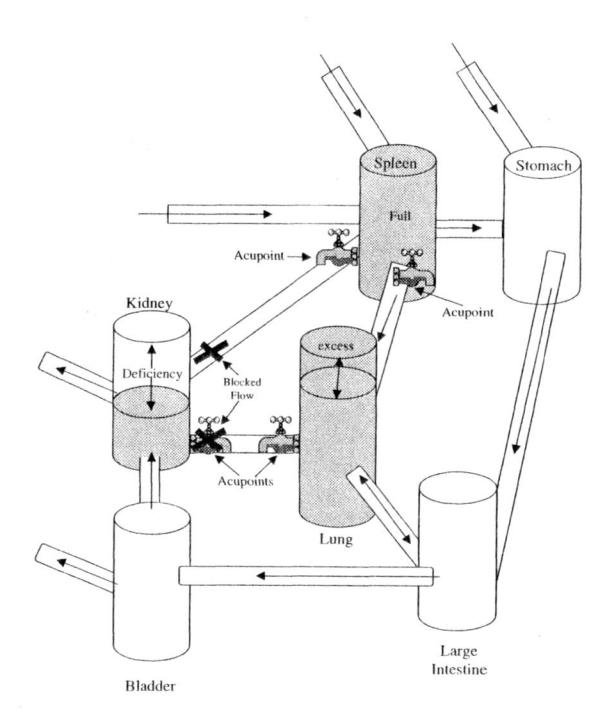

Figure 2.5. The Meridian-Blocked Valve Analogy. Wherever a pipe joins a cylinder there is a valve, the acupoint. Blocked valves cause the energy to back up creating an excess of energy in one or more of the upstream meridians, and a deficiency of energy in one or more of the downstream meridians.

they might be able to maintain their own health more effectively. Thie took the basic techniques that had been worked out in Applied Kinesiology and developed a new system that he called Touch for Health.[29]

His view was that too seldom in western society are we touched for health because generally touch was seen to have negative or sexual connotations. In fact, touching is one of the most healing things one human being can do for another. If I sit across a room and listen to your story or your problems, I can empathise with you. But how much more secure will you feel, and how much more will you feel my empathy if I am holding your hand? When I touch you, you can feel the sincerity of my words. You can feel my empathy and energy. Everyone knows that touch is a real experience.

Within the constructs of western medicine that prevailed when Thie was introducing his system, doctors were supposed to be cool, analytical, technical, white-coated and separate. They certainly were not supposed to touch someone in a feeling way, because that would potentially detract from their ability to diagnose objectively. Touch for Health was therefore seen as a radical fringe therapy of the early 1970s.

Despite considerable opposition, Thie wanted to teach lay people so they could balance their own health, the health of their family and their close friends. So he started to teach the basic principles of Touch for Health in workshops that could be taken over a couple of weekends. In essence, he taught the procedure known as The Fourteen Muscle Balance, which assesses the balance of energy in the 14 major meridians that are related to specific organs.

In this procedure, a muscle, representative of each meridian, is manually assessed for its state of balanced function. If the muscle was found to be weak, the basic techniques developed by George Goodheart (origin/insertion, Chapman and Bennett reflex points and meridian tracing), were then employed to strengthen the weakened muscle. Once all 14 muscles were balanced, meridian energies were also balanced, restoring the balance of Yin and Yang in the body. Often this very simple system could produce profoundly positive health outcomes.

Thie started teaching his system in California. Quickly it spread throughout the United States and from there to many other countries across the world. Now there are millions of people in over 50 countries who know about Touch for Health and who can practice it with great effect. Not only that but Touch for Health made the basic techniques of Applied Kinesiology available to ordinary people.

CLINICAL KINESIOLOGY

One of George Goodheart's most brilliant protégés, Dr. Alan Beardall, made several crucial discoveries that added additional tools to the developing field of kinesiology. While treating a famous marathon runner, Beardall discovered that individual muscles did not all function as one unit, but rather, that many muscles had functionally unique divisions. He found that although a muscle may test 'strong', when one or a combination of its divisions were monitored, individual divisions of this 'strong' muscle might test 'weak' or unlock.[30]

From 1975, through extensive anatomical study, clinical observation and testing procedures, Beardall not only identified these functional divisions within muscles, he went on to develop specific muscle tests for each division and isolated reflex points which differentiated these muscle divisions as unique functional units. He discovered over 250 specific muscle tests isolating divisions of the major muscles of the body and published his exciting findings in 1980.[31] He was eventually to publish five volumes of muscle testing instruction books[32] and from this body of knowledge Beardall developed a new kinesiological method he called Clinical Kinesiology.

Beardall was also the originator of the concept of the body as a 'biocomputer', which has proved to be such a powerful model for many aspects of the subconscious functions that can be tapped into by muscle monitoring.[33] The subconscious appears to process data in a binary way, indeed neurons running the muscles can only fire or not fire—lock or unlock. A lock in a muscle test thus indicates 'yes, I am in balance'—there is not enough stress to impede my function, while an unlock response indicates 'no, I am unbalanced'—there is too much stress for me to work properly.

More importantly, this simple 'yes' or 'no' response of the muscle is the summation of *all* the factors influencing the brain and central nervous system, from the level of your structural alignment to your nutritional and emotional status. As well, the subconscious readout of muscle function is the interface with the other energy systems of the body, including the meridian systems. As such, these 'yes' or 'no' responses can also indicate states of energetic balance.

Beardall also developed several other innovative concepts that have become fundamental in the application of all the kinesiology systems developed to this day. In 1983, while working with a patient, he noticed a unique phenomenon. When the patient touched a painful area with an open hand, the muscle he was monitoring suddenly weakened, a normal response indicating a 'stress' condition in the painful area. In a second test on the same area, however, the patient happened to touch his thumb and little finger together. Something very odd occurred. The muscle immediately strengthened and locked.[34]

In a flash of insight, Beardall recognised that the thumb and fingers had energy flows similar to the energy flows of the meridian system itself, and that muscle monitoring provided a means of assessing these flows. He discovered that the thumb acted like an earth or neutral, grounding the energy flows of the other fingers. Through extensive research, he found that these 'handmodes' represented another form of readout on the essential functions within the body.

Beardall established that the thumb and each finger represented a specific type of energy flow: thumb to index finger responded to structural stresses; thumb to middle finger responded to nutritional stresses; thumb to ring finger responded to emotional stresses; and thumb to little finger responded to energetic stresses such as meridian Ch'i imbalances.

Beardall also developed another technique central to current kinesiology, a means of retaining 'energetic' information over time based upon the sensory output of sensors in the hip joints. While he originally called this procedure 'pause lock', it is now called 'retaining mode', 'circuit mode' or simply, putting an imbalance 'in circuit' in other kinesiology systems. A description of this mechanism is beyond the scope of this book, but is more fully described elsewhere.[35]

So now, whenever he discovered an imbalance through testing a muscle, he could quickly ascertain the nature of the problem causing that imbalance by using his new handmode system. Was it emotional, nutritional, structural or energetic? Beardall's 'finger modes', along with the complementary technique of retaining this energetic information over time by 'putting it into circuit', are some of the most important tools used in modern kinesiology systems.[36]

Once the muscle tests, reflex points and concepts developed in Applied Kinesiology and Clinical Kinesiology, both chiropractic fields, reached the public through Touch for Health, there was a great flurry of creative activity as new kinesiology systems were developed by innovative individuals from a diversity of backgrounds.

KINESIOLOGY: USING MUSCLE RESPONSE.

From these beginnings, kinesiology has blossomed to become a diversity of different types of kinesiology-based treatments. These new systems were developed by people who saw the incredible potential of the techniques because generally, they were not locked within the rigid western medical and physiological models.

While in Academic Kinesiology, you are indeed testing a muscle for strength, in the more recently developed kinesiological systems, the muscle response is used primarily as a form of biofeedback. Hence, in these systems you are 'monitoring', not 'testing' muscle function. The redefinition of the term to 'muscle monitoring' is to denote that we are now accessing the integrity of the muscle response, and not its strength.[37]

The truly amazing aspects of muscle monitoring is that the response can indicate such a wide variety of possible stressors. The muscle being monitored may respond by unlocking because of a physical factor (a sore muscle, for example); because of a disturbance in the function of its related organ system (blocked or restricted lymph or blood flow); because of a disturbance in its associated meridian (blocked energy flow); or because of a disturbing emotion or thought.[38]

If we monitor a muscle and it is strong and locks, and then ask a person to think about their mother, the muscle may suddenly give or unlock. This indicates to the kinesiologist that something has interfered with the integrity of the neurological flow between the muscle and the central nervous system preventing normal muscle function. This interference may have come from whatever stress 'Mother' set up within this person's system.

Your conscious brain may tell you that you and mother get on famously. But when you consider that a stressor is not always conscious, and may often be held within the subconscious, which is also wired directly to the muscles, this previously undetected subconscious stress can be the factor that produces a block in the neurological flow. This informs both the practitioner and the client that there is a stress around their mother, most probably related to an unresolved issue that occurred when they were growing up.

This access into the usually inaccessible realms of your subconscious is one of the most powerful aspects of kinesiology as it is now practiced. Something that you think, can be instantly detected as a stressor within your physical-emotional being and it may be something your conscious brain was never aware of until the muscle response made it apparent. Further, the use of finger modes allows a kinesiologist to identify the exact nature of that subconscious stress. Thus kinesiology allows us to eavesdrop on our subconscious.

One of the first people to recognise this aspect of kinesiology was a health practitioner in Southern California, John Barton. After the death of one of his children, Barton realised that western medicine didn't hold all the answers and he turned down a scholarship to the Massachusetts Institute of Technology. Instead he launched into a career in holistic health, studying foot reflexology, acupressure, herbs and natural childbirth.

In the mid 1970s Barton saw a demonstration of Applied Kinesiology on television and was hooked. Kinesiology became his tool to determine how the body could be balanced through massage, acupressure, position-releasing postures, nutrition and emotions. Out of this vast body of research developed another new field, Biokinesiology.[39]

Another person who made a contribution in the 1970s was Dr Paul Dennison, a very dyslexic individual who was incapable of learning in the traditional educational system. Like so many others he started innocently enough by attending a Touch For Health course.

The instructor showed him 'cross crawl' or cross-patterning, which is marching on the spot moving opposite arms and legs in unison. He then demonstrated 'homolateral crawl' or marching on the spot with the same side arm and leg moving in unison. Dennison gained great benefit from these techniques and from the application of another Touch For Health technique called Emotional Stress Release (ESR).

In ESR, while the subject thinks of a stressful issue, gentle finger pressure is applied to the frontal eminences, the broad bumps on the forehead above the eyes. This appears to help return blood flow to the frontal lobes which are our thinking and new learning centres. When a person is stressed, blood flow is largely withdrawn from these regions and redirected to the subconscious survival centres. But when touch is applied to these points until subtle pulses are felt beneath the fingertips on the forehead, the emotional charge in the previously stressful situation is usually reduced or eliminated.

At the time, Dr Dennison was working with children with learning disabilities, and when he employed these same techniques with his students, he discovered their learning abilities also improved. Inspired by these changes, Dennison developed further applications of kinesiology to create a kinesiology system that he initiatially called Educational Kinesiology, but which is now called Edu-K or Edu-Kinesthetics, for working with children and adults with learning problems.[40]

He perceived that learning problems lay in improper coordination of brain activity and developed a series of movement exercises, many of which were based on standard yoga asanas or postures, to re-integrate brain function. To these movement exercises he added several acupressure techniques and several standard remedial education techniques. He called his synthesis Brain Gym.[41] When Brain Gym exercises are practiced regularly, they stimulated integrated brain function and thus greatly improved learning potential.

In the cascade of discovery, his system spawned yet another form of kinesiology, created by Gordon Stokes, Candice Callaway and Daniel Whiteside. Stokes had been Instructor-Trainer for Touch For Health in the United States and in an inspired collaboration with Callaway and Whiteside, produced a creative amalgamation of concepts from Edu-K, Touch for Health, Applied Kinesiology, other kinesiologies and psychotherapeutic practices. The partners called their system, Three-in-One or One Brain Kinesiology and applied it to dyslexia, learning problems and emotional stress that had not been resolved by other methods.[42]

In the One Brain model, unresolved emotional stress was the basis of most learning problems, as unresolved emotions were shown to have the ability to block our personal growth, our emotional and spiritual learning. The threesome went on to develop a much more in-depth emotional defusion technique based upon ESR, but which they named Emotional Stress Defusion (ESD).

The name change was important because it indicated that the new method was not just the release of emotions but it served to defuse and then reintegrate into our lives what had otherwise been unresolved emotional experiences. What was vital about this technique was that it facilitated greater choice. To get even deeper and be more precise about the nature of unresolved emotional issues, the group also added age recession techniques.

Coming in from an entirely new angle, in the early 1980s, Richard Utt added to the growing number of kinesiological systems by developing Applied Physiology, a model based on an in-depth understanding of both western physiology and the Law of Five Elements. Utt developed a kinesiology based acupressure application of the Law of Five Elements of Chinese acupuncture which he called The Five Houses of Ch'i.[43]

His system allows the practitioner to determine which of two equally valid energy pathways within the Five Element system would most effectively equalise the energy, release stress and thereby promote healing for the client. Utt also formulated the Seven Element Hologram which is based upon the Holographic Supertheory proposed by physicist David Bohm and neuroscientist Karl Pribram.[44] This is a single integrated kinesiological system capable of accessing all levels of the human hologram from the physical level of the muscles through the levels of emotion and thought, to the level of our attitudes—our essential beliefs.

As you can see by the incredible trajectory of this healing science, many other types of kinesiology have been developed and are still developing throughout the world. It is an incredible blossoming of knowledge. This science, which is a unique marriage of ancient eastern esoteric sciences with the physiology of the West, is now in a stage of tremendously exciting fermentation. Kinesiology provides access to the holographic or whole body: the mind, the spirit, the emotions and the physical being. In essence all the realms of being that can impact on our health.

As such it is a truly remarkable healing tool.

THE SUBCONSCIOUS RULES

Through the muscle monitoring techniques of kinesiology, the body can be asked direct questions. By body, we mean that integrated unit of the physiological, emotional, mental and spiritual realms of your being. 'You.' We underline that this access is possible because muscle response is predominantly controlled from the subconscious.

We think we run our body consciously, yet if you consider it from a physiological point of view, even when you are standing still there are hundreds of muscles in various states of contraction operating to keep you upright. Consciously, you are not involved but every second millions of bits of information are being processed in your subconscious.

The reason you are not aware of these five to 10 million impulses per second is because most of the information goes directly into the cerebellum, the basal ganglia and other subconscious parts of your brain. Only a small amount of that sensory data is passed into your conscious cortical areas for you to perceive. In a sense, what you perceive consciously is only a summary statement of everything that is happening subconsciously.

You tell your body to stand up. That simple instruction constitutes conscious input into the subconscious areas of your brain that run the motor system; they then issue instructions for your muscles to contract and synchronise in a way that allows you to stand up. This action requires millions of pieces of sensory data, yet all your conscious brain needs to know is the fact that you are standing up.

When you walk, the decision to move is conscious. Once you start walking, however, you can begin thinking about something else entirely. The body can go into auto-pilot, a sub-system or a subconscious program that interacts with the consciousness to some degree, but largely leaves you free to think about other things. This subconscious programming is extremely powerful because at times it can and must supersede conscious instructions. When we examine muscle responses, we see that the mechanism is set up in such a way that ultimately, it cannot be overridden by the conscious. When it comes to the more important program of survival, or of protecting the body from harm, the subconscious rules.

If, for instance, you consciously wish to be stupid and try to pick up a weight that would violate your physical integrity by loading so much tension onto the body that muscles and tendons would tear and bones break, the subconscious sensors measuring the increasing rate of tension would tell the subconscious control centres that damage is likely to occur. The subconscious would then turn the muscles off: overriding your conscious instructions. You can see this happen in any weight lifting competition. Just as a finalist is pushing the barbell above their head, they begin to tremble and drop the weight. Their subconscious has overridden their conscious desire to break the world record. It will not allow them to damage their structural integrity even to fulfill a consciously desired goal.

In a sense, what happened was when they reached the critical point, the tendon and muscle sensors said to the subconscious: 'Sorry, you have not trained long enough and hard enough to lift this weight. If you go any further, damage will occur.' The subconscious replies. 'Turn off all muscles causing this tension, and the bar is dropped.'

And have you ever noticed that the weight lifter appears to throw the bar to the floor? He really does throw it down, but not consciously. Again, what happens subconsciously is that signals are not only sent to the muscles that are pushing up, telling them to turn off, other signals are simultaneously sent to the muscles that push the bar away and down in order to release the tension as swiftly as possible and to keep the bar from falling on the weight lifter's head.

So while we think we are in charge of our physical activity, we are actually aware of very little of it. The vast majority is subconsciously driven and the subconscious has its own agenda: survival.

SURVIVAL FIRST

Scientific experiments have established that neuropathways are activated by the simple act of remembering an event. They are the same neuropathways that fired when you actually experienced the event.[45] While this aspect of recalling from memory powerfully loaded survival experiences is useful for our physical well-being, it can become an equally powerful impediment to our personal growth.

These mechanisms have their roots in our evolutionary origins. The traditional lifestyles of aboriginal peoples allude to the idea that mankind basically grew up as a social species who lived in small kinship groups and who spent most of their lives eking out a living from their environment, an environment which contained considerable physical risk. In prehistoric times, there was much more danger in the immediate surroundings. Real physical threat occurred on a day-to-day basis and because of these conditions, the brain evolved in a way that ensured survival.

It also evolved in a way that helped maintain emotional harmony, interaction and cooperation in small, dependent social groups, because an individual had a much better chance of survival by being a member of a group. This has left us with an emotional structure that is built around both physical and social survival. Taboos and rituals developed to facilitate our social survival as much as reactions to threat developed for our physical survival. While physical threat alone was necessary to initiate physical survival programs, mechanisms to survive emotional threat evolved to ensure cultural survival. Primary among the mechanisms that aid social survival is guilt!

The emotion, guilt, is programmed into us in a social context before we are capable of rational thought and hence it becomes one of our basic survival programs. When you do something that is considered outside the norms of your group, you are told or made to feel that you are bad. Children learn very early that when they are bad they are not liked, and love is often withheld. So quickly, children realise that when they do something bad, they feel bad. This is the essence of the Guilt Program. How many adults, including yourself, do you know who are often run by their guilt programming?

You can see that there are powerful subconscious emotional programs that drive our behaviour. Guilt is only one, but an important one. While the sight of a charging bull will trigger your physical survival program: Run!, unspoken disapproval can just as powerfully trigger your emotional survival program: Guilt!

This is particularly true of children who operate on a much more intuitive, feeling level. Unspoken gestures and vocal tone have much more power and meaning than spoken words which children largely don't comprehend. The power of these signals is that they activate or trigger strong emotions which are linked to similar, negative emotional experiences that have occurred in the past. When this happens the child is now *reacting*, not to the current circumstance, rather to their emotional experience of a similar circumstance in the past. The past becomes *now* for them and the emotion of the past dominates their current state.

To the brain, what it remembers is no different to what is actually happening in real time. A memory that you are experiencing currently, is, to your brain, your current reality. A situation that you are thinking about, even one that may not occur until the future, can also have the same impact or emotional charge to the brain. The brain responds to both real, remembered or imagined impulses in the same way—as if they were occurring right now. Brain time is Now Time!

This now-time programming triggered by past experiences is the basis of a muscle unlocking or weakening, when we merely think about a past experience or event. When a muscle is monitored and the person accesses a negative memory, the guilt or the other negative emotions, interferes with the neurological conversation that is taking place between the muscle and the central nervous system.

THE MUSCLE-EMOTION INTERFACE

How can something that I only thought or felt, particularly something from the past or that may only happen in the future, affect a muscle?

The subconscious area of the brain that controls or elicits our emotions is located in the limbic brain, the ancient brain developed in our evolutionary past. There are direct neurological connections between the limbic brain and the pathways that control our muscle tone and tension.[46] Why do you think your neck gets tight when you are anxious and worried? Why does your stomach churn? Why do purely mental events have such a telling physical effect?

It is because the part of the brain that controls our emotional and physical survival programs also subconsciously sets the tone of our muscular system. Therefore, the emotional tone of a person is directly reflected in their muscular tone. If you see someone walking down the street with head down, shoulders slumped, drooping mouth and downcast eyes—all states of muscle tone—you would probably correctly surmise that this person is depressed or unhappy. It is interesting to note that somehow western medical science has been largely blind to an observation of the effect of emotions on muscular tone that even young children make: 'Mummy, are you unhappy?' Our emotional states are very graphically echoed in our physical postures.

Clearly, because kinesiology monitors subconscious muscle tone, it is directly linked to the emotional centres that are setting that tone. When monitoring a muscle, it is possible to get in touch with the interface between the neurological physical body, and the emotions and thoughts that affect that

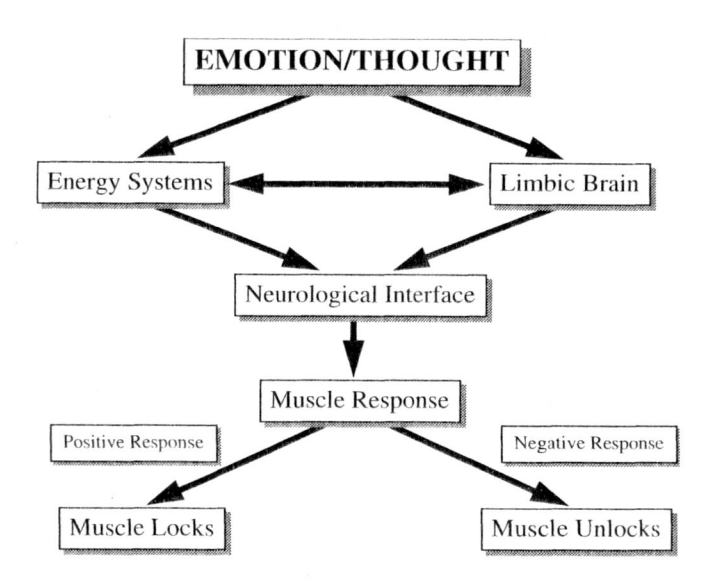

Figure 2.6. The Emotional-Muscle Interface. Emotions and thoughts may affect muscle function through two pathways. One is through the Limbic brain and its affects on muscle tone. The other is via the energy systems and their affects on the physiology of muscle response.

body. Further, the muscle also monitors the interface between the physical body and the energetic systems of Chinese acupuncture. If you recall, the Chinese recognised that each energy flow was affected by specific emotional states. What kinesiology adds is the physical response linking energy and emotions. Figure 2.6 illustrates this relationship, while Appendix A gives a table of meridian-related emotions.

EMOTIONAL STRESS DEFUSION

As we've explained, one of the most powerful techniques in kinesiology as it is practiced today is Emotional Stress Defusion, or ESD, the technique that allows us to alter the blood flow patterns in the brain. To spell out the reason why this is important: Under stress the brain redirects blood flow, which contains vital oxygen and glucose, to those areas of the brain that are most important for survival.

Under threat, the limbic centres become extremely active and access the back brain cortical areas where our memories of what happened in the past are stored. These areas, therefore, demand high levels of blood flow.

The blood flow to areas in the front of the brain that are involved with our associational thinking, our conscious thoughts, is temporarily shut down so our thoughts do not interfere with our ability to react.

Threatening circumstances require you to react. Not to think about action.

When you are in a potentially threatening circumstance, you must act instantly. This instant action, is really a *re-action*, or a re-enactment of a survival program that has been successful in the past. When your brain becomes aware of threat, within 1/500th of a second the limbic brain reviews all of the experiences you have had that closely match the one you are undergoing. Without your conscious awareness, the limbic brain then chooses the past program that had the highest survival value in similar circumstances. This program is then replayed and directs your behaviour, serving as a reference, so you can re-enact the behaviour that enabled you to survive in the past.

For instance, a little girl knocks over her glass of milk at the dinner table. Her father, who has had a bad day at the office, over-reacts and yells at the child: 'I can't believe you have knocked over the milk again! You stupid girl!' Because she is still at an age when she is largely irrational, she cannot understand that her father's outburst is actually based on his emotional state, which had little to do with spilled milk. True, he did yell at her, but rationally he was not intending to threaten her.

What the child's limbic brain perceives from this verbal assault and his angry tone, however, is a threat to her survival. She begins to cry, her posture becomes submissive and she starts to shake, all limbic responses for survival. Her father, seeing her response, realises he has overreacted and suddenly softens. He takes his daughter into his arms, pats her head and tells her: 'It's OK sweetie. Don't cry.'

Because of the emotional intensity of the event, this experience may become a pivotal emotional survival program of how this woman should react when men are angry and yelling at her. It becomes her way of deflecting male anger.

Now, as an adult woman she may find herself reverting to this childish behaviour whenever she is yelled at by a man. She becomes a consummate helpless woman, needing constant consolation from dominant males. This can add to what psychologists define as 'learned helplessness'. In her current life, this woman may have an argument with her boyfriend. He raises his voice. His vocal tone and intensity trigger her three years old 'Angry Daddy' tape, which activates the emotional survival program to submit and become helpless to reduce the threat.

It might have been an effective program for a young child, but it now impedes her ability to act like an adult woman and resolve differences in a mature, responsible way. In effect, she is responding as a three-year-old and she expects her male partner to console her as her father once did.

As time goes by this woman begins to recognise that this behaviour is truly not serving her in her relationships with men. What to do about it? She has heard about a kinesiology practitioner who is said to work well with entrenched emotional issues. She decides to make and appointment to see him.

EXPERIENCING KINESIOLOGY

After a brief outline of muscle monitoring and the general techniques that will be used in the consultation, the woman and her therapist discuss the reason she has come and what outcome she is seeking.

'I'm sick and tired of falling in a heap every time my boyfriend and I get into an argument and he raises his voice. I feel like a child. I'm sick of being so totally unable to express my point of view.'

To evoke the emotional context of that experience, the kinesiologist asks her to think about the last argument she had with her boyfriend. He monitors a muscle to ascertain if there is any subconscious stress around this issue. The muscle unlocks, indicating there is indeed unresolved subconscious stress around the issue. While the woman continues to think about her problem the kinesiologist touches the ESD points on her forehead and remonitors her muscle. It now locks. A change in response.

What has happened? Thinking of the stress created a frequency of imbalance. Holding the ESD points on the forehead also activates a frequency. If the frequency of her stress matches the frequency of the ESD points, the muscle will now lock. This is very much like tuning your radio. Every station has a specific frequency. Between stations there is just static, but once you match the frequency of the station with the frequency of your receiver, suddenly there is a change. The music.

In the energetic body, each type of thought you have generates its own specific frequency or vibration. When you hold specific acupoints, of which the ESD points are just one example, you also activate a frequency. If the frequency of your thought is that of emotional imbalance, it will match the frequency of the ESD points, hence there will be a change in the muscle response.

What the practitioner now knows is that the issue is emotional in nature and is causing an imbalance in the woman's body function. The energetic detective work begins: In kinesiology and many complementary health fields, we are much more interested in the origin of a problem than in the specifics of the problem as it now presents. What then is the origin of this emotional imbalance?

In biocomputer terminology the issue is now 'on line' and the practitioner can hold the data, the information of the energy imbalance, in a working file via Beardall's ingenious 'retaining mode'. The frequency of the stress is now on the biocomputer.

To ascertain the time of the origin of this emotional stress the kinesiologist may have the woman state, 'present' and monitor the muscle. No change. No frequency match. She says 'future' Again there is no muscle change. Then she says, 'past'. Now there is a change which indicates that the origin of the issue, which he knows to be emotional, is in her past.

Here the practitioner can employ the very important technique of Age Recession in which the practitioner monitors the muscle while the client states different ages; starting with the current age and working back towards birth. He asks her current age? 'I'm 32.' No match. No match all the way back to 'five to birth?' Then the muscle unlocks.

He now knows that the cause of the emotional response in the current circumstance originates from something that happened to the woman between birth and the age of five. The muscle response pinpoints age three.

The woman repeats, 'age three' and as she does so her limbic brain, in a miracle of processing refined through millennia of 'survival first' evolution, immediately inspects all her experiences at that age for their emotional content. Simultaneously it is also assessing how they relate to the current issue. In the subconscious, what is triggered from memory is 'now' and those same neuropathways that were activated during the original event become active once again.

Seeking further information via muscle monitoring the kinesiologist now applies the techniques that allow him to assess who was relevant at the time, a male? A female? It is an entirely logical process. The male, as it happens, turns out to be Daddy.

What specific emotion did the interaction with Daddy almost three decades before leave as a trace in this woman's subconscious? The practitioner now directly applies the Law of Five Elements to locate the meridian most out of balance by touching the point of alarm for each meridian. Because the energy flow in each meridian is disturbed or unbalanced by a different type of emotion, the alarm point that unlocks the muscle being monitored when touched reveals the nature of the emotion associated with the issue.

Touching the alarm point for heart meridian gives a muscle response. The kinesiologist has his client state 'hate' and monitors the muscle. No response. 'Insecure', again no response. But when she states 'anger' the muscle unlocks.

The practitioner now knows the emotional issue is with her father at the age of three, and involves 'anger'.

The woman also knows, as she has observed and 'felt' her body's response to the questions. She may now begin to become conscious of the origin of her current problem. 'Oh yes. I do remember that when I was young, whenever my dad was angry and yelled at me, I would fall to pieces.'

What has happened is that the woman's initial thinking about the current issue, activated the old limbic program about males yelling and this triggered a deep subconscious recall of her original encounter with her father's anger: the initial experience of male anger and her subconscious behavioural survival response. The same response she is constantly re-enacting in her adult life.

How many adults do you know who at times act extremely childishly? What you are looking at is a rerun of one of their childhood emotional survival programs. The person doing the behaviour can even realise they are acting like a child but still, cannot help themselves and stop.

The practitioner may now apply the ESD technique to assist this woman to resolve the causal issue which is now on-line consciously. By simply holding two acupoints, Gall Bladder 14s, the gentle acupressure overrides the effects of the subconscious emotional stress the woman is now experiencing.

Holding these acupoints on the frontal eminences, redirects the blood flow from the deep limbic centres forward into the frontal lobes of the brain which permit you to look at life's experience from a point of view of learning. In other words, this woman should now be able to see that 'what happened, happened'. She also finds herself with new rational choices'. What can I learn from what happened? What was life's lesson in that circumstance for me ?'

As the kinesiologist holds the points and the woman just relaxes, she may or may not have sudden recall of that early life event. Some people recall infinite detail of an experience that they have not contacted in decades; some people may become emotional, to the point of tears. Some people feel very little. Emotional Stress Defusion experience varies with each individual and with each issue dealt with.

After a period of time, the practitioner will detect that the subconscious and conscious review of the past has defused the stress from the original event, indicated by synchronous pulsing in both points on the forehead. The woman's brain has finished the process of emotional defusion on this issue.

With more muscle monitoring the closure of the procedure is to review the major tenets of the presenting issue: 'Age three'; 'males', 'daddy', 'anger'. The muscle now remains locked/strong with each question. The stress on that issue at that age has been defused including the stress at the subconscious level.

The practitioner then monitors the muscle as he states ages from three back to her current age, 32, no further muscle response, the issue has been cleared back to the present. He now has her think once again about that last argument with her boyfriend. The muscle locks, indicating that the 'stress' in this current situation has also been resolved.

He may then ask her, 'I'd like you to think of the issue again and tell me how you now feel?'

After a moment of reflection she says 'It's weird, I just can't feel the charge in the argument, even though I can still see us having it.'

You cannot change what has happened to you in your life. However, with kinesiology, what you can change is how you feel about what happened to you, even if you were unaware of what caused the feeling in the first place.

This greatly simplified treatment story demonstrates that kinesiology can be an effective technique to resolve long-standing emotional problems. But it must be emphasised that because each person has had unique experiences that have contributed to the evolution of their personality, every individual's experience of kinesiology will be different.

A FAR-REACHING HEALING SCIENCE

Kinesiology is a potent and remarkable system that enables a practitioner to work with a wide range of issues. While it can work exceedingly well with the defusion of emotional stress, it may work equally well with the elimination of muscular pain and weakness. It can also be effective in the elimination of allergies and food sensitivities, as well as loosening the grip of self-destructive habits such as obsessions and addictions.[47]

When viewed from a conventional western point of view, the range of application of this new science seems almost impossibly wide. It almost seems miraculous. But it must be remembered that it is miraculous that I, who was never supposed to be able to walk again, am able to walk.

The reason kinesiology can have such wide-ranging effect is based on several factors: The first is that it is an energetic model that states that energy reflects physiology, and that energy affects physiology. Second, it is based on a model of health in which the Body-Mind seeks an innate sense of balance, but that sometimes this Body-Mind needs assistance to re-establish that balance. Third, the Body-Mind actually leads the practitioner to the source or origin of the problems creating stress. It is through the remarkable biofeedback mechanism of muscle monitoring that the subconscious can be directly contacted, and just as directly divulge its secrets.[48]

Thus the kinesiologist is not the dispenser of healing knowledge to the client but rather the facilitator of the body's own wish to be healed and whole. Even as a long time practitioner, I am still awed by the process I engage in every day in my practice and even more so by the outcomes. Part of this fascination is that because every person is unique, every treatment is utterly individual. I never find myself doing the same thing twice. Each treatment is a personal journey for both the practitioner and the client.

In many ways, the practitioner operates more as a detective than a diagnostician. In fact in kinesiology, we do not diagnose at all, we simply follow the trail of clues that the body provides us through the muscle response.

What is, in some ways, even more significant is the person's muscle response not only directs us to the cause of their problems but then is capable of also directing the therapy to resolve these problems.

In many ways the advent of kinesiology in the late 20th century indicates that the healing arts have come full circle. Ancient eastern energetic healing arts have melded with western physiological healing sciences. Mind and body are being reunited and the person who seeks healing is empowered with the responsibility for his/her own health. The future of kinesiology seems to hold boundless promise. However, at present it is in its formative stages and while there is much excitement and enthusiasm in the field, it is still developing.

New discoveries are constantly being made and new applications developed. At the same instance it is so new, that there has not yet been enough time to establish standardised training for practitioners. Up to this point kinesiology training has only been available through informal short courses, which has left the synthesising and implementation of much of this knowledge to the individual student. The result of such piecemeal training is that there is a wide diversity of expertise represented by people calling themselves 'kinesiologists.'

In Australia and other parts of the world currently, kinesiological training is being consolidated into schools and colleges which present integrated programs of learning. As well, the Kinesiological Associations in many countries are presently developing accreditation procedures for kinesiology practitioners. This means that in the near future kinesiologists will undergo more formalised and standardised training and the accreditation process will guarantee to the public a high level of professional service.

While these standards are being established personal recommendation is perhaps the best method of locating a suitable practitioner for your needs. Appendix B is a list of associations and centres providing information on kinesiology practitioners both here in Australia and overseas.

PART TWO

How to have a fully functional brain

Our deepest fear is not that we are inadequate.
Our deepest fear is that we are powerful beyond measure.

It is our light, not our darkness that most frightens us.
We ask ourselves, who am I to be brilliant, gorgeous, talented and fabulous?

Actually, who are you not to be?
You are a child of God.
Your playing small doesn't serve the world.

There's nothing enlightened about shrinking
So that other people feel secure around you.

We were born to make manifest the glory of God that is within us.
It's not just some of us. It's everyone.
And, as we let our own light shine,
So we consciously give other people permission to do the same.

As we are liberated from our own fear,
Our presence automatically liberates others.

Marianne Williamson, A Return to Love.

INTRODUCTION

The first part of this section introduces you to the amazing terrain of the human brain.

For most of us, there are at least some areas of function that we find difficult. To understand why this is so, we need to appreciate how the brain works and this requires a knowledge of the major structures involved in the processing and storing of information, and in the phenomenal synthesis of these processes which is thinking.

It is a fascinating journey into this remarkable inner world and like all canny travellers we will begin the adventure into the unknown by studying a map.

Though complex, the map is essential to understanding the full implications of the journey you are about to take deep into yourself.

We acknowledge that Chapter 3 represents a very steep learning curve because it outlines the principles of neuroanatomy, a science that asks you to take a multi-dimensional look at what is largely an abstract concept. The Brain. That mysterious mass beneath your skull.

Neuroanatomy also requires the learning of a whole new language to explain the exchanges that occur in all the functioning parts; the interactions of the hundred billion neurons that make up the human biocomputer.

If, at this point, you find this chapter too challenging, we encourage you to skip forward.

At any time you can return to the fascinating information outlined here by using the index.

Chapter Three

MAPPING A MARVELLOUS ENTITY

BRAIN STRUCTURE AND FUNCTION

The 1990s are being called the Decade of the Brain because although we have explored most of the planet and much of our planetary system, we have only just begun to explore the universe of the brain: the hundred billion or so neurons that make it the most complex structure on earth. Dr James Watson, co-discoverer of the double helix of DNA, rightly called the brain the last and greatest biological frontier.

But how are we to understand the incredible complexity of these hundred billion neurons which in turn, are each connected to thousands of other neurons? The structure rapidly becomes so complex that we cannot hope to follow the pathways of impulses even with the most sophisticated instruments.

Human beings have attempted to make computers to duplicate the brain's functions and as we become more and more adaptable in our ability to use these machines so we try to make them even more like our own brains. We now have computers that can perform parallel processing and batch processing, which is a measurable advance on the old analogue processors. Analogue processing mimics the logic functions of the brain in that it processes one thing at a time in a logical, linear, sequential way. These analogue functions cannot accommodate what the human brain can achieve so easily via the more creative aspects of what we call Gestalt processing.

Gestalt processing can consider many different things at once and reach a conclusion based on that universal sampling. It is the truly creative aspect of the brain, and even the most powerful supercomputers on the drawing board today pale into insignificance when compared to the brain's ability to work with metaphor and analogy, to see a logical sequence of events and then, to go beyond, and take an incisive leap of insight. The insight might not seem to follow and yet, somehow the hunch will be correct.

Such is the wonder of the human brain.

It seems that the more the scientific community learns about the capabilities of the human brain the more amazed we become. We are constantly finding ourselves at a new threshold, marvelling that each advance only reminds us how little we know.

One of the bigger questions brain researchers are now seeking to unravel is how the brain achieves such rapid integration of so many complex functions. Where does this integration of information, memory, learned responses and the ability to act almost automatically, actually take place?

We can identify different parts of the brain, and can stimulate them electrically to produce certain responses. But the brain is not made up of parts operating independently; there is an integration process at work that takes brain function to a higher level again. What has not been found is where in the brain this integration takes place.

Every time scientists think they have it pegged a new mystery arises. As clever as the human brain makes us as a species of reasoning survivors, the complexity of its functions continues to elude us.

THE NEURON,
Where It all Begins

Understanding brain function requires a basic understanding of its simplest element, the neuron or nerve cell. Neurons are cells specialised to transmit electrochemical impulses throughout the body. The human nervous system is thought to consist of more than a trillion neurons, or about the same as the number of stars in the Milky Way.[1] It suggests an awesome complexity.

While no two neurons are the same, all consist of three basic parts: dendrites which are tree-like branching filaments from the cell body; cell bodies which contain a nucleus and cellular machinery; and the axon or primary transmission line, which leaves the cell body to deliver its message elsewhere in the nervous system.

There are three types of neurons: sensory neurons, association or interneurons, and motor neurons. They vary greatly in the relative proportions of dendrites, cell bodies and axons.

Sensory Neurons bring information from all parts of the body to the central nervous system—the brain and spinal cord.

The dendrites of sensory neurons are connected to various types of sensory receptors, ranging from simple, naked nerve endings that report pain, to the highly complex receptors of sight and sound. Each type of receptor is adapted to receive a specific type of sensory stimulus, whether it be stimulus from the photoreceptors of the eyes or pressure of touch from sensory receptors in the skin.

When a stimulus of any type that registers above a threshold value is received by a receptor, it will cause it to 'fire', and this firing initiates a nerve impulse to travel down the usually long and well insulated high-speed sensory dendrite to the cell body, which lies just outside the spinal column.

The impulse then continues into the spinal cord, moving along the sensory axon. In some sensory neurons, the dendrites and axons, which may measure only a few hundredths of a millimetre in diameter, can be very long. When a two metre tall man stubs his toe, the sensory neuron carrying the pain signal to his brain must stretch a distance close to 1.8 metres.

Once the impulse enters the brain, it connects to other sensory neurons that relay the message to other brain areas. In only a few cases do sensory neurons connect directly to motor neurons that carry the message to move muscles.

Another notable characteristic of sensory neurons is that the sensory axons can branch, giving them the ability to send signals into other neural networks and thus spread the message even more widely.

Interneurons. The majority of sensory axons end on the dendrites of interneurons, or association neurons, whose axons go to yet other interneurons. These systems can often become great networks and account for more than 99 percent of all the neurons in the brain.[2] After these interneuron networks 'consider' the sensory information, one or more of the interneuron axons connecting to the dendrites of a motor neuron will fire. Thus is the decision to act on incoming sensory data initiated. Move your hand. The stove is hot!

Motor Neurons generally have shorter, highly branched dendrites which enable them to receive input from hundreds, or sometimes a thousand or more interneurons. Once the input in the cell body reaches threshold, the nerve impulse then rolls down the axon to innervate other motor neurons which relay the message to the muscles of the body to contract. Before you know it, your hand is off the hotplate.

To increase the speed of impulse conduction, the long dendrites of sensory neurons, and even their axons in some cases, are ensheathed by a whitish phospholipid segmented insulation called myelin. When the myelin sheath is destroyed, as in Multiple Sclerosis, the neural messages may go astray. Myelin gives the white matter of the brain and spinal cord its characteristic colour and name. In contrast, unmyelinated nerve fibres and cell bodies appear greyish and make up the so called grey matter of the brain.

The end of each axon branches like the tentacles of a squid, and each tentacle ends in a bulb, the axonal end bulb. The end bulbs of many tentacles may appear to make 'contact' with the dendrites or cell body of another neuron, or the end bulbs of each tentacle may appear to 'contact' the dendrites or cell bodies of different neurons, allowing the message from one axon to be delivered to a number of other neurons.

But the axonal end bulbs do not actually touch the dendrites of the next neuron. Instead, there is a minute gap or synapse between them. Measuring only 40 millionths of a millimetre across, the synapse plays a crucial role in controlling the flow of information in the nervous system (see Fig. 3.2a).

When the electrochemical nerve impulse arrives at the axonal end bulb, it causes the release of chemicals known as neurotransmitters. Neurotransmitters 'ferry' the message across the synapse to the dendrite membrane on the other side. The dendritic membrane has specialised 'docks' or receptors to receive the neurotransmitter ferry. These docks (the neurotransmitter receptors) are attached to channels through the neuronal membrane (see Fig. 3.2b). When the neurotransmitter ferry docks it can cause the ion channel to open wide, or

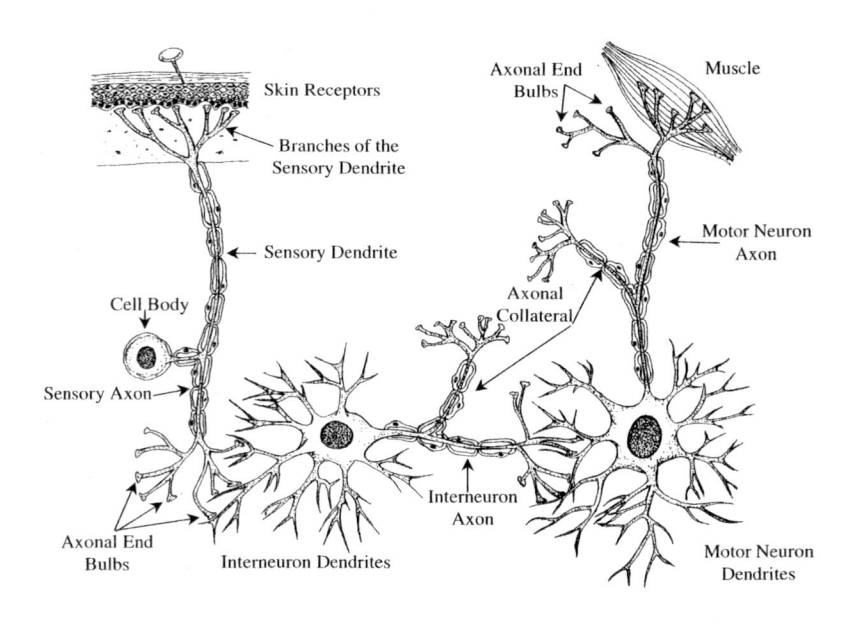

Figure 3.1. Types of Neurons and their Structure. The dendrites of the sensory neuron on the left connect to the receptors in the skin and carry the sensory information to the interneuron in the middle. The axon of the interneuron would normally connect to one or more other interneurons before making contact with the dendrites of the motor neuron on the right. The axon of the motor neuron then carries the message to contract to the muscles. The motor neuron axon and also most interneuron axons have collaterals or branches which distribute the information widely.

to close tightly depending upon the type of neurotransmitter and the type of receptor.

But how can this be? Since all nerve impulses are the same, how can one impulse cause muscles to contract and another to relax? How can one impulse make you excited and another calm you down?

The key to this distinction lies in the type of neurotransmitter and receptor involved. Neurotransmitters and receptors come in two varieties, either excitatory or inhibitory. The docking of an excitatory neurotransmitter causes the dendritic membrane to prepare to fire by opening the sodium ion channels, allowing positive sodium ions to enter the cell and thereby decreasing its polarity or charge. All nerve membranes have a resting potential of approximately -70 millivolts, or a greater negative charge on the inside than they do on the outside (see polarised dendrite membrane in Fig. 3.2b).

To maintain this polarity, cellular energy is used to actively pump positive sodium ions out of the cell body. A decrease in the membrane potential of the cell body of only 11 to 15 millivolts can result in sodium ion channels being popped open electrically, allowing the sodium ions to pour into the neuron and reversing the charge inside from negative to positive. The reversal in polarity, or depolarisation, begins the nerve impulse, which, once initiated, then rolls down the axon to its end bulbs resulting in the release of a

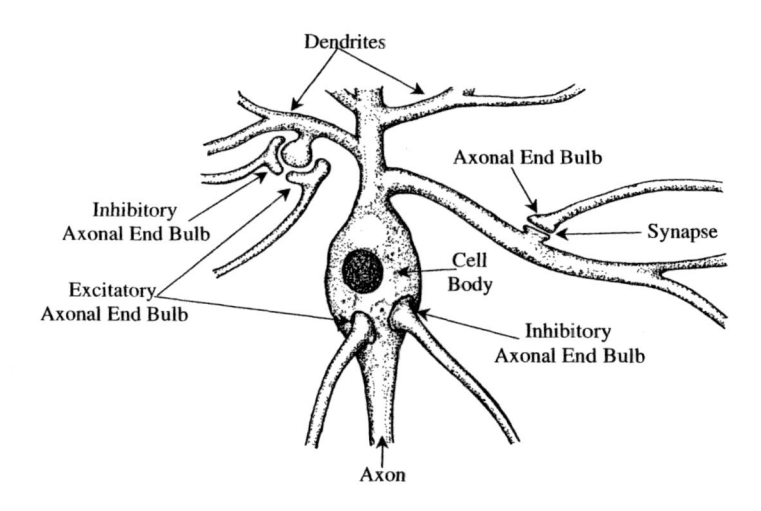

Figure 3.2a. Synapse of Axonal End Bulbs on the Dendrite and Cell Body of a Neuron. Note: The Inhibitory and Excitatory axonal end bulbs synapsing on a single dendritic spine and on the cell body often lie side by side. Whether that dendrite fires or not depends on the amount of inhibitory and excitatory neurotransmitter released.

neurotransmitter at the next synapse (see axon end bulb in Fig. 3.2b).

You can think of the neurotransmitter (NT) ferries as messengers: excitatory (+) NT ferries carry the message to 'fire', while inhibitory (-) NT ferries carry the message to 'stop'. The message to fire is relayed by opening the gates to the sodium ion channels caused by the docking of (+) NT ferries on

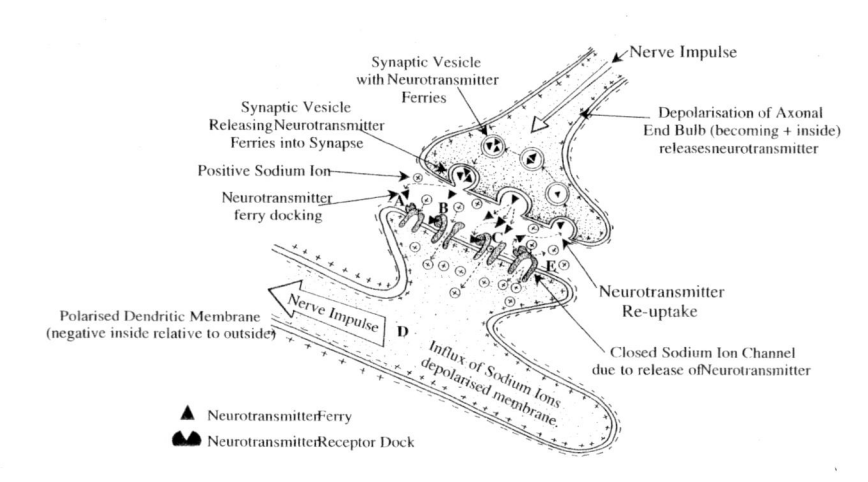

Figure 3.2b. Neurotransmitter Release initiates nerve impulse in Dendrite of downstream Neuron.
A. *Neurotransmitter ferry docking on receptor of closed sodium ion channel.*
B. *Docking of neurotransmitter on receptor opens sodium ion channel. Sodium ions begin to rush into the dendrite, depolarising the membrane.*
C. *Continued release of neurotransmitter ferries keeps ferries in the receptor docks and sodium ion channels open resulting in more sodium ion influx further depolarising the dendritic membrane until threshold is reached.*
D. *Threshold depolarisation of dendritic membrane electrically opens all sodium gates in that part of membrane allowing massive numbers of sodium ions to rush in initiating a wave of depolarisation (negative to positive inside) that begins to roll down the dendrite toward the cell body. This is the nerve impulse.*
E. *Neurotransmitter ferry leaving receptor dock and being taken up by the axonal end bulb for re-use. Sodium ion channel closes preventing further depolarisation. Sodium-Potassium pump begins immediate re-polarisation of the membrane by using energy to pump three sodium ions out for each two potassium ions pumped in, resulting in a resting potential with an excess of sodium ions outside and a negative charge inside (See part of dendrite in front of nerve impulse not yet depolarised)*

the (+) receptors, or the message to stop, is relayed by closing the gates to these channels—the docking of (-)NT ferries on their (-) receptors.

Thus when enough (+) NT ferries have docked and opened enough sodium ion channels, threshold is reached and a switch is thrown electrically opening all sodium ion channels on the membrane. In a sense this signals 'fire, fire, fire!' and the sodium rushes in creating a wave of depolarisation that rolls down the axon to the next synapse releasing the (+) NT ferries to relay the exciting news about what happened at the receptor:

'Ouch, I stubbed my toe' is relayed to the next neuron, and the next, until the brain is informed of what happened. Then, after considering the event, the decision to do something about the situation is likewise sent back to the muscles by a similar chain of 'fire' commands carried by (+) NT ferries at each synapse.

However, if it was all 'fire' and no 'stop', we would be hyper-excitable, twitching humans. This is where the (-) NT ferries and their inhibitory messages come into play. When the (-) NT ferries dock on their receptors, they close and lock the gates, preventing sodium ions from entering the neuron, and maintaining the polarised state. This signal says in effect, 'The message stops here!'

Does this mean that if (+) NT ferries dock and open the gates, the next downstream neuron fires? And that if the (-) NT ferries dock and close the gates the downstream neuron doesn't fire? Could it be this simple?

Not quite. Most neurons have excitatory and inhibitory end bulbs sitting side-by-side on the dendrite membranes and on the cell body (See Figure 3.2a). Thus there is a constant competition between the (+) NT ferries opening gates and the (-) ferries shutting them.

It is an additive function: If more (+) NT ferries dock than (-) NT ferries, enough gates will open to reach threshold and bang! The nerve impulse is off and rolling down the next neuron. If the reverse happens and more (-) NT ferries dock, the gates are closed and the message stops.

Since many neurons in the brain may have 1000 to 10,000 synapses with up to 1000 other neurons[3], and these thousands of synapses contain mixtures of both excitatory and inhibitory neurotransmitters and receptors, whether an individual neuron fires or not is anything but simple. If the excitation is enough to add up to a fire, the same summing or integration process is repeated at the synapses of the next neuron and so on.

Consider the scale of the operation. Throughout the nervous system, the levels of integration vary, from the simple axon-dendrite pair of a simple reflex arc, to the complex integration of millions, or even billions of neurons in the neural nets that are involved in the mental act of thinking.

Dendritic growth and branching are not static processes. They don't occur just once or twice in your life, like growing teeth. Based largely on usage, they are in a constant state of flux. As long as there is regular stimulation, the dendritic branches and synapses keep actively branching out, forming new synapses to transmit this new information more efficiently. New learning or the laying down of new memory results in a flurry of branching and synapse formation.

Over time, what were massive webs of interconnection are usually pared back to a few more permanent connections which maintain the link to particular target neurons. In such a way our access to memories and learned behaviours becomes ever more efficient.[4]

It was long presumed that the process of aging caused a loss of neurons in the brain. Older brains had less weight and mass than younger brains. Increasingly, however, the still contentious evidence is suggesting that it is not cells, but rather dendritic connections that disappear over time. According to brain researcher Gary Lynch, from our 20s onwards we are losing glutamate synapses in the cortex which are the primary excitatory neurotransmitter in the brain. By the time you are 70, you have probably lost 20 percent of these synapses.[5]

This description of the microworld of the neuron was a necessary briefing before we entered the macroworld of brain structures. The function of the macro-elements ultimately depends upon the function of individual neurons because the large brain structures are really nothing more or less than massive networks of interconnected neurons which are stimulated into action, or turned off, by neurotransmitters secreted often by other massive neural networks.

It is important to remember that while I will present parts of the brain as separate entities that perform specific functions, the truth is not always so clear cut. The phenomenally complex interactions at the micro-level of neurotransmitters and synapses between these apparently separate structures is what allows them to act in concert. In the cerebral symphony of thought and action these elements are key players.

THE BRAIN AS A THREE-TIERED STRUCTURE
The Reptilian Brain, The Limbic Brain and the Neocortex

The brain is a three-tiered, stratified structure. This concept of serial structure was first proposed by the neurologist, Dr. Paul McLean who called it the triune brain. Meaning 'three in one', the name is apt because what we can see is that evolution has added new structures to the primordial brain.[6]

Figure 3.3 shows us that the brain has a central stalk, the medulla, the brainstem and diencephalon. Together, these constitute the deep part of the central brain known as the reptilian brain, so-called because fish and reptiles have similar brain structures, and little more.

The Reptilian Brain is the body's caretaker, it is responsible for homeostasis which runs such functions as breathing, heart rate, temperature and the orderly operation of the intestines—all those things that keep the body ticking over on a physiological level.

The Limbic Brain. Beyond the reptilian brain is a newer layer called the palaeomammalian cortex. More commonly it is known as the limbic brain because it comprises the very deepest and oldest parts of the cortex and is linked to other subcortical areas. Cortex means an outer layer of tissue—'skin or bark'- and the limbic cortex was in fact the skin or outer covering of the old reptilian brain. Today the limbic brain is recognised as the area that modifies the instinctual drives which are initially generated in the reptilian brain.

The limbic brain is therefore the director of the reptilian brain and its primary focus is survival. Its operation is subconscious.

The Neocortex. In the more recently evolved mammalian species, there is an increase in the size of a third layer of the brain, the neocortex, or new cortex. It has expanded over the top of the old reptilian and limbic brains, effectively encasing them. Humans have the greatest development of the neocortex as well as a correspondingly complex development of the limbic brain. Humans and Cetaceans (whales, porpoises and dolphins) are the only mammals with relatively similar-sized and complex cortical structures. The neocortex is there in a dog's brain, but it is smaller relative to other brain parts and is quite smooth. A rat's cortex is smaller still, and very smooth (see Fig. 3.4).

The characteristic wrinkling of the neocortex provides more surface area,

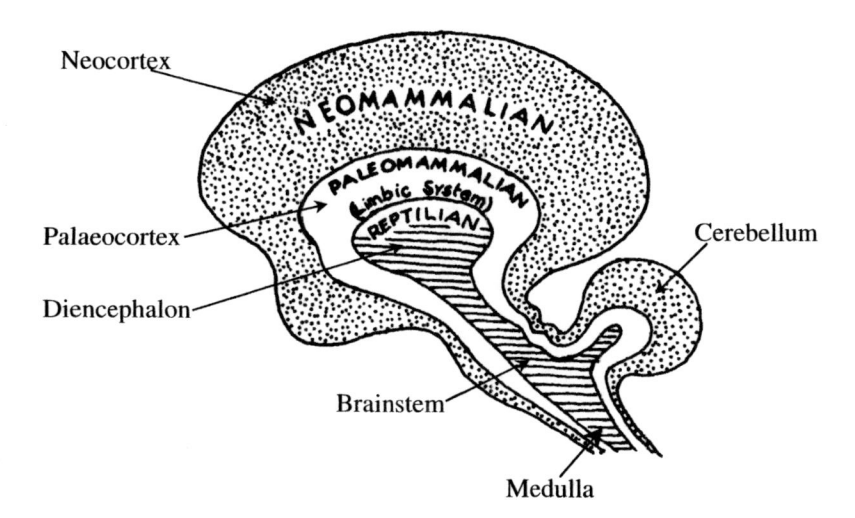

Figure 3.3. The Triune Brain. The ancient reptilian brain covered by our ancestral mammalian cortex now totally encased in the neocortex of modern man.

more room for more neurons. In the human brain this provides a huge surface area that contains billions of neurons. The neocortex is where we do our thinking.

THE HIERARCHY OF THE TRIUNE BRAIN

In this hierarchy, each layer plays its own unique role, but the basal physiological functions of the reptilian brain are modulated and controlled by the output of the emotional limbic brain, which in turn, can be controlled by the neocortex or thinking brain.

The limbic brain is the subconscious emotional processing centre whose major role is to look out for the survival of self and species. It directs the urges to mate, procreate, defend or submit. It says run if you can, fight if you can't or, stay where it is safe. It is also the part of the brain that elicits the nurturing response and controls and modulates all the basic built-in drives such as eating, drinking and sexuality.[7]

To give you a more graphic idea of how this triune brain works, picture

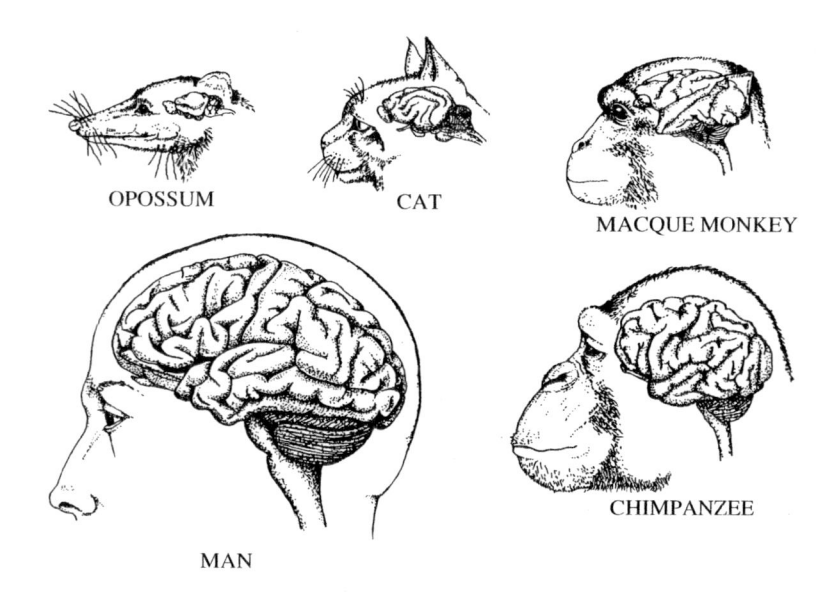

Figure 3.4. The brain cortices of different species. Note the size and convolution of the cerebral cortex increases dramatically from primitive mammals, the Opossum, to Man. The convolutions provide greatly increased surface area to accommodate greater number of neurons.

yourself at a party where you look across a room and see someone you find particularly attractive.

The limbic brain receives the information directly from the eyes, the nose and the ears in a rather coarse-grained way, then responds to the data by noting that there is an attractive, potential mate in the near vicinity. The instinctive drives and the direct limbic input concerned with procreation, will probably create an immediate subconscious urge to have sex with that person.

Now what happens in the brain of a thinking human being? In one who has a neocortex? The cortex begins to consider this impulse and the feelings that are being aroused, and incidentally, that are beginning to be expressed physiologically by the reptilian brain in the form of dilated pupils and feelings of arousal in various parts of the body.

But just as you start to walk across the room to say something to this person your partner steps in and asks who you are looking at? Your palms sweat, your mouth goes dry and you fumble for words. You are caught in the conflict between your limbic-driven desire and the cortical brain's response, which is to cut in and remind you sexual desire is not an appropriate response at this time and in these circumstances.

The neocortex, has strong but not definitive control over what happens next. It is as though partners are exchanging the lead in a kind of dance. At one point the logical, rational brain might be in charge ('Not now, this is not appropriate'). Then, quite suddenly, the other emotional, irrational, part of our brain takes over ('But I want that person—now!'). That might lead to doing something we might later regret. Ideally, the cortical structure has the ability to control and modify limbic response to suit your culture.

All cultures have a cortical 'scaffolding' constructed around the primary limbic drives. The limbic system might produce a particular urge, but the scaffolding then decrees how that drive will be expressed. Witness how young men from different cultures go about attracting a mate, and the different taboos of different societies. In each society there has evolved a framework of acceptable ways to express basic limbic drives. Social structure is then basically a cortical function, and losing touch with those social mores—letting an impulse escape and losing our cool—basically means losing cortical control.

THE SMALL BRAIN

There is another part of the brain called the cerebellum, Latin for 'little brain' (see Fig. 3.5). The cerebellum is the outbudding of the old part of the brainstem and orchestrates all of our co-ordinated, automatic physical activity, such as balance or equilibrium. It receives information from the cortex about what activity you want to perform and helps the basal ganglia, a structure deep in

84   A Revolutionary Way of Thinking

the brain, to organise the sequence of activity to perform this act. It organises, co-ordinates and smooths the flow of action, refining it so that the final action becomes the streamlined act intended by the cortex.

The cortex gives the direction: 'I want to ride a bike'. At your first attempt you are awkward and have trouble balancing. You fall off. For a while you are teaching the cerebellum and the basal ganglia the sequence of activities you want to perform. But once learned, this motor memory appears to be imprinted in the cerebellum.[8] Even years later, riding a bike will present little difficulty because your cerebellum remembers how to do it.

When you are touch-typing, you will find you can do it even if you are thinking about something else because, having learned the skill, the cerebellum can basically run your fingers. I once had a secretary who could type at 90 words a minute while having a conversation. She would occasionally glance at the paper she was typing from then keep talking. She could do it because her little brain was running her fingers while her big brain, the cerebral cortex, was running her mouth. All she had to do was pause occasionally to take in some visual data.

The cerebellum appears to store our motor memory of reflexive automatic actions. Once these motor patterns—learning to walk—have been stored, you never have to think about the actions again. Playing tennis is the same. After you learn all the basic moves and become proficient, moves that require

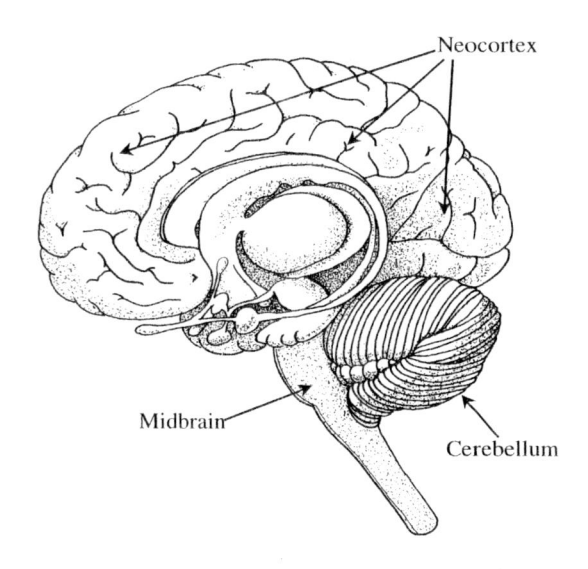

Figure 3.5. The Cerebellum. The cerebellum is the little brain beneath the larger cerebral cortex that is largely involved in the interpretation of sensory feedback from the body and the integration and co-ordination of movement.

fine and precise control are imprinted and can be reproduced automatically.

Training in any sport or activity is about getting those initial movements exactly right so that the cerebellum is programmed correctly. That is why if you learn something incorrectly, it is so difficult at a later time to learn to do it correctly. It is also arguably why it is worth getting a coach and learning how to do it right the first time because it is so much harder to override bad habits once they have been encoded into the cerebellar circuits.

THE STRUCTURE OF THE CORTEX

The cortex sits on the brainstem like a mushroom cap sitting on its stalk. The brainstem, as we have explained, is the reptilian brain. At the top of the stem is the limbic brain. Over it, and flowing down on both sides, is the cerebral cortex, a mass of convoluted tissue more commonly known as the grey matter.

One very obvious feature of the cortex is the deep longitudinal fissure that appears to divide the brain in half. It marks the division between the right and left hemispheres of the brain. These two hemispheres are anatomically very similar and for a long time scientists were at a loss to know what types of functions they performed.

The two hemispheres are further divided into areas known as lobes. Lobes

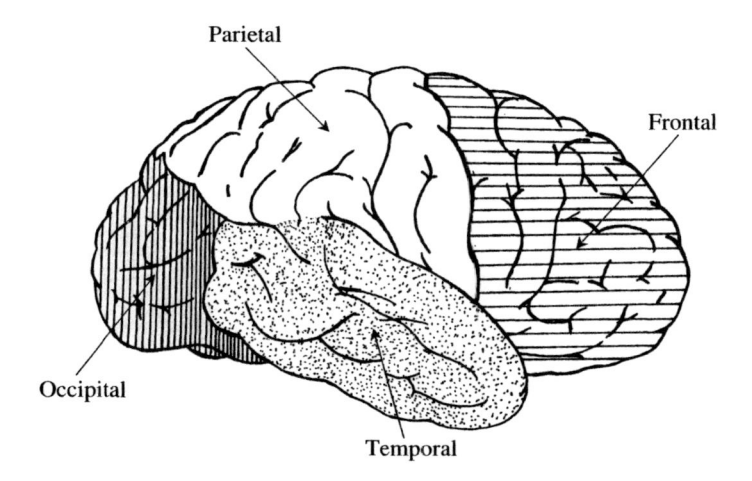

Figure 3.6. The lobes of the brain. The frontal lobes account for almost half of the brain while the parietal and occipital lobes make up the back half of the brain. The temporal lobes extend forward from the junction of the parietal and occipital lobes to line each side behind your eye.

86 *A Revolutionary Way of Thinking*

are technically the functional regions of the brain and they too display deep grooves, which divide them into four distinct areas or lobes (see Fig. 3.6).

One groove runs from the region near the top of the ears to the crown of the head. This is the central sulcus, or central groove. The central sulcus divides the frontal lobes from the large expanded area of the brain sitting behind the ears. Technically this area is known as the parietal lobes.

Another groove runs horizontally across the back of the brain just above the base of the skull. This fissure separates the parietal lobes above from the occipital 'base' lobes below. The temporal lobe is separated from the frontal

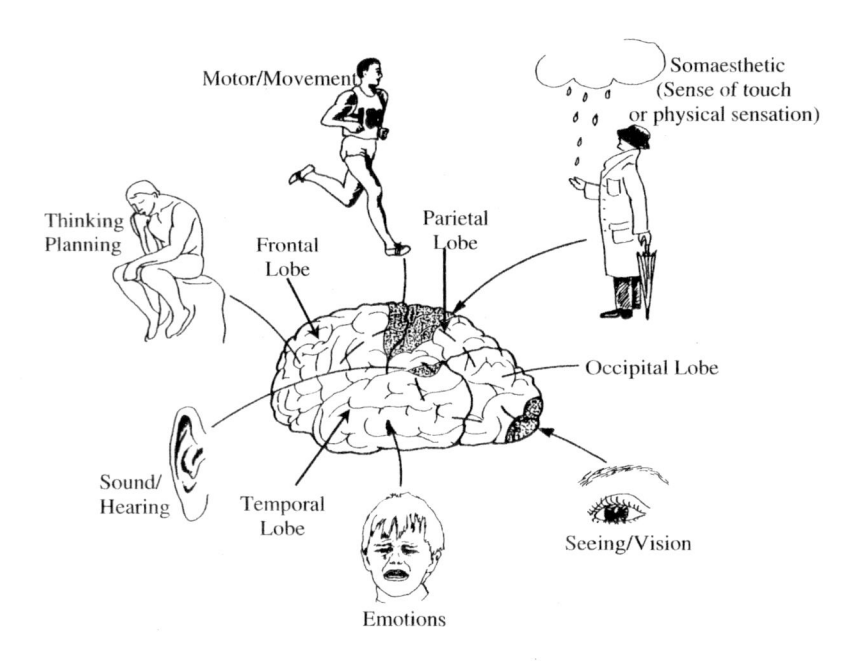

Figure 3.7. A graphic representation of cortical functions.

lobes by the lateral cerebral sulcus, and less distinctly from the parietal and occipital lobes by the parieto-occipital sulcus.[9]

The Frontal Lobes are the areas of the brain where we do our planning, thinking and reasoning. They also control all voluntary movement. For example, when you decide to move your right finger it is the frontal lobes that instruct the body to perform this action. There is a specialised region in the frontal lobes that produces speech by way of organising and sequencing all the muscles required to speak. The frontal lobes also control voluntary eye movement, enabling you to look about.

The Parietal Lobes receive and process sensory data. If you step on a pin this is the area of the brain that registers the pinprick. It is also called the somaesthetic area because it perceives all physical sensation and interprets touch and body image and awareness. These lobes also have the capacity to store memories of touch and body experience.

The Occipital Lobes are the site of vision. They receive and process visual data, creating our conscious visual images. This area also stores our memories of past visual experiences.

The Temporal Lobes are where we hear and interpret music, speech and language. A specialised area in the posterior of the left superior temporal lobe is the site where our thoughts are turned into words. Another specialised area, the hippocampus, a part of the limbic brain, is the centre for short-term memory, and this lobe stores the memories of our emotions. Memories, emotions and hearing are all located in this same region, a proximity that explains the evocative power of music.

The function of each lobe is graphically represented in Figure 3.7.

THE AMAZING TERRAIN OF THE HUMAN BRAIN

The cortex of the human brain has been mapped. The initial mapping was done by the German neuroanatomist Korbinian Brodmann, who explored the brain on an anatomical/architectural basis. He divided the brain into 52 areas, now known as Brodmann's Areas and although it was first published in 1909 his work remains a standard map of the brain that is often still referred to today.[10]

If we look at Brodmann's map (see Fig. 3.8) we see the brain is now divided into areas that relate to different functions. Brodmann constructed his map by looking at the structure, arrangement and grouping of similar types of cells in the cerebral cortex.

In the 1940s and 50s the neurosurgeon Wilder Penfield mapped much of the brain using electrical stimulation of the brains of conscious patients during brain surgery. Achieved with the co-operation of patients undergoing brain surgery, the process allowed him to take a very close look at some localised areas that seem to be very strongly related to function. Because brain tissue has no pain receptors, the skull can be opened while a person is under only a local anesthetic and fully conscious. In this way scientists have been able to insert fine electrodes into specific parts of the brain, stimulate these areas with a mild electric current and ask the patient what they feel.[11]

By such means researchers discovered that structures located either side of the central sulcus and known as the precentral and postcentral gyri are respectively involved with the control of movement and the reception of sensory stimuli. Gyrus means 'ridge' and these two ridges run down the cerebral hemispheres, just in front of and at the back of the ears. They are otherwise known as the primary motor cortex and the primary sensory cortex (see Fig. 3.10).

The primary motor cortex is the place from which instructions are issued to voluntary muscles. If you want to move your right index finger there is an exact point in the left primary motor cortex that directs the action. When the point is electrically stimulated, the right index finger of a patient will move, even though he will say he is not moving it. Whenever the primary motor cortex is stimulated, some part of the body will twitch or move and the part

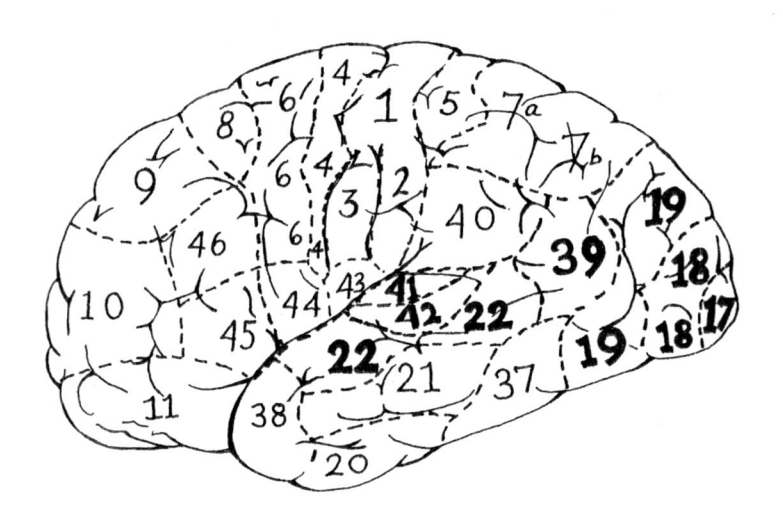

Figure 3.8. Brodmann's Areas of the cortex. Based on the cytoarchitecture of the brain Korbinian Brodmann divided the cerebral cortex into 52 functional areas. The numbers on the brain above are the Brodmann numbers which are still commonly used today.

that moves depends on what point receives the stimulus. Scientists were able to show that the control of the body parts is indeed topographically arranged[12].

For instance, in the primary motor cortex, the thumb is controlled from a point located right next to the point that controls the index finger. The ring finger is at a point beside the little finger and so on. Then follow the areas that control the wrist, the forearm, the elbow, the upper arm and the shoulder—all laid out in the brain just as they are in the body.

Likewise, the primary sensory cortex is also topographically arranged with sensory stimuli from adjacent body areas lying next to each other in the sensory cortex. When you stub your big toe, the way the brain knows it is your big toe and not your thumb is by the area of the sensory cortex that receives the impulse from your big toe.

The area of the sensory cortex at the end of the pathway from the big toe lies beside those coming from the second toe, the third toe, the foot, the ankle, the calf, the knee and so on. Again, the brain receptors imitate the arrangement of the body and what this uncanny mirroring allows is for the brain to project back to where the impulse was first registered. The sensory experience is only registered within the brain. The brain then uses projection to externalise that experience, and assign the source of that experience to the big toe.

An even more interesting aspect of the primary motor and sensory cortices is that within each, those parts of the body that require the finest motor control and have the greatest degree of sensation, are represented by proportionately greater areas.

In Figure 3.9 we see a visual representation of the scales of the different sensory centres in the brain. You can see the enormous areas given to the hands, lips and tongue while that for the torso is extremely small. The rest of the body too is quite small in terms of its sensory receptors. But look at the feet!

The brain would certainly perceive a blow to the trunk but the skin on a bare back may fail to pick up the fine texture of fabrics. By contrast, the

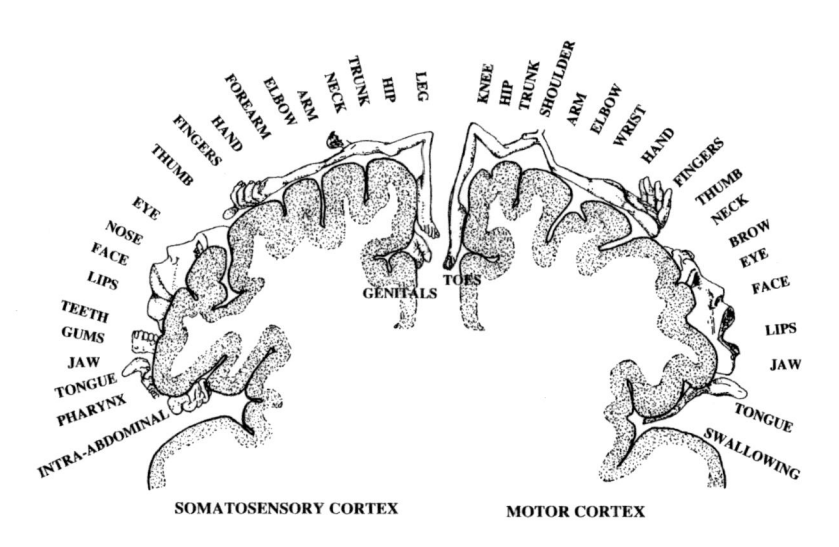

Figure 3.9. The topographic representation of motor and sensory function. Shown here as motor and sensory homunculi or little men drawn with body regions proportional to the area of motor or sensory cortex devoted to that body part.

fingers would give very precise information about fabric texture and the tongue would be even more acute. Part of the reason that objects in the mouth feel so large is the enormous number of sensory receptors on the tongue. The tongue is able to locate the tiniest hair, seed or fishbone and will not leave it alone until it is removed from the mouth.

In the motor homunculus, the genitals are given little space because relatively little motor function takes place there. The legs and arms are also small. So is the trunk of the body, which only performs gross motor functions. But the hands, lips and tongue again, are enormous because of the precision of motor function that they need to perform. Consider the large number of muscles you use to speak or make a facial gesture.

All of this makes complete sense because obviously, it would require more brain cells to operate a function that requires finer motor skills or interpret more precise sensory perception. The greater the degree of motor function or sensory perception at a particular area of the body, the greater is the space it takes up in the brain.

SIGNIFICANT SITES OF PERCEPTION AND PROCESSING

Brain mapping added dynamic detail to the knowledge of the function of various brain areas (see Fig. 3.10). By the end of the last century, functions were found to be localised in various parts of the brain. The two World Wars of our century provided many soldiers with head injuries that had damaged specific areas of the brain. By correlating the specific area damaged with the corresponding loss of function, the lesion studies provided, and continue to provide, valuable information about the functions of various brain areas.[13]

One major discovery was that the occipital lobes were found to be largely involved with vision. The parietal lobes are involved with touch and the memories of sensations. Going into more precise detail, the mapping revealed that the back part of the frontal lobes is involved with motor movement. But that this area was even further subdivided into the premotor cortex and the primary motor cortex.

The premotor cortex appears to organise and stage the sequence of movement. The frontal lobes give the instruction to tap your foot, but it is the premotor cortex that organises the sequence of muscles needed to perform this action. This sequence is then forwarded to the primary motor cortex which activates the individual muscles in the order required to perform the action of toe tapping.

A large area of the frontal lobes, which comprise almost half of the brain, has no known motor function. It does not respond to stimulation by producing any particular movement in the body. Called the association areas of the prefrontal cortex, it is now understood to be the place in which we perform free-thought associations or abstract thinking.[14] The upper lateral areas also house our working memory and areas along the middle and bottom of the frontal lobes—the inferior medial prefrontal cortex—are known to be involved in the process of creating our emotions.[15]

Looking into the temporal lobes, we discover that the top and medial (inside) temporal lobe is the place where we hear and taste, respectively. Another major temporal lobe function is the perception and interpretation of sound and the memory of what was heard. Around those hearing sites are still other areas where emotional memories are encoded, alluding again to a close regionalisation of sound and memory.

Brodmann's Areas. An important aspect of cortical function that we need to understand is how the different ridges or gyri in Brodmann's Areas relate to other specialised functions. In Figure 3.10 it can be seen that some individual gyri appear to perform specific functions, while in other areas of the cortex several gyri together perform a specific function.

One gyrus in the frontal lobe, Brodmann Areas 44 and 45 and named Broca's Area after the great 19th century neuroanatomist Pierre Paul Broca, organises the muscles that allow us to make the sounds of speech.[16] To be able to speak, we need to be able to control the breath, the tension in the vocal chords and the

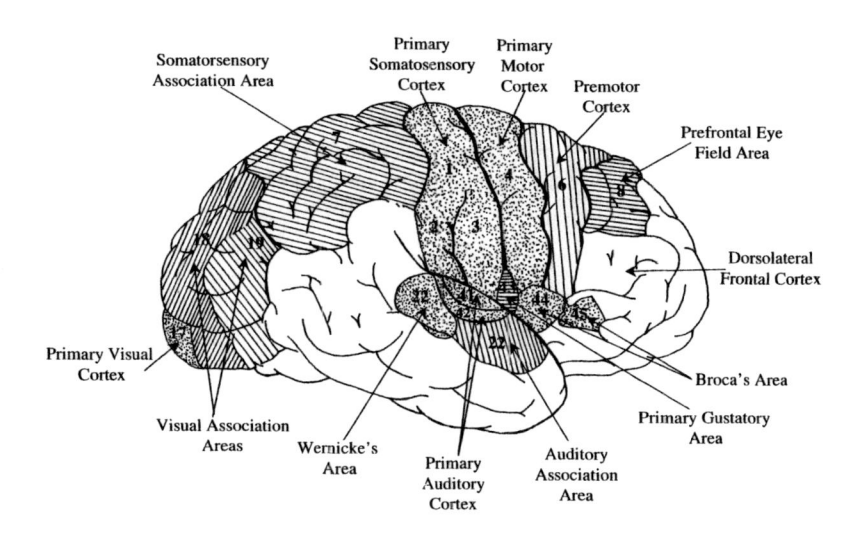

Figure 3.10. Major functional areas of the brain. The cortical areas identify with specific sensory and motor processing and their associated Brodmann numbers. The dorsolateral frontal cortex is the site of working memory to be discussed in the next chapter.

shapes of the muscles in the throat, as well as the tongue and the lips. All must come into play in a particular sequence before we can utter a sound.

Another gyrus, the posterior part of Brodmann Area 22, has similarly been named after the 19th century neuroanatomist Carl Wernicke, who discovered it. It is the all-important area where we develop our thoughts. Located at the juncture of the temporal, parietal and occipital lobes Wernicke's Area is the site that turns our thoughts into words that we may speak, and words that we read or hear, into thoughts to think about.[17]

Many other gyri appear to work together to perform other more complex functions. Brodmann Area 17 has been found to undertake the initial organisation of visual image formation which is then built upon in Area 18 to create a sharp static image. Parallel processing of the same visual input in Area 19 adds motion, colour and three-dimensional position in space to create a seamless unified visual perception.[18] Visual information entering your eye, thus goes back to these gyri in the occipital lobes, and in both a multi-layered and parallel sequence, the information is melded into what we 'see'.

THE SITE OF MENTAL PROCESSING

The Cortical Columns

The enlarged neocortex is structured differently from the older palaeocortex (of the limbic brain) in that it displays six layers or strata. The ancient cortex has only three. It has been found that the six layers have a distinct functional arrangement. Based on topographical logic it was once believed that these layers should operate in horizontal associations, but they don't.

Newer research has shown that vertical columns bisect all six layers forming distinct processing units called cortical columns. These are not circular columns in the architectural sense, rather long three-dimensional slabs up to 0.5 mm wide and variable in length.[19] Each cortical column is concerned with a specific type of function, and as functions vary in complexity so the columns vary in size. And sometimes several columns may be involved in performing a single more complex function. Along the sensory cortex, each column is concerned with sensory input from a particular region of the body.[20]

From figure 3.11 you can see that the six layers of the cortex contain many different types of neurons. Some specialise in connecting horizontally across a layer, some in connecting adjacent layers, and some interconnecting all layers, much like the large pyramidal neuron in the centre. While only a few connecting neurons, or interneurons, are shown, it is by the interconnecting neurons that the sensory input to the cortex is integrated with the output from the cortex to other parts of the brain and the rest of the body. Indeed, since the job of the cortex is integration or decision-making based upon integration of sensory and

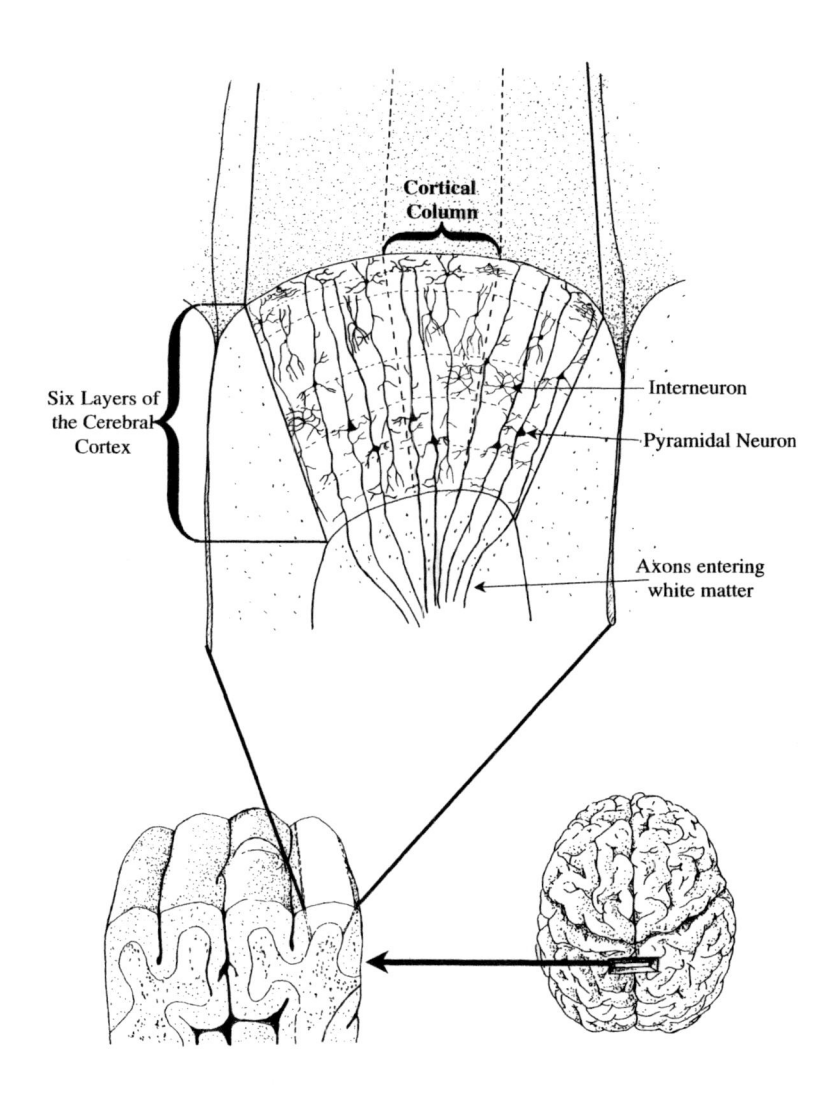

Figure 3.11. **Cortical Columns.** *Vertical slabs of cortex consisting of all six distinct cell layers, called cortical columns, are the functional units of the cerebral cortex. Some of the cells like the large pyramidal cells have dendrites that extend through almost all layers and axons that exit the grey matter to become part of the white matter tracts carrying information to other parts of the brain and body. There are also innumerable interneurons connecting the cells within each cell layer and between the layers.*

mental input, interneurons make up the vast bulk neurons in the cortex.

Most of these neuronal connections are restricted to the grey matter of the cortex, although some axons, like the pyramidal cells, project out of the cortical columns to become part of the white matter of the brain. It is these white matter tracts that transmit the decisions made in the cortex into the deep, subconscious brain nuclei and all the way down the spine.

Since the cortical columns are the processing modules that relate to specific types of cortical functions, they are the centres for the Gestalt and Logic lead functions. The *lead* functions provide a point of entry into an inter-linked set of cortical and subcortical modules performing our mental function.

The cortical columns in the right hemisphere usually perform global, spatial functions and inductive reasoning—Gestalt functions, and are the seat of our intuition.

The cortical columns of the left hemisphere usually perform linear, sequential and analytical functions—Logic functions, and are the seat of our rational thought. Linking these two complementary types of processing together in various combinations allows us to perform the vast number of functions of which the human brain is capable.

When you read words on a page, cortical columns that perform various Gestalt lead functions involved with the decoding of symbols will be activated by the visual stimulus of those words. This will in turn activate other cortical columns, housing Logic lead functions involved in understanding the meaning of words and their grammatical relationships.

The cortical columns can be likened to the processing units of a computer, which can be linked together in many different combinations to perform different functions. But computers remain crude machines when compared with the human capacity to link two random pieces of information into insightful reasoning. Indeed, many of the great scientific advances have resulted from people linking disparate pieces of information in a new way.

Albert Einstein was the classic creative processor. Even he said that the foundation of his Theory of Relativity resulted from 'thought experiments'. He could mentally place himself at the tip of an accelerating light beam and see what happened within his mind's eye as he approached the speed of light. What this visionary journey enabled Einstein to realise was that as he approached the speed of light—300,000 kilometres per second, his body got bigger and bigger, a phenomenon that makes no sense in logic but an idea that became one of the greatest-ever advances in science.

From his Gestalt experiment, Einstein was able to go back to his logical, rational processing brain and work out the mathematics to prove that what he had experienced as an abstract idea was theoretically valid. He used the facility that a computer does not yet have to gain the insight and then used Logic to manifest it as mathematical equations which could be tested. Such is the wonderful dexterity of cortical function.

THE HEART OF THE MATTER

White Matter and Grey Matter
The brain itself is made up of two distinct types of brain tissue or matter. They are the grey neuronal cell bodies, and their extensions, the dendrites and axons, which when highly insulated with myelin appear white.

WHITE MATTER
The Routes of Integration
White matter is basically the wiring of the brain. It conducts information as though along high-speed cables. This mass of white matter, like so many fibre-optic cables, connects the hundred billion neurons of the cortex and subcortical centres of the brain. This means there is a consequent need for at least a

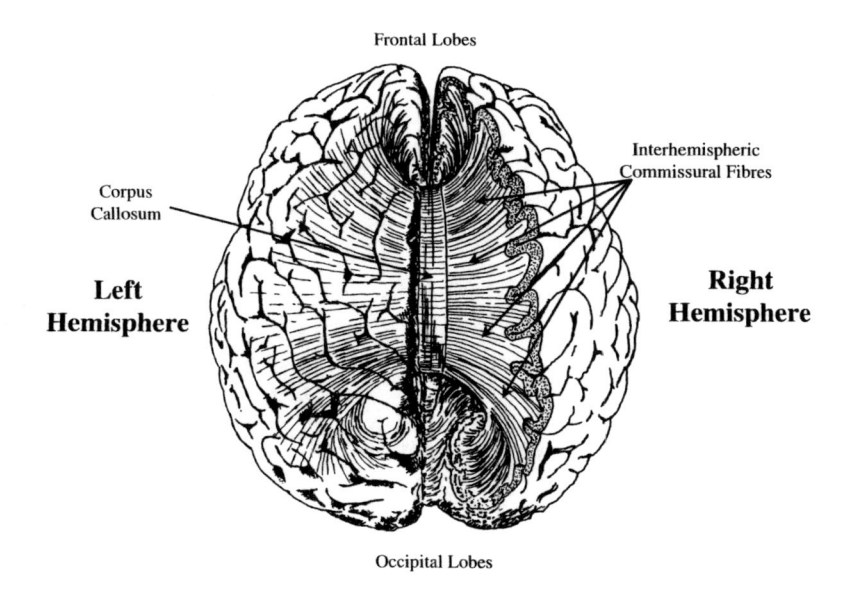

Figure 3.12. The Corpus Callosum—expanded view. On the right side of the diagram the cortex has been removed so that you can see that most of the interhemispheric fibres that cross the corpus callosum connect a cortical column of one hemisphere with cortical columns in exactly the same area in the opposite hemisphere.

hundred billion 'wires' or axons. There are even more when you consider the thousands of millions of neurons that also connect into other parts of the body.

White matter is made up of three different types of fibres: Commissural Fibres, Association Fibres and Projection Fibres.

Commissural Fibres run from the right side to the left side and the left to the right, connecting the two cerebral hemispheres. The largest group of these fibres passes through the corpus callosum (meaning 'white body'), a very distinct feature in the brain. It is approximately a one centimetre wide slab of axons of the commissural neurons that form the major connection between the two cerebral hemispheres, which are otherwise divided by a deep longitudinal fissure.

As you can see in Figure 3.12 on the previous page, the interhemispheric commissural fibres connect across the corpus callosum from an area in one hemisphere to exactly the same area in the opposite hemisphere. Thus the dendrites and cell body of commissural neurons in the right hemisphere have axons passing through the corpus callosum to end on the dendrites of neurons

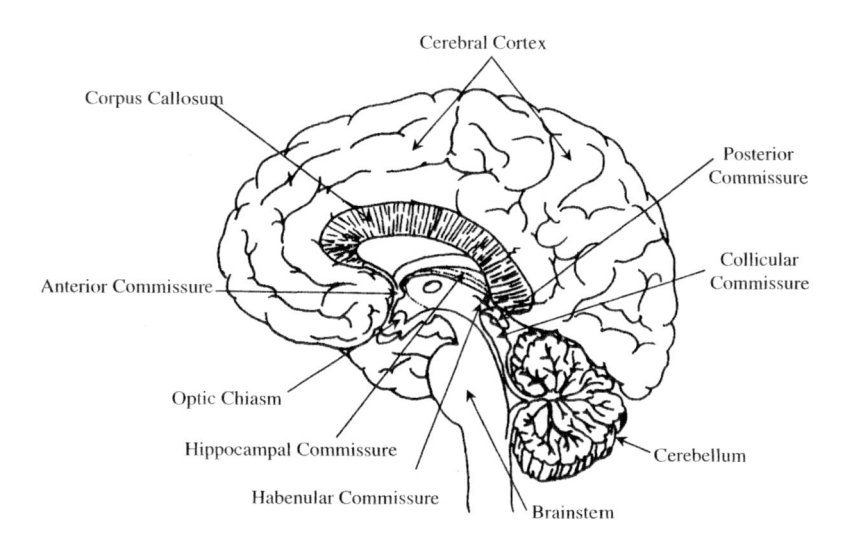

Figure 3.13. The Corpus Callosum, Anterior Commissure and other Commissures of the brain—cross sectional view. The fibres crossing through the corpus callosum connect most cortical areas in one hemisphere with the same areas in the opposite hemisphere. Whereas the Anterior Commissure connects areas in the anterior, inferior and medial temporal lobes in one hemisphere with the same areas in the opposite hemisphere. A number of other minor commissures connecting the right and left hemispheres can also be seen.

in exactly the same location in the left hemisphere. Likewise, there are commissural cell bodies in the left hemisphere whose axons pass back through the corpus callosum to end on the dendrites of neurons in exactly the same location in the right hemisphere.

While the numbers of fibres running through this structure almost defy imagination, the two-to-eight hundred million neurons passing through this structure form what is comparable to the fibre optic cables connecting the highly sophisticated telephone switchboards of the commissural neurons in each hemisphere. When the right hemisphere needs to communicate to the left hemisphere, the information must pass through this centre for the two sides to integrate their activity.[21]

Each cerebral hemisphere has a specialised capability to interpret and process specific types of information. However, on many occasions, information processed in both hemispheres must be integrated to provide a higher level of function. For example, when you are attempting to solve a problem in higher mathematics, something that involves both analytical abstract thinking as well as an understanding of spatial arrangement, the awareness of the spatial layout of the problem is led largely by centres in the Gestalt (generally the right) hemisphere, while the abstract reasoning is performed largely by centres in the Logic (generally the left) hemisphere. To get the correct answer, both hemispheres must co-ordinate and integrate their activities, a function dependent upon intact function of the fibres crossing the corpus callosum.

In my work, I have a task called 'picture arrangement' in which subjects are challenged to use both processes simultaneously. They are given pictographs of scenes that make up a story sequence and asked to arrange the pictures to interpret the sequence in which the events occurred. Gestalt function will recognise the pictures, while the understanding of the sequence of events is a Logic process. To perform such tasks well, you ideally need a full access to the interhemispheric connections crossing the corpus callosum.

The interhemispheric fibres crossing the corpus callosum are indeed one of the most important integrative pathways in the brain and one of the major concerns of this book.

A much smaller but equally important integrative pathway, the anterior commissure, connects the right and left anterior temporal lobes and subconscious brain nuclei like the amygdala, which are the site of much important information processing and integration for each hemisphere. The anterior commissure also plays an important role in unifying the emotional responses of the two sides of the brain.[22]

Smaller, but equally important commissural bundles, also visible in Figure 3.13, include the hippocampal commissure connecting the right and left hippocampi (which will be discussed later in this chapter), and the habenular, posterior and collicular commissures. The posterior commissure is comprised of axons of interhemispheric fibres connecting the superior parietal lobes involved in the integration of physical sensations. The fibres passing through the habenular commissure connect right and left nuclei of other midbrain areas providing integration of subconscious processing, while fibres in the collicular commissure automatically synchronise eye, head and neck movement to provide a stable base for vision.

Notice that the commissural fibres do not run diagonally, only right to left and visa versa. How then do the areas in the back of the brain, such as the visual areas, communicate with those in the front of the brain—those areas that 'think' about what you have seen? This is the role of the association fibres.

Association Fibres are a group of white matter fibres running between the front and back of the brain (see Fig. 3.14). The brain performs many different types of functions at widely separated sites, some being in the front of the brain, some in the back. The association fibres facilitate this integration.

The association fibres vary in length; some are short, U-shaped fibres running only between two adjacent gyri, or ridges, while others are considerably longer, running all the way from the occipital lobes at the back of the brain to the frontal lobes. The axons of the cell bodies of the occipitofrontal

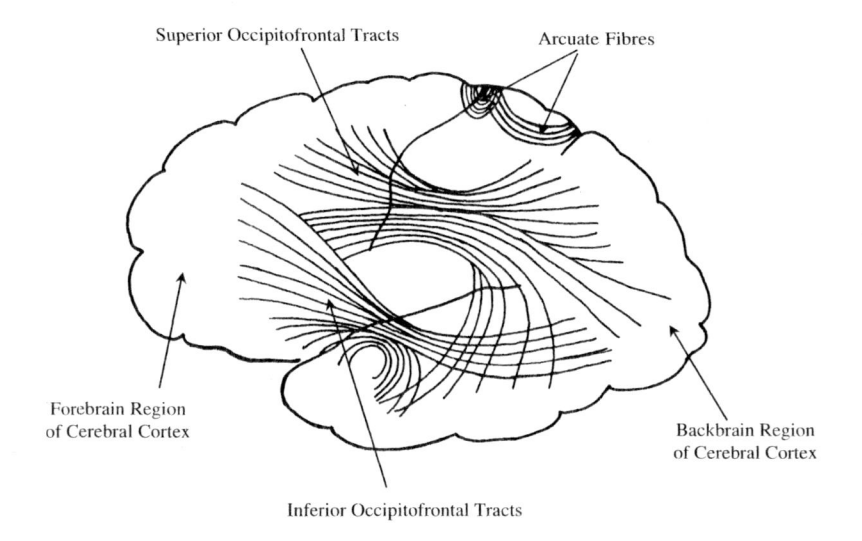

Figure 3.14. Association Fibres. Association fibres are principally of two types. 1. Long fibres connecting the front and back areas of the same hemisphere such as the occipitofrontal tracts and 2. Short U shaped fibres linking adjacent cortical areas in the same hemisphere such as the Arcuate fibres.

tracts in the primary visual areas of the occiput, where visual perceptions are formed, extend all the way to the pre-motor areas controlling the eye muscles, which enable you to look at items of interest. Many of the short, U-shaped association fibres connect adjacent cortical columns into functional units. When you think of something to say, the cortical area that generates your thought is connected to the cortical area that organises your speech, via this type of short tract.

The Projection Fibres are the third type of fibres that make up white matter. They project from deep within the brain's subconscious core up into the conscious cortical areas and are the fibres by which our subconscious emotions enter our consciousness. Likewise, the axons of cell bodies in the cortex project deep into the subconscious limbic system and other subconscious areas to relay your conscious desires to the part of the brain that carries out these desires (see Fig. 3.15).

Other projection fibres lead from the motor cortex down into the spinal column providing voluntary control of movement. When you want to walk, your cortex develops the commands to perform this activity and these commands are transmitted via projection fibres called the corticospinal tracts all

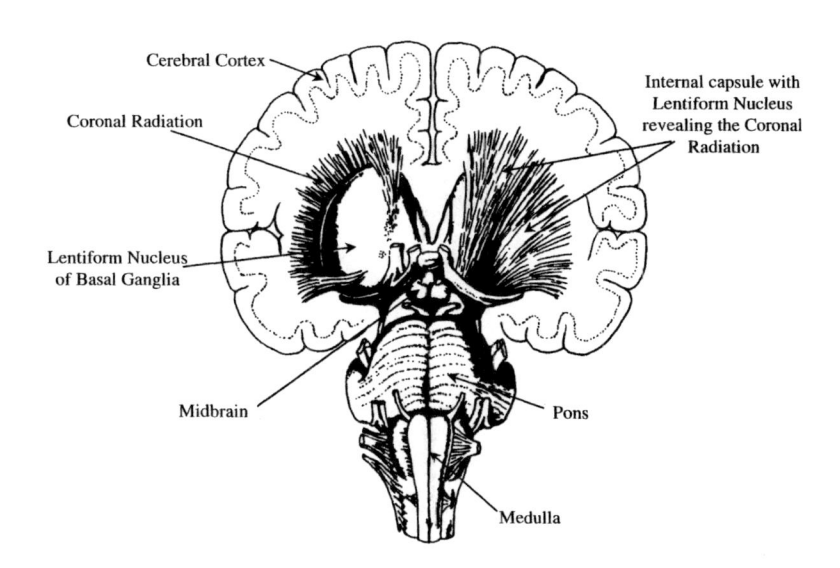

Figure 3.15. Projection Fibres. Projection fibres of the internal capsule and the coronal radiation into the cerebral cortex are the major integrative pathways linking the cortical and subcortical areas of the brain. View is from the bottom of the brain with the cortex cut away.

the way to the spinal level where they synapse with the alpha motor neurons to the muscles that need to move.

By the reverse, sensory projection fibres also run from your extremities and the torso, up into the brain. When you stub your toe, it is the fibres that project from the spinal column, into the sensory areas of the cortex, that allow you to identify the type and degree of this sensory experience.

THE GREY MATTER
Where all the decisions are made

Grey matter is made up mostly of interneurons connected in vast neural nets or webs. Both the dendrites and axons of interneurons are usually unmyelinated, as they are both generally very short and have no need for the high speed conduction of the sensory and motor neurons. Myelin takes up considerable space and if all the interneurons were myelinated, there would have to be far fewer of them. While we have just discussed the role of white matter, which is made up largely of the myelinated dendrites and axons of sensory and motor neurons, it is the unmyelinated cell bodies and dendrites of the grey matter that provide the sites of integration of information (see Fig. 3.16).

The actual sites of integration are the synapses on the dendrites and cell bodies of each neuron, as it is the adding up of all the excitatory and inhibitory

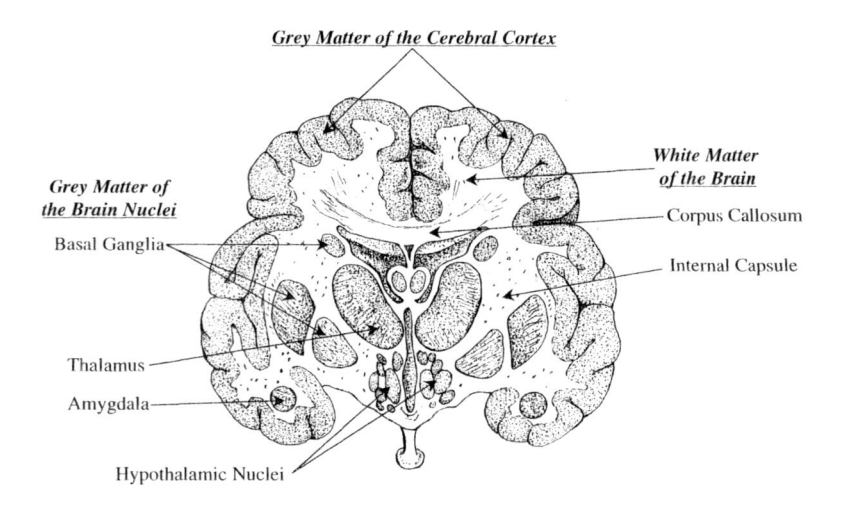

Figure 3.16. Distribution of Gray Matter and White Matter in the Brain. Grey matter is present as the superficial cerebral cortex and the deep brain nuclei suspended in the white matter. The white matter represents highly myelinated axons and dendrites connecting all areas of the brain.

inputs to each neuron that constitutes the integration of information in the brain. The 'decision' to fire or not to fire, and either pass the information on to the next neuron in the network, or to initiate some new action, are both based on the integration of synaptic input.

The grey matter thus integrates the sensory information transmitted to it via white matter. Decisions are made within the grey matter based on information received both from the environment via sensory neurons, and also by retrieval from memory via other white matter tracts. These decisions are then transmitted by yet other white matter tracts to other areas of grey matter for further processing or, are sent down white matter tracts of the spinal cord to the muscles for action.

Picture a boss working in his office. He receives information via the telephone or fax, then uses the intercom to discuss matters with his middle managers. He then makes a decision which he sends out as a memo to his employees to perform a particular action. In this scenario, the boss is like the neuronal grey matter. The telephone and fax are the sensory white matter fibres carrying information to him. The middle managers are other related grey matter areas of the brain that provide additional information needed for

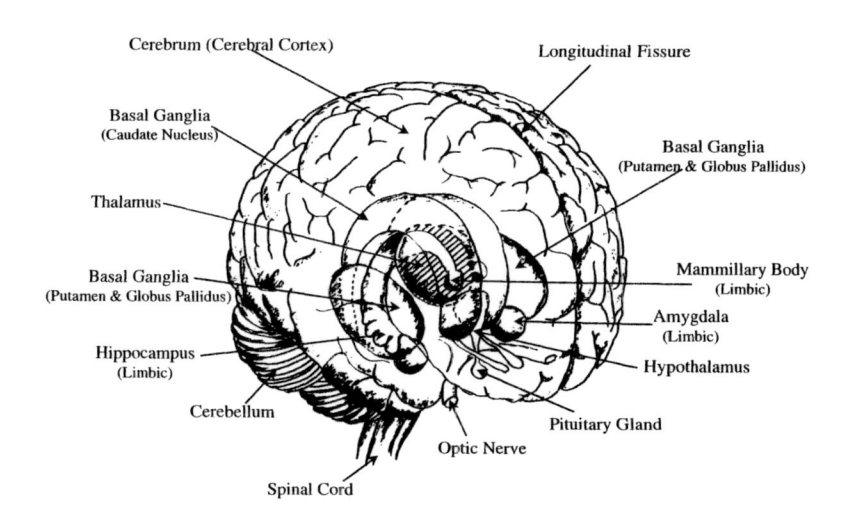

Figure 3.17. The Brain Nuclei. The Human Brain looking through the right cerebral cortex at the deep brain nuclei. These subcortical structures are buried deep within the white matter. Some of these structures are the basal ganglia, the thalamus, components of the limbic system (hippocampus and amygdala), and the hypothalamus from which the pituitary gland is suspended.

good decision-making, and the motor tracts are the memos telling the employees, or, in our analogy the muscles, what to do.

Grey matter may take two forms: The superficial layer that covers the convoluted cerebral and cerebellar cortices, and the brain nuclei and ganglia, which appear as islands of grey matter deep within the white matter (see Figs. 3.16 & 3.17). The superficial cerebral cortex is the site of conscious processing and thinking, while the brain nuclei and ganglia, lying below the cortex and deep within the white matter, are the site of subconscious filtering and processing of information.

Whereas the functional units of the cerebral cortex are the cortical columns, the functional units of the subconscious are the various brain nuclei and their subnuclei. Anatomically the brain nuclei are a diverse group of midbrain and limbic processing centres that orchestrate our physical and emotional responses to life. For instance when a life threatening circumstance occurs, the sensory input to the amygdala, one of the limbic brain nuclei, may elicit the emotions of fear, while the hypothalamus, another set of subconscious brain nuclei, dilate your pupils, cause your mouth to go dry and your muscles to tense.

THE ORIGINS OF THE SUBCONSCIOUS

We are aware of some of the processing in the cortex because it gives rise to conscious perceptions and conscious thought. But we are totally unaware of much that happens in many other areas of the cortex, the palaeocortex and all the processing in the subcortical brain nuclei, because it occurs below consciousness, or subconsciously.

In the next section of our voyage, we will briefly discuss the parts that really make us tick, the mysterious areas of the subconscious.

The Basal Ganglia

A group of paired deep brain nuclei that play a crucial role in the integration and organisation of co-ordinated motor activity are called the basal ganglia. Along with the cerebellum, the basal ganglia act to turn the desired conscious activity into reality. These are one of the largest groups of brain nuclei consisting of the corpus striatum, which is itself divided into the caudate nucleus, the tailed nucleus, and the lentiform nucleus. Lentiform means lens-like.

The lentiform nucleus itself is divided into an outer part, the putamen, and a medial or inner part, the globus pallidus, which is in turn divided into external and internal segments. The over-arching caudate nucleus is also divided into functional regions, the head, body and tail. While the putamen and globus pallidus are primarily concerned with running predetermined motor programs, the caudate nucleus appears to have cognitive as well as motor functions.[23]

The basal ganglia are mainly concerned with learned motor activities that become automatic such as walking, running and throwing a ball. When you want to perform a new activity, the conscious 'thinking' association areas of the prefrontal cortex in a sense 'asks' the head of the caudate nucleus to work out a motor sequence for this activity. This portion of the basal ganglia will then devise a motor pattern of how this new activity might be accomplished, and transmit that sequence back to the cortex. The cortex will then consider this sequence and if satisfied, direct the motor cortex to run this muscle sequence. If the outcome is not exactly what the cortex wanted, this process may be repeated with the head of the caudate working out a modification of the previous motor program until the outcome is what the cortex desired.[24]

You decide to learn to play golf. From watching others and your coach's instructions, you 'know' how to hit the ball. The motor sequence to hit the ball however, is a collaboration between the frontal cortex's 'idea' of hitting the ball, and the motor program devised by the caudate nucleus. The first few times you run this motor program, the outcome, a topped ball that dribbles off the tee, or a slice into the woods, may not have been the outcome desired.

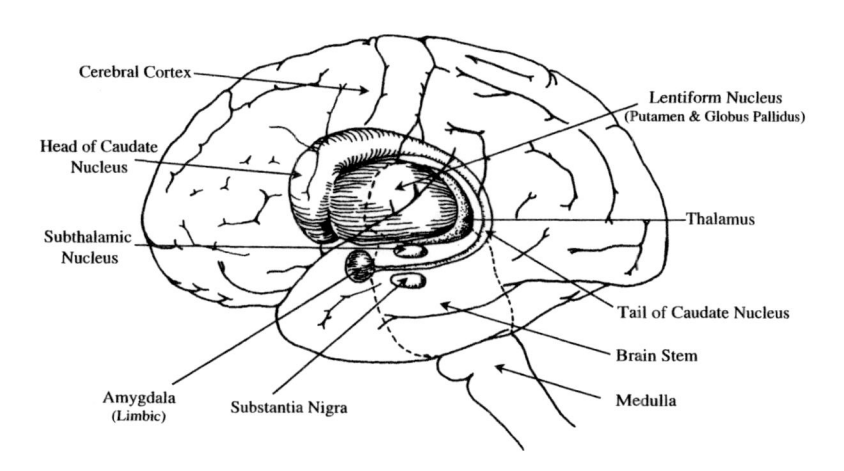

Figure 3.18. The Basal Ganglia. This view is looking through the cerebral cortex at the components of the basal ganglia deep within the brain. The lentiform nuclei of the basal ganglia enclose the more medial thalamus, and lie above the subthalamic nucleus and substantia nigra of the mid brain. Although structurally part of the basal ganglia, the amygdaloid nucleus is functionally part of the Limbic System.

So your cortex asks the caudate to modify that motor sequence to correct the previous errors.

One of the major obstacles to properly hitting the ball in the first place, actually resides in the body of the caudate nucleus. This region holds a semi-automatic motor program to look up and see where the ball is going to go, as this part of the caudate controls eye movements via its feedback loop to the prefrontal eye fields of the frontal cortex. And as everybody who has ever played golf knows, it is essential to keep your eye on the ball until the club actually strikes the ball, then look to see where it is going.

Once you have the head and body of the caudate working together to produce the desired outcome—a consistent tee shot straight down the fairway, then in a sense, this motor program is down loaded to the putamen, which in conjunction with its partner the globus pallidus now run this program on command. Now your brain is free to consider in what direction and how hard you need to hit the ball to place it near the pin.

Unfortunately, for many golfers, the basal ganglia are also very richly connected to the limbic system, our emotional centre.[25] Thus emotional states can affect muscle tension which can in turn, affect the timing of the motor sequences that are run. This is why even a professional golfer may suddenly start slicing the ball. Their perfectly good putamen 'hitting the ball' program is being interfered with by limbic emotional input to the caudate and globus pallidus, changing the timing of their swing. Since these limbic emotions are subconscious in origin, the person just can't understand what's wrong with their game.

This also explains why a sportsman or woman can get to the very brink of winning a championship and blow the final shot. Because they became emotionally stressed by the importance of the moment, this stress and the subconscious emotions generated in the limbic system, affected the basal ganglia program, resulting in a muffed shot or a ball that didn't get over the net.

True professionals are those people who prevent the stress from interfering with their basal ganglia programming and play through to win because they actually have two sets of practice programs—one without stress, and the other with the stress gained in other championship competitions, known as state conditioned learning. Obviously, if you have not been at the brink of winning a major tournament before, you could not have conditioned the practice program that prevents interference from your emotional state. Champions train to maintain their cool, both mentally and physically.

This is the reason why very few athletes ever win the big tournament the first time they play through to the final round. They have not yet conditioned their basal ganglia programs to handle the stress at that level. It is also why, whenever an athlete gets angry with himself for missing the last shot, he is likely to miss the next one as well. His anger interferes with his normally accurate basal ganglia program.

What you do, is decided by your cortex. How you do it is largely a subconscious process, one that is often affected by our subconscious emotional states.

Likewise, when you throw a ball, you don't consciously know how you manage to perform the activity. You just do it. But if you watch a child learning to throw a ball, you can almost see the child's cortex ask his basal ganglia to work out the motor sequence called 'throw the ball'. The child already 'knows' how to throw the ball from watching others, but does not yet have the motor program to do so.

Upon the request of the prefrontal cortex, the caudate nucleus develops a sequence that is sent back to the motor areas of the cortex to tell the hand: 'Grab the ball. Go back, back, back. Stop! Now bring the arm forward. Now, let go of the ball.' The first time the child does this, they may let go of the ball too soon, or too late. The cortex, upon seeing this mistake, asks the caudate nucleus to re-write the original program to overcome this problem. The corrected program is then down-loaded into the putamen for future use.

After the pattern is encoded in the putamen, throwing a ball becomes something that can be done without conscious effort. You merely tell your brain to run the 'throw the ball' program and the shoulder, arm and hand will perform the sequence of the action in one smooth motion.

Once an action is stored as motor memory it can then largely be run by the subconscious. You simply ask for a prearranged pattern to be run and it happens. From a survival point of view such storing of learned motor behaviour is very efficient because it frees up cortical function to concentrate on other activities of more immediate importance. That is also why, when you are walking down the street you can think about what you want for dinner rather than having to concentrate on watching your feet. You don't have to worry because you learned to walk a long time ago.

As a child however, it took all your conscious effort just to balance on two feet. As soon as a toddler stops concentrating on walking and is distracted by something else, they are likely to fall. But once the child gets the right sequence encoded in their subconscious motor memory, they never have to think about walking again.

While I have just discussed the subconscious role of the basal ganglia in controlling our automatic movements, it must be realised that when you are born, you already have many pathways 'hard-wired' into your motor system. If you take a baby just out of the womb and hold it vertically so that its feet touch the ground, its legs will go through walking movements. What the basal ganglia do is modify and fine-tune these pre-existing programs.

Also, the basal ganglia do not work alone. All motor patterns rely upon

106   A Revolutionary Way of Thinking

subconscious input from the cerebellum to smooth out and co-ordinate muscle activity. The cerebellum does this via feedback of millions of impulses that it receives each second from the subconscious sensors in the muscles, joints and fascia of the body which tell it exactly what the body is doing. Thus, along with the cerebellum, the basal ganglia act as the interface between the sensory and motor systems permitting us to perform complex movements with little or no thought about how we are doing it. This allows us to focus on what we *want* to do, not *how* we have to do it.

The Thalamus
Two nut-shaped collections of nuclei, (thalamus means 'nut' in Latin), lie immediately on either side of the centre of the brain. The thalami play a major role as the relay station for all information transmitted to and from the body. The thalamus on each side, is the final processing station where all sensory input, except olfactory (smell) input, is relayed or filtered before transmittal to the cortex where it may becomes conscious. Figures 3.19 a&b show the major nuclei of the thalamus and the areas of the cortex receiving output from these thalamic nuclei.

This arrangement allows still unconscious messages to be stopped before they become conscious. Because the thalamus acts as a junction box, if survival is at stake, it can, if necessary, filter information that is still below

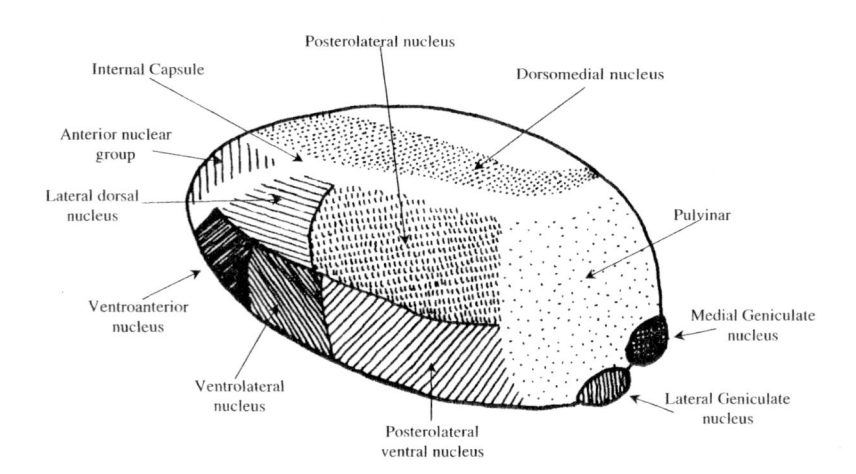

Figure 3.19a. The Thalamic Nuclei. The ventroanterior and ventrolateral nuclei relay motor messages from the basal ganglia and cerebellum to the Premotor and Motor cortices. The posteromedial ventral, central medial and other medial nuclei are internal and therefore not shown.

conscious awareness. Your subconscious therefore has the ability to filter what is being sent to the cortex. This filtering is important for your survival. Say you stepped on a pebble with a bare foot, and simultaneously, your other foot landed on a jagged piece of glass. The subconscious brain centres, like the thalamus, will receive that information, and before your are consciously aware of it, will cause you to take the appropriate action to move your foot off the jagged glass and not the pebble.

The glass is ultimately more threatening to your well-being so that message will take precedence. You may even be unaware of the existence of the pebble. On the other hand, in the absence of the piece of glass, your whole attention would have been focussed on the pebble.

In war, it is well-known phenomenon that soldiers are often horribly wounded but have no knowledge of it because their whole drive is directed toward surviving. The message of pain, often grievous pain, only got as far as the subconscious, which in effect says: 'Forget the pain! You have to survive!' It is only because the fibres carrying pain and other sensory information, project into the subconscious areas of the brain, like the thalamus, and then are secondarily relayed into the conscious areas of the cortex, that this survival mechanism can work.

Research has shown that not only is the thalamus a major relay centre for

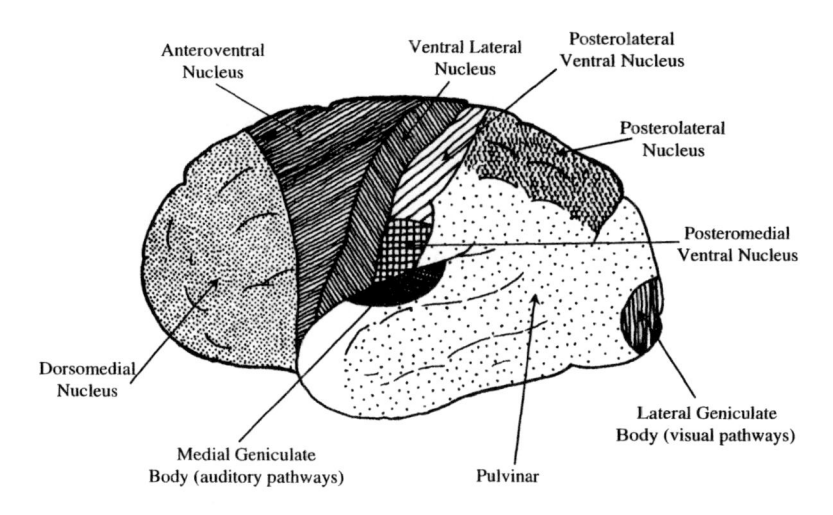

Figure 3.19b. Projections of the Thalamic Nuclei to the Cortex. The areas of the lateral cerebral cortex into which each thalamic nucleus projects fibres relaying sensory information. The anterior nuclear group projects fibres only to the cingulate gyrus which is on the medial surface and not shown.

information, but that conscious awareness of crude sensations; pain, touch and temperature, begin in specific thalamic nuclei and are then relayed to specific areas of the cortex where more detailed conscious perception is formed.[26]

As you can see in Figure 3.19a, there are knobs on the inside of the thalamus called the medial (middle) geniculate nuclei, and on the outside called the lateral geniculate nuclei, which are the relay stations for incoming signals of sight and sound. The medial nuclei are the thalamic portal through which all incoming sound signals enter the auditory cortex to be decoded as speech, music or just plain noise.

Likewise, visual input from the retina first comes back to the lateral geniculate nuclei and, then via optic radiation fibres, passes back to the visual cortex in the occipital lobes. In several layers of processing, this visual input is converted into conscious visual perceptions or images.

As well as receiving sensory input, motor sequences from the basal ganglia and cerebellum are forwarded to two specific nuclei of the thalamus. These thalamic nuclei relay this motor information to the pre-motor cortex and/or primary motor cortex, which send signals to activate the individual muscles via the corticospinal tracts running down the spine.

While the anterior nuclear group is anatomically part of the thalamus, functionally it is involved with the transmittal of information that form our feelings and is part of the limbic system.[27]

The Hypothalamus
Another set of the deep brain nuclei that must be considered in order to understand brain function is the structure whose name means 'under the thalamus' (see Fig.3.20). It takes up an area about the size of the tip of your little finger and constitutes less than 1 percent of the brain by volume and only 0.3 percent by weight.[28] Together with the thalamus, the hypothalamus makes up a part of the brain called the diencephalon. But where the thalamus acts as a junction box for incoming and outgoing messages, the hypothalamus takes overall control of the homeostasis of the body, hopefully ensuring that all systems to do with bodily functions are operating harmoniously.

The hypothalamus achieves this in two ways. Containing about 24 individual nuclei it is in charge of the autonomic nervous system (meaning, almost automatic). The hypothalamus receives a constant stream of subconscious sensory information from your viscera, or internal organs, informing it of the current status of function.

After eating that Christmas dinner and having stretched your stomach, visceral stretch receptors in the stomach's wall send a stream of messages to the hypothalamus about this new state. The hypothalamus responds by sending signals via the sympathetic part of the autonomic nervous system, back to the stomach to tell the glands to secrete acid and for the stomach to churn and begin the digestion of this indulgent feast. Receipt of these same visceral messages from the stretched stomach activate other hypothalamic nuclei that then give rise to the 'I'm full' sensation informing us not to have yet another piece of that yummy Christmas pudding.

From similar feedback from other parts of the body and brainstem the hypothalamus also controls heart rate, blood pressure, respiration, intestinal peristalsis, body temperature and the more basic drives of hunger and thirst. It has master control of body metabolism because it is in charge not only of

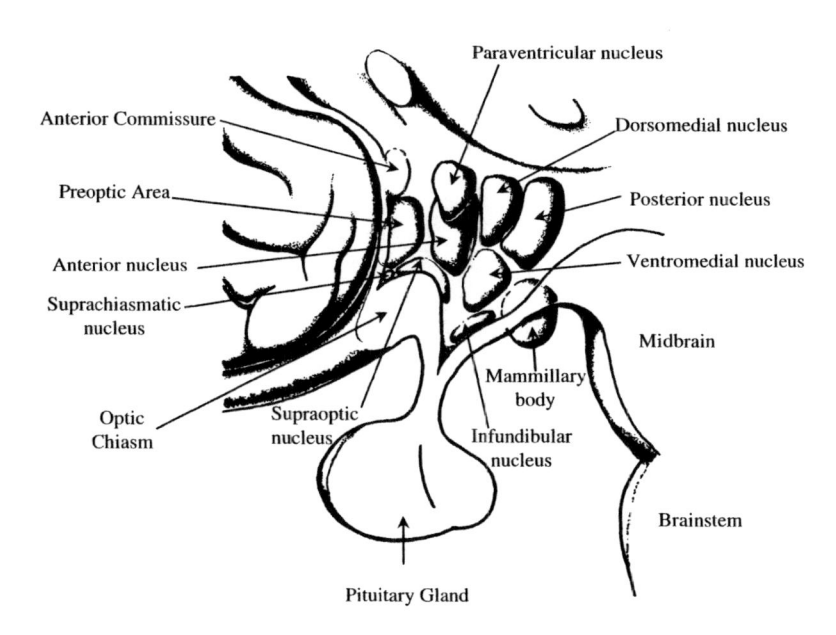

Figure 3.20. Hypothalamic Nuclei and the Pituitary Gland. The hypothalamus is composed of a group of approximately 24 nuclei located in the white matter just above the optic chiasm. The pituitary gland hangs from the bottom of the hypothalamus by a stalk called the infundibulum.

the autonomic nervous system, but also of the nearby pituitary gland.

For many years the pituitary gland was mistakenly called 'the master gland' because endocrinologists had rightly detected that by producing chemical substances called hormones it controlled the function of the other endocrine glands. These glands in turn control our basic metabolism and physiological function. The pituitary gland however, turned out not to be much of a chief at all when it was later discovered that it was in fact being controlled by the hypothalamus.

Releasing or inhibiting factors or hormones issued from the hypothalamus are sent the very short distance to the pituitary gland instructing it to send out other hormones regulating most of the other glands in the body. These chemical messages convey information about what hormone to release from which gland; when to start releasing it and when to stop. The whole show is thus determined by the hypothalamus.

In a sense, we can think of the hypothalamus as the composer of a symphony of bodily functions, the pituitary gland as the conductor of the musicians (the glands), and their remarkable orchestration as the equally amazing outcome: The symphony of homeostasis.

There are also other nuclei in the hypothalamus involved in the expression of very strong emotions, such as rage, fear, punishment and reward. It directly controls the physical and physiological expression of these states, a function that also relates very obviously to survival. When specific nuclei in the hypothalamus are stimulated they produce states of anger or pleasure and scientists have managed to trigger these outcomes in experiments with laboratory animals (see Fig. 3.21).

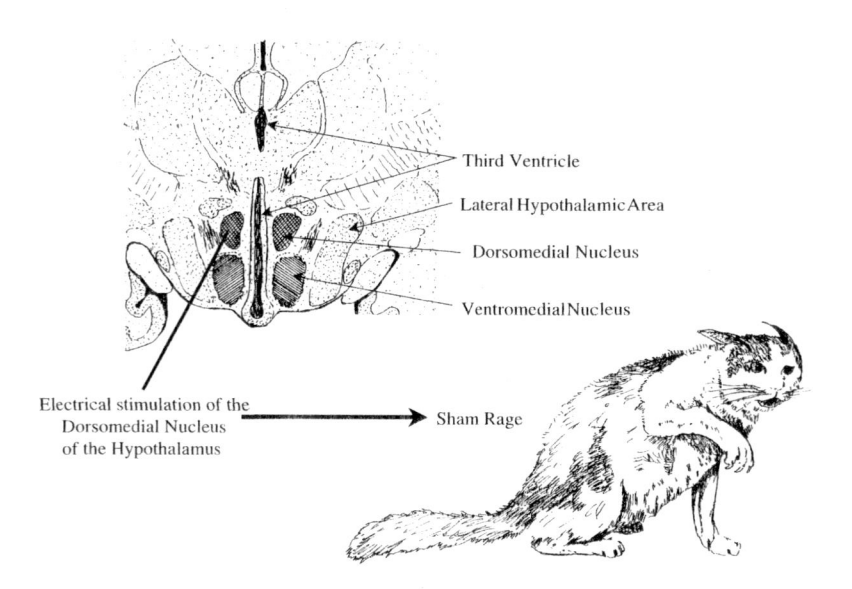

Figure 3.21. Sham rage in a Cat. Electrical stimulation of the Dorsomedial Nucleus or bilateral destruction of the Ventromedial Nuclei results in a cat demonstrating 'sham rage'; all the physical signs of rage and aggression, but which cease immediately when stimulation stops.

When the rage centre in the dorsomedial nucleus of the hypothalamus of a cat is stimulated by a fine electrode, the cat's fur will stand on end, the claws will be bared, it will hiss and growl and the back will arch to make the animal appear bigger as if it were preparing to fight for its life. In 1925 Walter Cannon, one of the fathers of modern physiology, called this electrically stimulated behaviour 'sham rage' because it lacked the elements of conscious experience expressed in natural states of rage. Turn the current on, the cat displayed all the external features of rage. But turn off the current, and the cat was instantly placid.[29]

In other experiments, animals allowed to press a bar to electrically stimulate the pleasure centres in their own brains will keep pushing on the lever until they die, ignoring other impulses to eat or drink or have sex.[30] Pleasure is a seemingly addictive state in the brain. More naturally, it is a product of an emotional state that has its origins in another brain nuclei, the amygdala, which is the actual mediator of many of our basic emotions.

Thus the hypothalamus and its control of our physical homeostasis is under the control of our emotions. In fact, one of the major roles of the hypothalamus is to produce the physiological expression of our emotions called 'feelings'. At the physical level, blushing is the physiological involuntary response generated by the hypothalamus to the emotional state of embarrassment. Even more ephemeral feelings, the warm glow in your chest, the dilated pupils, and your heart going pitter patter, are all created by your hypothalamus in response to the emotion, love.

THE LIMBIC SYSTEM

Where emotions arise

The limbic system, also known as the limbic brain, is the centre of our subconscious emotional processing. It contains areas that give birth to our emotions, lay down and retrieve our memories, and look out for our survival. The fight or flight response originates here, but is expressed in the body by the hypothalamus.

Anatomically, the limbic system is the cortical rim surrounding the diencephalon at the head of the brainstem. Limbic means rim or border. The cortical components of the ancient cortex are known as the limbic lobe and comprise the cingulate gyrus lying just above the corpus callosum, the orbitofrontal and subcallosal gyri of the basal frontal lobes, as well as the dentate and hippocampal gyri and the parahippocampal, entorhinal and perirhinal cortices of the medial temporal lobes (see Figs.3.22a & b).

In addition to the cortical limbic lobe, the limbic system also includes subcortical areas, the mammillary bodies of the hypothalamus, the amygdaloid bodies of the basal ganglia, the anterior thalamic nuclei of the thalamus, and the septal nuclei of the basal forebrain (see Figs. 3.22b & 3.23). Even though anatomically these structures belong to other parts of the brain that have more to do with physical sensation and movement, they are functionally linked together as the emotional centre of your being.[31]

The components of the limbic system are linked and interact in an amazingly complex way and although I will talk about function of individual parts of the limbic system, I want you to remember that all of these components, at many levels, are working together simultaneously. The output of these complex interactions are our feelings, emotions and memory.

In Figures 3.22a and 3.23 you can see that the cingulate gyrus is a band of tissue lying above the corpus callosum that functions as the major relay centre for the limbic system. Many of the messages coming from the subcortical limbic nuclei are relayed through the cingulate gyrus on their way to the cortex. Likewise, cortical messages to the subconscious limbic system, are delivered via the cingulate gyrus. In a sense you can consider the cingulate gyrus as one of the major interfaces between the conscious and the subconscious.

In particular, the anterior cingulate (Fig. 3.22a) appears to be the site where our emotions, feelings, attention and working memory flow together. In the

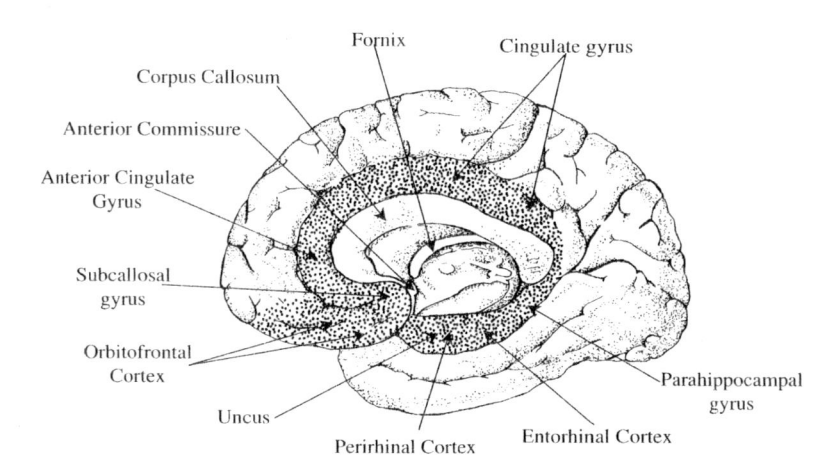

Figure 3.22a. The Limbic Lobe looking at the medial (inside) surface of the right cerebral hemisphere. The cingulate gyrus virtually encircles the corpus callosum with the subcallosal and orbitofrontal gyri extending forward along the inferior medial surface of the forebrain. Extending forward from its posterior end the parahippocampal, entorhinal and perirhinal cortices form the medial surface of the temporal lobe.

words of Antonio Damasio author of *Descartes' Error*, this is 'the fountainhead' where body and mind interact.[32]

Also located within the anterior cingulate is a centre that suppresses our feelings of anger and rage. Destruction of these centres releases the rage centres in the septal and hypothalamic nuclei resulting in animals and people becoming vicious, and subject to fits of uncontrolled rage.[33] Whenever you suddenly lose your temper and express extreme anger or rage, the anterior cingulate has momentarily lost control of these deeper, more primitive limbic areas, and the feelings are largely delivered to your consciousness via this important relay station.

Now, consider that to experience even a simple feeling, all of the following events take place at the same time:

The hippocampal formation, which comprises the dentate and hippocampal gyri together, is a central processing unit for memory and our on-going awareness of events. Input to this area, whether from the senses (seeing someone you dislike or like) or other brain areas (thinking about someone you dislike or like), is appraised for its relevance and compared to other data that is stored in memory.

If incoming information is of relevance, ('Gosh, I dislike him, he's such a bore!'), it will be held in short-term memory and compared with what is

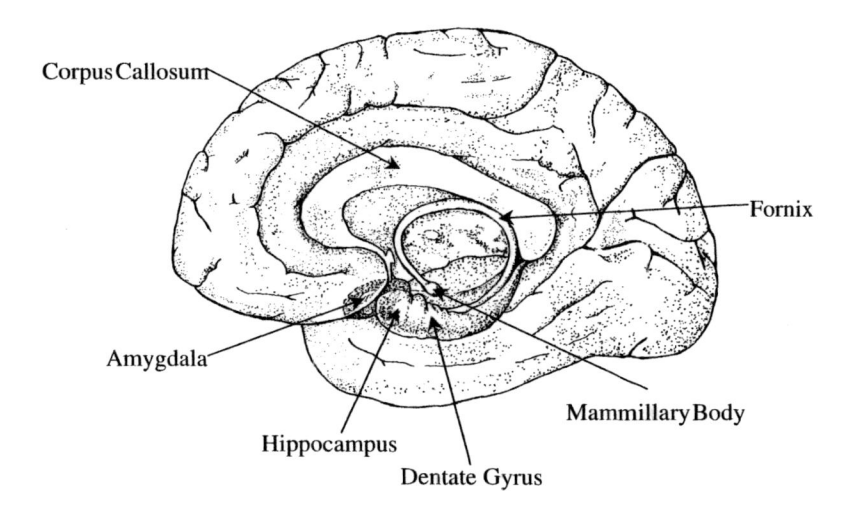

Figure 3.22b. The Limbic Lobe with the parahippocampal, entorhinal and perirhinal cortices peeled away to reveal the hippocampal and dentate gyri beneath. The hippocampal and dendate gyri are the in-turned edge of the medial temporal lobe which can only be seen by removal of the overlying medial temporal lobe structures.

already known, ('He never stops talking about himself'). If it is of great importance it may even be prepared for permanent storage in the long-term memory areas of the cortex, ('That's a face I'll never forget!').

At the same time the information held in the hippocampus will be made available to the surrounding parahippocampal, perirhinal and entorhinal cortices, which appraise this information against the matrix of previous experience in all the senses: sight (of his face), sound (of his voice), smell (his body odour), touch (he's always slapping me on the back) and taste (if relevant). Via its interconnections with all of the association areas of the cortex, the amygdala and temporal lobe, emotional associations are made and reactions to this information in any of the senses are registered by the entorhinal cortex and sent back to the hippocampal formation for further consideration.[34]

Meanwhile, the same information is being processed by the amygdala—the seat of our subconscious emotions. Output from these subconscious emotional centres to the hypothalamus and prefrontal cortex generates respectively,

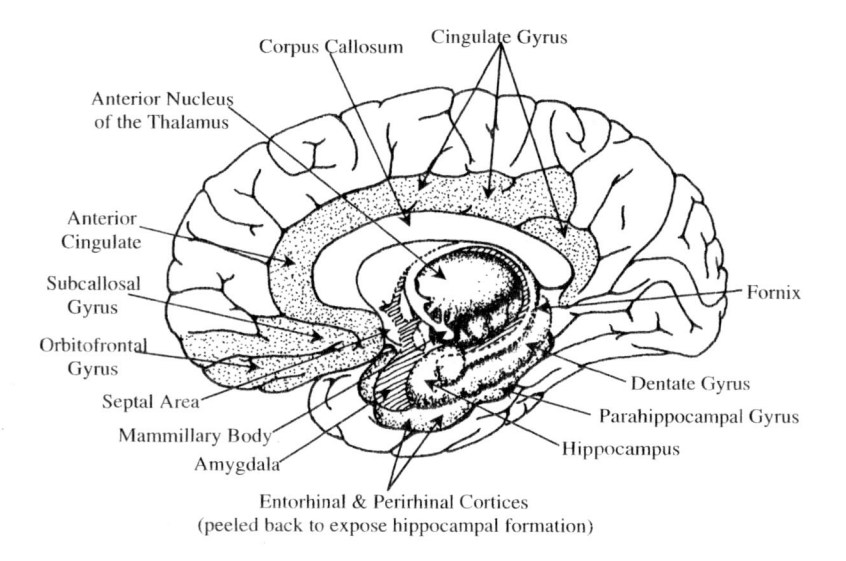

Figure 3.23. The Limbic System. *This subconscious processing system is composed of the limbic lobe areas of the cingulate, subcallosal and orbitofrontal gyri, the septal area, and the medial temporal lobe structures, the entorhinal and perirhinal cortices, the parahippocampal and dentate gyri, hippocampus and its major output pathway the fornix; it also includes the subcortical anterior nuclei of the thalamus, the mammillary bodies and amygdalae.*

our feelings and conscious awareness of the experience. In a way, these subcortical brain nuclei assign the emotional content to the information, which is then experienced as specific feelings in the body and emotions by the higher cortical areas.

Subconscious emotions, often triggered by memory, thus initiate a physiological cascade from the hypothalamus of both autonomic nervous system signals and hormonal flows that create our physical sensations of these emotions resulting in conscious feelings. The result of all these simultaneous subconscious processes, is that you become consciously aware of a subjective feeling. 'I really don't like this guy'.

The final area of the limbic system to be considered here is the mammillary bodies. These small bumps on the bottom of the brain gained their name from the perception of early anatomists who perceived them to be breast-like, albeit tiny. They are involved in two quite different areas of function. On the one hand, the mammillary bodies play an important role in the storage of conscious memory as they are a major relay station for output of the short-term memory centres in the hippocampus to the anterior thalamus and anterior cingulate, which in turn, have rich connections to the association memory areas of the cortex.[35]

On the other hand, the mammillary bodies also receive input from the taste areas of the brain and control our behaviours relating to eating. This includes the licking of the lips and salivation when perceiving food. And via its interconnections with the amygdala and hippocampus, it activates our emotional response to a particular food.[36] No sooner have you looked at, or even just thought about, chocolate ice cream sunday, than you find yourself salivating and licking your lips in anticipation of a taste treat, all behaviours and sensations run by the mammillary bodies.

So what may seem to be a sudden unconscious emotion or impulse clearly has its roots in a complex processing that takes place deep within the brain and involving many, many structures.

The limbic system also plays an important role in the expression of our basic behaviour. Research has shown that stimulation of certain hypothalamic nuclei and specific nuclei of the amygdala result in expressions of rage or fear, while stimulation of areas of the cingulate gyrus, hippocampal formation, hypothalamic and anterior thalamic nuclei and other nuclei of the amygdala produce pleasure or docility.[37] Such centres have been named 'punishment' or 'pain' centres, and 'pleasure' or 'reward' centres, and are critical to learning, because the major motivation to learn is based on reward or punishment.

Because the limbic system assumes such a primary role in the formation of emotions such as pain, pleasure, anger, rage, fear, sorrow, sexual feelings, docility and affection, it is sometimes referred to as 'the emotional brain of man.' Indeed, the limbic system is involved with many expressions that make us human, namely, emotional behaviour and feeling states.[38]

It is also by the widespread connections of the limbic system to the hypothalamus, basal ganglia, thalamus and cerebral cortex that our emotions have such profound effects on our visceral or gut functions (ulcers); muscle tone and posture (tight neck, hunched shoulders); aversion to noxious sights, sounds, tastes and smells and the overall feeling states that define our moods.

WHERE MEMORY AND EMOTIONS MEET

The two limbic structures most directly involved in our memory and emotions are the hippocampus and the amygdala. While I have alluded to some of the functions of both of these structures above, and will discuss them in some depth in the next chapter, I would like to take you on a brief tour of these fascinating limbic areas.

The Hippocampus

Because the hippocampus is known to be involved in the processing of memory, it is a site critical to learning. Researchers discovered this function through observing what happened to people who had sustained accidental damage to this particular area of their brains. The theories were confirmed by the case of a man known to science only by his initials, H.M.[39]

H.M. was a young man who suffered intractable or uncontrollable epilepsy. He was fitting continually. In a bid to give him some sort of a life, in 1953 brain surgeons excised sections of his anterior temporal lobe, including the hippocampi on both sides. When he had recovered from the operation, the fitting had been controlled, but H.M. was found to have completely lost his short-term memory.

His long-term memory and intelligence were intact but because he had lost the capacity to assimilate new information, he could no longer learn. Apart from a very few acts which he learned through endless repetition, he has not been able to assimilate anything new since the early 1950s. It was, granted, an extreme way for science to learn what function this part of the brain performed.

Extensive evidence supports the view that the hippocampal formation, the hippocampus, subiculum (located between the hippocampus and dentate gyrus) and dentate gyrus, are indeed essential for processing information in short-term memory, particularly the consolidation of memory traces for transfer to long-term memory. The effects of operations such as in the case of H.M. and lesions resulting from head injury have shown the hippocampal system to be in charge of laying down and retrieval of our conscious memories.

The hippocampus in each temporal lobe has an arm, the fornix, which arches up to lie just below the corpus callosum before diving deep into the brain ending in the mammillary bodies which protrude from the bottom of the brain.

As you can see in Figure 3.24, the fornix has commissural fibres, or wiring, that allows the left hippocampus and right hippocampus to communicate with each other and thus to co-ordinate activities. Evidence suggests that the left hippocampus is involved in symbolic digital processing and auditory short-term memory, while the right hippocampus is largely involved with visuospatial processing and visual short-term memory.[40] It is obvious why the two need to be linked and that linkage is provided by the hippocampal commissure.

If communication breaks down between these two centres you can undergo an experience such as going blank during an exam. The auditory part of your brain will be repeating the question over and over again but you cannot seem to access your visual long-term memory: all the facts that you studied to learn. A similar situation occurs when you see a face that you know you know but

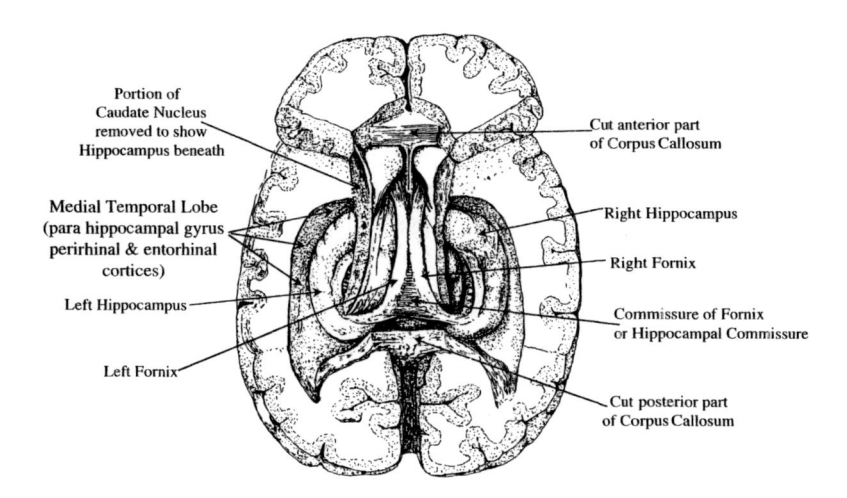

Figure 3.24. The Hippocampus, Fornix and Hippocampal Commissure. Note that the whole top of the cerebral cortex on both sides has been removed, the corpus callosum cut away and the basal ganglia largely removed to expose the hippocampus which makes up the most medial, ventral upturned edge of the temporal lobe. The Fornix is the major output pathway of the hippocampus to the mammillary bodies and via radiations from the fornix to many areas of the limbic system and the cerebral cortex. Note the commissure of the fornix, the hippocampal commissure, by which the right and left hippocampi communicate and integrate their activity.

can't put a name to it. The face is visuospatial information while the name belongs to your auditory function. Communication breakdown across these vital commissural fibres may compromise our function.

The Amygdala
This name means 'almond-shaped' and defines a set of nuclei that lie in the medial temporal lobe between the hippocampi and the basal ganglia. While anatomically, they are the bulbs on the end of the tail of the caudate nucleus of the basal ganglia, functionally they have become integrated with the limbic system and are now known to be major subconscious emotional processing and integration centres. The amygdalae are primarily responsible for our deepest emotions of fear, rage, pain and pleasure, and our reactions to punishment, as well as our behaviours relating to species survival, sexual arousal and the desire to nurture the young and helpless.[41]

The amygdala processes incoming data and sorts it for emotional content or, in another light, for its impact on your survival. It is particularly attuned to alert you to events that are potentially negative to your survival. Danger or threat produces fear and fear alerts your system to the fact of the danger. Suddenly your whole system gets ready to fight or flee for your life. The amygdala is the sentinel that triggers the fight or flight response.

Recent research has shown that the amygdala plays a pivotal role in storing emotional memories, the expression of fear and the perception of emotional expression in other people. When the amygdala is damaged, people lose all fear and are unable to interpret the meaning of facial expressions in others.[42] When subjects were shown a series of photographs of different facial expressions while they were being scanned with Positive Emission Tomography (PET), the blood flow increased, indicating increased activity, in the amygdala. The increase in blood flow in the amygdala paralleled the increase in intensity of fear expressed in the photographs. This response occurred even though the subjects were consciously unaware of the expressions, as they were busy trying to identify the gender of each face.[43]

While the hippocampus records memory of objects and events as facts, the amygdala appears to assign the emotional content to these facts. Indeed, a major impetus to memory is the emotional relevance of the object or event, without which it is likely to be quickly forgotten. The fascinating role of the hippocampus and amygdala in memory will be discussed in the next chapter.

Events that are threatening or perceived as punishment are therefore encoded into memory along with the emotional content assigned to these events by the amygdala. Because memories of an event may be strongly bound to the strongest emotion aroused during the event, we can often react in irrational ways to recurring or similar circumstances in our lives. A new trigger may recall a powerful emotional experience associated with a similar trigger in the past, and these emotions can then be brought back in full force. Witness phobias.

Another example is the young child who stumbles over words and is laughed at when asked to read to the class. The embarrassment caused by this event is perceived as a punishment by the amygdala. When attempting to read out loud as an adult, the remembered pain of embarrassment may come flooding back resulting in loss of integrated brain function. The only thing a person in this situation wants to do is flee: to run from the punishment.

Even though the amygdaloid memory of punishment associated with reading is based upon a childhood experience and totally outside the person's conscious awareness, the fearful prospect of standing up in front of people to read or speak may make the adult break out in a sweat and go weak in the knees. Because the amygdala remembers the first awful outcome of an activity and has encoded a strong negative emotion with that activity, it will do all it can to prevent you from putting yourself in the same circumstance again. In this case, the amygdala perceives reading in front of people as punishment and says, 'Forget it!'

Once those amygdaloid punishment circuits are encoded they can override our conscious desire to do many things that we might sincerely want to do. The fear that was encoded in childhood often cannot be easily overridden, so people may end up being controlled by their subconscious punishment programs. In some circumstances, events in the present trigger subconscious reactions from the past, issues totally irrelevant to the present circumstances, yet these reactions can still run the show.

An innate understanding of this process is the reason tight-rope walkers, trapeze artists and horse riders are all encouraged to get back on the rope, trapeze or horse immediately after they have taken a fall. Any event that has created fear will first be held in short-term memory before being passed into long-term memory. In the interim (before the fear has been indelibly linked to the fearful stimulus, the fall) there is a chance to overwrite the event by replacing it with a new, successful experience. Doing it again can put the person back in charge.

'Have another go' is therefore a very worthwhile phrase for parents to repeat when teaching their children new skills. And a teacher, with any awareness of this process, would step in before the child at the front of the class is laughed at and mortified by fear. With a little support, perhaps by stopping for a while and then gently encouraging the child to succeed in reading, the fear could be short-circuited before it becomes a lasting imprint. Persistence of negative emotional imprinting can last long after the original event that triggered it—even a lifetime.

It is in this area of brain function that kinesiology is powerful because it can defuse these old emotional patterns and release people to make new choices for themselves in their present life circumstances.

Overall, amygdaloid function has a great deal to do with the process of learning. If excitement is encoded around it, learning can become a joy. A fearful encodement can produce the opposite result.

As challenging and complex as the information presented in this chapter has been, it must be realised that this has been just a brief overview that leaves out many of the details of what really happens. This is a mere summary of the much more difficult and complex science of neurology and neuropsychology. And as new information about the workings of the brain is being revealed almost daily, it is really a 'best guess' about what all these parts of the brain do from the perspective of what we know today.

For all that we have explained in this chapter about the wonders of the brain, what remains unknown is even more awesome. This great and astounding mystery is what keeps me, and so many other researchers in the field so fascinated and captivated by the quest to push on further into the amazing universe of the human brain. A total understanding of its wonders, however, may remain forever beyond our grasp.

Chapter Four

THE REMARKABLE REACH OF MEMORY

WHAT DOES THE BRAIN DO? IT LEARNS AND REMEMBERS

The facility of memory truly is amazing as it gives us the ability to remember information from events that have taken place throughout our life, and hence to learn from life's experiences.

Most of us can recall memories from our childhood, little vignettes that come back to us in almost infinite detail. A man I know who is in his seventies was a Latin scholar in his youth. About 25 years ago he visited the basilica of St. Peter's in Rome and was delighted to discover that he could still read the Latin inscription that runs around the base of the dome. He could translate the instruction: 'You are Peter and on this rock you will build my church and I will give you the keys to my kingdom.'

Even now, when he is talking about that visit to the Vatican, you can see him looking up into his mind as if he were looking up at the dome and moving his eyes, as if he were reading the inscription again.

Memory is even more astounding when we begin to investigate how it works. Many decades of research have been dedicated to unravelling the mechanisms of memory but like so much else that concerns the workings of the brain, we understand very little. To quote Endel Tulving, a prominent memory researcher: 'Memory is one of nature's most jealously guarded secrets. At the beginning of the second century of its scientific study, it continues to baffle, frustrate, and mystify those who would explore it'.[1] The outline that follows in this chapter can therefore only be an overview of the much more incredible memory function of the human brain.

To focus on what we mean we need to define the terms we will be using:
Memory can be defined as the capacity of storing, retrieving and acting

upon knowledge. Or, as the ability to recall thoughts. It is a crucial function for learning because learning cannot occur without memory.

Learning can be defined as the ability to acquire knowledge or skills through instruction or experience. Or, as the ability to modify our behaviour in response to new experience based on our memory.

Obviously, to learn something we must have an experience and then be able to remember it. Experience that does not stay in our memory will not modify our behaviour. Experiments with animals have shown that sensory experience that causes neither pain nor pleasure is almost never remembered.[2] For memory to occur, there has to be some relevant impetus, relevant to the animal's survival or relationship to its environment. If there is no relevance to survival or relational meaning, the brain does not commit it to memory.

An everyday event to illustrate this process occurs when we are reading a book and come across a word that we swear we've never seen before. We look up the word in the dictionary to find the meaning. The word now has meaning to our mind. It now has relevance. A short time later, browsing in a bookstore we are surprised to suddenly 'see' this previously unknown word. Obviously it has always been around but until it had meaning for us it remained 'unseen'.

While much of what we know about memory is based on experiments with animals, in a broad area of learning the human mind makes an interesting distinction from that of an animal. For humans, remembering something you have learned can be a pleasure in itself. It does not necessarily need to be associated with survival to have relevance. The human mind takes pleasure in recognising or remembering ('Oh, I know what that means!'). Knowing is tantamount to a reward which is a pleasurable stimulus to the brain, and hence the joy in playing memory games like *Trivial Pursuit*.

And just as the eastern mystics have been suggesting for thousands of years, mere thought can cause associations with pain and pleasure.

If you think a negative thought, all the punishment centres in your brain will be activated despite the fact that there is no real threat in the immediate vicinity. If, on the other hand, you think of something pleasant, you can experience pleasurable sensations, including smiles, because you have stimulated the pleasure centres in the brain.[3]

You begin to realise just how intricately memory is woven together with the facility for learning and this will be discussed in more detail in the next chapter. Meanwhile, to better understand how we remember, we need to set out what is currently known about memory.

WHAT IS KNOWN

While memory was originally conceived as a single monolithic system in the brain, research over the past decade, and especially in the past five years, has suggested quite a different picture. It now appears that memory functions are multiple and widely distributed across the brain. Instead of a single monolithic system, our memories seem to be created by an integrated set of subsystems, each making its own unique contribution to this amazing function that largely defines our identity.

Not only have a number of different types of memories been identified, but with the aid of fantastic new imaging devices such as Positron Emission Tomography (PET) and functional Magnetic Resonance Imaging (fMRI), the neural substrate or brain areas performing these different types of memory are rapidly emerging.

The different types of memory fall into roughly two categories: conscious and subconscious. Although experiments may demonstrate conscious and subconscious memory as separate functions—focussed in different parts of the brain, in our normal mental activities, these two types of memory are integrated into the seamless experience we just call remembering.

THE NEURAL SUBSTRATE OF CONSCIOUS MEMORY

The creation of conscious memory is centred in the hippocampal system of the medial temporal lobe, as so graphically demonstrated in the case of H.M. Since surgery removed this part of his brain in 1953, H.M has not been able to encode any new conscious memory about the days of his life. Other cases of brain damage examined via PET, fMRI scans, and electrophysiological recordings, have all confirmed that this system plays the central role in formation of our conscious memories.

The hippocampal system is widely used to refer to a system of interrelated brain regions that play a central role in memory and learning. It is comprised largely of parts of the ancient cortex in the medial temporal lobe lying deep within the brain. It lies alongside the brainstem to which it is richly and reciprocally connected. The major components of this system are the hippocampus and the structurally contiguous dentate gyrus, the subiculum and fornix, and the limbic lobe structures of the parahippocampal gyrus, entorhinal and perirhinal cortices (See Figs. 3.22b & 3.23).

While the hippocampus is the central processing unit of this core memory module that contains our short-term memory circuits, the dentate gyrus and subiculum are major input-output centres that send and receive information to and from other parts of the brain.[5] One component of the dentate gyrus, the hilus, may even filter information that passes through the hippocampus, thus altering our on-going awareness.[6] It is via these centres that data that is being held in short-term memory in the hippocampus can be modified or developed more fully.

While the subiculum receives major output from the hippocampus and has extensive reciprocal connections with many areas of the brain, including areas of the cortex, it is also the origin of fibres in the fornix that ultimately innervate the hypothalamus. Through these later pathways information being held in the short-term memory circuits of the hippocampus can result in the physiological responses we call 'feelings'.

The fornix is also the major output pathway of the hippocampus, providing information held in short-term memory to other areas of the limbic system and cortical association areas for further processing, or to be laid down as long-term memory.[7]

The other components of the hippocampal system are the folds of the limbic lobe surrounding the hippocampus, including the parahippocampal gyrus and entorhinal and perirhinal cortices (See Figure 3.22a). These limbic lobe structures mediate the two-way flow of information between the cortex and the limbic system.

Pathways from the parahippocampal gyrus and perirhinal cortex provide a conduit for information from the memory areas of the association cortex to the hippocampus. This information travels via the entorhinal cortex. Indeed, the entorhinal cortex is the final convergence zone for cortical inputs into the hippocampus.[8]

In this way the information held in the short-term memory circuits of the hippocampus can be compared with 'referents' that are being held in long-term memory areas of the cortex. These 'referents' help to define and give meaning to the hippocampal content.

The entorhinal cortex also plays an important role in linking many of the subconscious sensory and emotional centres, such as the anterior cingulate gyrus to the hippocampus.[9] While the role of the perirhinal cortex is less well understood, it appears to play a similar role in linking the amygdala and hippocampus to the association areas of the cortex which hold long-term memory.[10] Thus, data held in hippocampal short-term memory circuits, can be evaluated for its emotional significance to survival by the amygdala and further, for comparison with past emotional associations stored in the cortex. The end result is that neutral facts held in short-term memory may become emotionally coloured by being referred to our past experience. This process can add greatly to the relevance of these facts.

What these limbic lobe structures appear to facilitate is a way in which data held in short-term memory may be referenced against past experience and knowledge. The hippocampus provides the connections from the long-term memory areas of the cortex allowing specific data to be identified and made more meaningful.

Other connections between these structures, the hippocampus and the emotional centres of the brain, give relevance to information held in the short-term memory, and further determine whether this information will be 'remembered' or lost to our conscious experience. The reciprocal connections of these limbic lobe structures to the long-term memory areas of the cortex, also provide the hippocampus pathways by which new information can be laid down or encoded as long-term memory in these cortical areas.[11]

Although not structurally part of the hippocampal system, the nearby structures of the amygdala—the emotional centre, and the hypothalamus—the feeling centre, are also extensively and reciprocally wired to the hippocampal system.

Indeed, it is through these connections that 'relevance' is largely assigned to information held in the hippocampus. With special emphasis on the survival responses of fear and anxiety, the amygdala appears to supply the 'emotional colour' while the hypothalamus supplies the 'gut feelings' associated with previous experiences.[12]

These same connections between the hippocampal system and the largely subconscious amygdala and hypothalamus form the nexus between our conscious and subconscious memories.

We are conscious of the moment-to-moment content of the hippocampus. In fact, this is largely our awareness of the present moment. The hippocampal system, however, is only involved in the *processing* of sensory experience and memories as declarative 'facts'. It is a car, a yellow Ford. The memories evoked by the emotional association with this 'fact' and the gut reactions to a yellow Ford, are largely subconscious responses. We usually only become consciously aware of the source of these emotional and gut reactions after we have already experienced them. That is, if we become conscious of their source at all. How many times have you had an experience, then wondered why your feeling state has suddenly changed?

An event from my life provides a poignant illustration: When I was in my twenties, I fell helplessly and hopelessly in love with Phyllis. We were sure, as all young lovers are, that our love would last forever.

The inevitable happened. She broke my heart by leaving me for another man. During the time I knew her, Phyllis happened to drive a yellow Ford. After the breakup, and for years after, whenever I would see a yellow Ford of the same year and model, I would suddenly feel my heart ache and my gut tighten.

At the neurological level, my hippocampus merely brought a recent visual experience—a certain model yellow Ford, into my conscious awareness. Outside of my consciousness, this same visual stimulus had triggered my amygdaloid memory of the emotions associated with that yellow Ford, and my hypothalamic-controlled gut reaction to this emotion.

126 A Revolutionary Way of Thinking

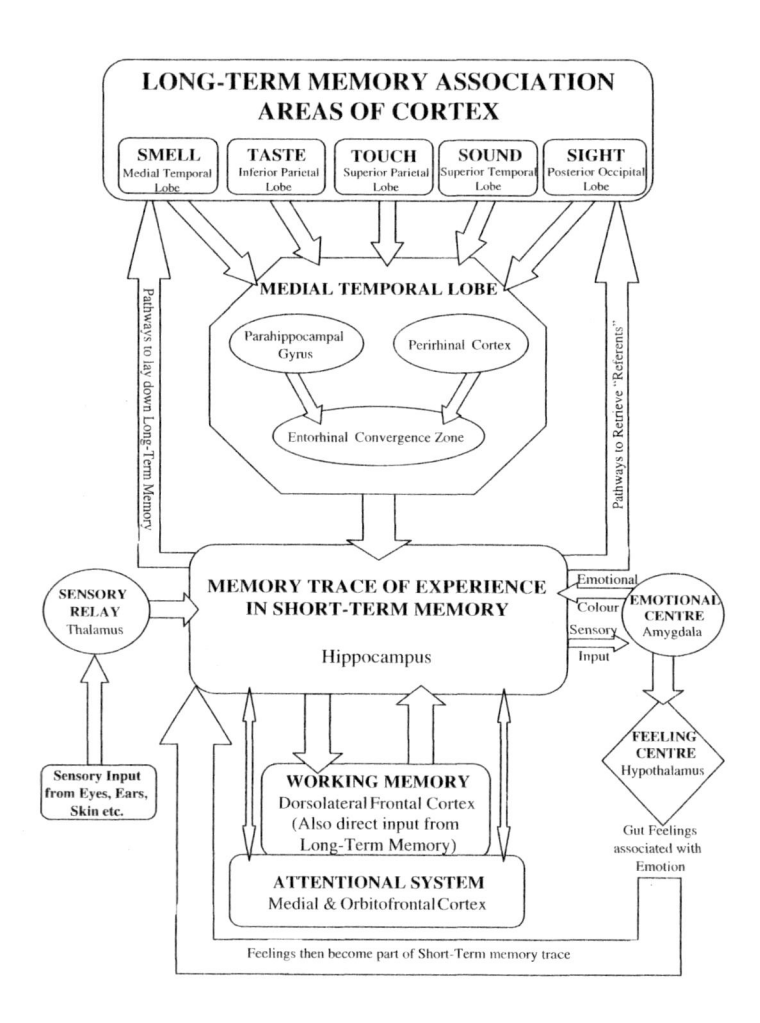

```
                 LONG-TERM MEMORY ASSOCIATION
                        AREAS OF CORTEX
   ┌─────────┬─────────┬─────────┬─────────┬─────────┐
   │  SMELL  │  TASTE  │  TOUCH  │  SOUND  │  SIGHT  │
   │ Medial  │ Inferior│ Superior│Superior │Posterior│
   │Temporal │ Parietal│ Parietal│Temporal │Occipital│
   │  Lobe   │  Lobe   │  Lobe   │  Lobe   │  Lobe   │
   └─────────┴─────────┴─────────┴─────────┴─────────┘

              MEDIAL TEMPORAL LOBE
         ┌──────────────┐  ┌──────────────┐
         │Parahippocampal│  │  Perirhinal  │
         │    Gyrus      │  │    Cortex    │
         └──────────────┘  └──────────────┘
              Entorhinal Convergence Zone

   ┌─────────┐    MEMORY TRACE OF EXPERIENCE    ┌─────────┐
   │ SENSORY │     IN SHORT-TERM MEMORY         │EMOTIONAL│
   │  RELAY  │                                   │ CENTRE  │
   │Thalamus │         Hippocampus              │Amygdala │
   └─────────┘                                   └─────────┘
                                                      │
   ┌─────────┐                                   ┌─────────┐
   │ Sensory │      WORKING MEMORY              │ FEELING │
   │ Input   │   Dorsolateral Frontal Cortex    │ CENTRE  │
   │from Eyes│   (Also direct input from         │Hypothal.│
   │Ears Skin│    Long-Term Memory)             └─────────┘
   └─────────┘                                   Gut Feelings
              ATTENTIONAL SYSTEM                 associated with
              Medial & Orbitofrontal Cortex      Emotion

         Feelings then become part of Short-Term memory trace
```

Figure 4.1. A Schematic Model of the Memory Systems of the Brain. The memory traces of experience generated either from sensory experience or memory are brought into consciousness in the hippocampus. Referents from long-term memory are used to define on-going sensory experience, which if found to be relevant may be laid down as new long-term memory. Sensory input is also relayed to the amygdala which provides the emotional colour of the experience and also activates feelings by the hypothalamus. These feelings, in turn, are incorporated into the memory trace in the hippocampus. Information from both the hippocampus and from long-term memory are available for conscious processing in working memory where they may be contemplated.

The response persisted so strongly that many times I would find myself thinking—'Why am I suddenly feeling like this?' Then I would realise that a yellow Ford was in my field of vision. 'When am I ever going to get over her?'

The line between our conscious awareness and our subconscious experience and memory is very, very thin. While the subconscious memories often play a significant role in our conscious experience of the current moment, the extent and nature of that role is often 'hidden' to our consciousness.

In summary, the hippocampal system appears to subserve three distinct functions with regard to our memory: (See Fig. 4.1).

- The first is the processing of on-going or recent events, either sensory or mental, that are relevant or useful for the moment, but which may not be stored as longer term memory. These immediate and short-term memories appear to be based largely upon the function of the central processing unit, the hippocampus.
- The second function is retrieval or recall of information stored in long-term memory. This appears to rely on the medial temporal lobe connections to transport the pieces of past experience from the association cortex storing each type of sensory experience (the visual component, the auditory component, the olfactory component, etc.), to the hippocampal system where it is reconstructed as the 'memory' of the experience.
- The third function is the laying down or encoding of new long-term memory of information held in the short-term memory circuits of the hippocampus.

This summary does, however, overlook one of the most important aspects of memory.

Why do we bother in the first place? Why do we remember one experience and not another? Why are some experiences forgotten almost as soon as they are over, yet others last a lifetime?

Here we enter the murky water of emotional relevance and feelings which appear to reside in two largely subconscious structures, the amygdala and hypothalamus. It must be noted that these two structures alone are not responsible for relevance. Rather, they activate other subsystems and reward and punishment centres that give us the reason to remember. If an experience is associated with neither pain nor pleasure, it seldom leaves a trace in our consciousness.

REWARD AND PUNISHMENT

The major factor controlling formation of memory in the brain is emotional relevance in the form of reward and punishment. It is said that when we store information, the affective quality of the data determines where it is put and how well it will be remembered. 'Affective' means feelings or emotions, sensations that are interpreted in the brain as pleasant or unpleasant, satisfactory or unsatisfactory or, by the textbook definition, as reward or punishment.

Why you store these memories in the first place, is, as we have discovered, a decision of the limbic system; in particular the hypothalamus, amygdala, hippocampus and certain areas in the forebrain that contain primary and secondary centres for reward and punishment.[13]

Reward. When you do something that gives a positive outcome, like finding a delicious patch of wild strawberries, it constitutes a reward. This activates receptors within the reward centres of the brain which provide the impetus to 'remember' the location of that patch of berries. Scientists were at first amazed to find opium receptors throughout various areas of the brain, especially the areas involved with the experience of pain and pleasure.[14]

Why would the brain create opiate receptors? Since the action of opium and its derivatives, morphine and heroin, are to block pain and generate feelings of well-being—even euphoria, it would appear that the brain must manufacture compounds similar to the extract of poppies to the same end. In 1973, a morphine-like substance was identified in mammalian brains and it was shown to reduce pain and anxiety. These first natural brain opiates were called 'enkephalins' (from the Greek word meaning 'in the head'), and were found not only in areas associated with pain, but also in areas associated with well-being and pleasure.[15]

Since then, a number of other natural brain opioids have been discovered, with a major class called 'endorphins', meaning 'endogenous (or made in the body) morphine'. The endorphins were found to not only reduce pain and anxiety, but also to create feelings of well-being. In high enough concentrations they produced euphoria. The role that brain opiates (which I shall collectively call endorphins), play in the reward system of the brain is now being unravelled.

Figure 4.2 shows the reward system includes the deep brainstem nuclei, the substantia nigra (black substance), from which arise a series of dopamine secreting neurons linking the hypothalamus, the nucleus accumbens, and areas in the prefrontal cortex.[16] The nucleus accumbens is a primitive structure in the basal forebrain that is one of the brain's key pleasure centres. The dopamine-rich areas of the prefrontal cortex appear to be involved in the control of impulsive and irrational behaviours.[17] Broadly, feelings of well-being and pleasure arise from the release of endorphins into the brain's reward centres and cause either an increase in the levels of the neurotransmitter dopamine, or enhance its action.

The dopamine nerve pathways originating in the substantia nigra contain axons that form synaptic connections within each of the reward areas of the brain. When endorphins are released, they appear to bind to dopamine receptors increasing the release of this neurotransmitter in these synapses. The increased dopamine levels activate the neural networks of the nucleus accumbens which generate the mental sense of well-being, and then, the hypothalamic nuclei control the accompanying physiological responses that we recognise as the 'feeling' of well-being. At the same time, the release of dopamine into the prefrontal cortex appears to quell restlessness and helps us to focus on the task at hand.[18] Overall we feel great.

It is believed that this reward system arose early in the evolution of animals because it provides impetus to reinforce behaviour essential for survival. As higher animals began to interact with their environment in more complex

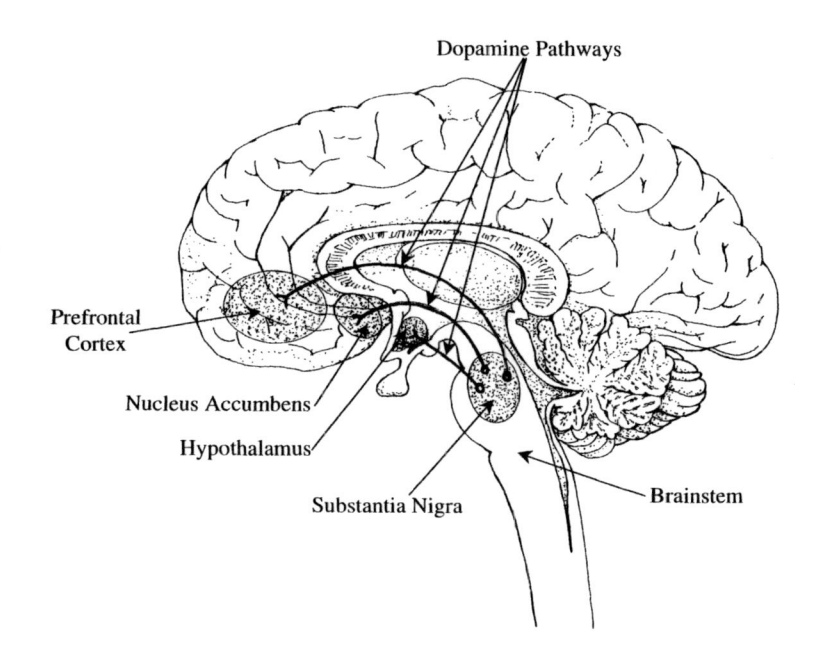

Figure 4.2. Reward System of the Brain. Consist of a series of dopamine secreting neurons originating in the substantia nigra and going to three major reward centres: Hypothalamus, Nucleus Accumbens, and Prefrontal Cortex. Release of dopamine in these reward centres gives rise to the sensations of pleasure and well-being, and when strongly stimulated—euphoria.

ways, this same reward system provided the impetus to remember information of survival value—to recall the location of the patch of delicious berries.

The endorphin-dopamine reward system appears to exert extraordinary power over learning and memory by providing the proverbial carrot for making survival-oriented choices. Thus any time you perform an act that gives you pleasure, the brain has just released endorphins to stimulate your opiate receptors and initiating what Kenneth Blum termed 'the brain reward cascade'.[19]

The same reward centres appear to be short-circuited by drugs of addiction. Drugs—from nicotine and alcohol, to heroin and cocaine—appear to exert their addictive effects because they mimic endorphins, increasing dopamine release or inhibiting its uptake, and in effect turning these powerful reward centres on.[20] In the case of drugs of addiction, the reward now drives self-destructive, rather than survival-oriented behaviour. A recent suggestion is that both alcoholism and Attention Deficit Disorder may be rooted in inherited deficits of dopamine receptors in these reward systems.[21] This concept will be discussed in greater depth in Chapter 9.

Punishment. Experiments using electrodes to stimulate various brain centres have shown there are also potent punishment centres. The most powerful of these is found in the area of the basal forebrain surrounding the third ventricle or cerebral aqueduct.[22] Called the periventricular gray matter, when stimulated either by direct sensory experience, electric shock, or by feedback from other brain centres such as the amygdala, this area releases chemicals and neural output to other brain areas, creating fear and unpleasant physical sensations. This gives the powerful signal not to repeat this behaviour again.

Other experiments which electrically stimulated other brain centres in animals, have demonstrated that secondary punishment centres are contained in the amygdala and hippocampus.[23] A serious limitation exists in these experiments because electrical stimulation elicits responses from only the very limited and isolated brain areas immediately surrounding the electrodes. In the intact, functioning brain, inputs to both the primary and secondary punishment centres come from many different parts of the brain, particularly those areas where emotions arise.

Current evidence suggests that the amygdala is the primary source of emotional states and that these emotional states determine the flavour of our experience, good or bad.[24] It is this emotional colouring that makes the experience positive or negative, and also determines the intensity of the experience.

It appears that the amygdala issues the primary punishment alert to the system in the form of emotional intensity and that the intensity activates the primary punishment areas in the periventricular grey matter. This area in turn, activates secondary areas in the hypothalamus, which then elicit the physiological response to potential punishment: the racing heart, the sweating palms, dilated pupils and fear of pain. Similar activation of secondary punishment areas in the hippocampus provide the relevance to lay down memory of the associated event. The amygdala is, therefore, the first adjudicator of punishment.

Memory of an event appears to be entirely dependent upon the reward or punishment associated with the event. No reward or punishment—no memory. This alludes to the critical importance of *emotional loading* in the process of laying down memories in the brain. As we go through the days of our lives, if there is no reward or punishment associated with an event, then there is no particular reason to remember it.

In memory, neutral experiences subside and this process is important to understand when we look back at our childhood and seem to be able to recall only the peak experiences of reward—receiving a prize at school or winning a race, and punishment—of getting into trouble for something a sibling did.

You may still be able to vividly remember receiving your school prize. More likely you can still 'feel' how unfair it was to have been wrongly blamed for something your sibling did. You can still feel the hurt of the injustice. In contrast, the mundane day-to-day events of childhood disappear entirely from our conscious memory.

In memory, a negative stimulus will always override a positive stimulus. You will tend to more easily remember the negative events and this is because the amygdaloid circuit is negatively oriented. In terms of survival it is much more important to recall negative events. Remembering vividly the feeling of these events, we can avoid or check threatening situations in the future. In terms of our emotional structure this can be a handicap because in memory, it can appear that negative or punishing events outweigh the positives that have happened.

For example, a friend may have provided hundreds of benefits (rewards). But that friend needs only to let you down once (punishment), for you to remember them in what is basically a negative light.

CONSCIOUS MEMORY:

Long-term and Short-term Memory
You might well ask, isn't all memory conscious? After all it's only information that I consciously recall from memory that I can claim to remember. In a following section you will find that for the retrieval of certain types of information the answer is a definite no. Not all memory involves our conscious awareness. But since the bulk of past research has centred on conscious memory, I will first discuss the properties, mechanisms and types of conscious memory before proceeding on to consider the more recently investigated subconscious memory.

What we commonly think of as memory is the retrieval of information about facts, objects, events and the associated elements of these events. These elements can be explicitly recalled, verbally described or used to govern our behaviour. The term *declarative or explicit memory* is used to encompass such forms of memory readily accessed by conscious recall. While declarative memory used to take only two forms—short-term and long-term memory—current neuropsychological research points to additional types of declarative memory.

Immediate Memory. Almost all incoming sensory experience—be it auditory, visual, olfactory and gustatory—is registered, albeit very briefly. For just a fraction of a second that incoming data will be held in short-term memory circuits associated with each sense. This faculty is called immediate memory or sensory store.[25]

Here it comes under the scrutiny of parts of the prefrontal cortex, the amygdala, parts of the thalamus and the hippocampus, which then decide whether the data has any real relevance for us. If it does, the information will be shifted into short-term memory circuits of the hippocampus. If the data is deemed to have no relevance, it will be instantly overwritten in immediate memory and leave no trace. And if the information never even reached short-term memory, you certainly cannot recall it.

This is what happens if you are driving down the road going past many parked cars. As each car comes into your visual field, it will be momentarily registered. But as the next car comes into view, this new data will overwrite the data on the previous car. Unless you pass a car that has some relevance to you, such as, 'It's a red Toyota just like *my* new car!', you will be totally unaware of the models and colours of the other cars that you have passed. They are just part of the stream of visual information.

Short-Term Memory. Short-term memory, also known as primary memory, appears to be more biochemical in nature, and here, memory traces persist for a slightly longer time. Once the information in immediate memory is deemed 'relevant', it appears to initiate *long-term potentiation* of neurons in the short-term memory centres of the hippocampus.

When a fact, object or event is held in these circuits, the emotional content associated with that fact, object or event, potentiates (activates) circuits within the hippocampus. The release of neurotransmitters at specific synapses activates the retention of this information.[26]

Long-term potentiation appears to result from the pairing of a stimulus, or information held in short-term memory circuits, with input from axons originating in the reward and punishment centres of the brain. This input takes the form of the release of excitatory neurotransmitter from the end bulbs of these axons into synapses of the hippocampal short-term memory circuits. The excitatory neurotransmitter facilitates the dendritic membranes of the hippocampal neurons, making them fire more easily the next time the information is presented. Every time this information is rehearsed, it becomes easier to remember. The short-term memory circuits have been established. But just how long this potentiation will last depends on the intensity of the associated reward or punishment and the duration of rehearsal. It may be minutes or weeks.[27]

Short-term memory is what gives us the ability to remember a telephone number and to dial it within the next few minutes. If, however, we are asked to repeat the number an hour later, we would be unable to do so because this data did not have strong associations to either reward or punishment.

But then, we might meet someone we find really attractive and 20 years later, if we meet that same person again, we'll remember their name. This is because the initial emotional intensity led to long term potentiation to hold the name in short term memory long enough for it to be committed to long-term memory.

Generally, for information to be maintained in these short-term memory circuits, it has to be consciously rehearsed and reinforced. Everyone has had the experience of going into a telephone box, without a pen or a piece of paper, dialling the information service and requesting a phone number. The operator gives you the number but to retain it long enough to be able to dial the number you must start repeating it; 'Five-three-six-four-five-eight-one. Five-three-six-four-five-eight-one. Five-three-six-four-five-eight-one.'

What happens to the number if a passerby, knocks on the phone booth and asks you for the time?

If it is a number that you will only use once, you are unlikely to remember it for more than a few moments, because it has only a little rehearsal and even less relevance. But if the number is relevant to that attractive person you just met and want to see more of, it is likely you'll be able to remember the number for months—maybe even years. This occurs for two reasons: the first is that the pairing of a strong emotion with the number leads to powerful potentiation of the hippocampal circuits. The second is that you will probably think about that person a number of times after the initial meeting, reactivating the associated memory of their telephone number.

In learning something like primary school multiplication tables, we have to keep the data active in the short-term memory circuits by rote repetition of the figures over and over again. What happens next is a little-understood neurophysiological process called consolidation. Consolidation means that if information in short-term memory is repeated often enough, and is relevant enough, or, if it is loaded with enough emotional content, it is somehow packaged for transfer into long-term memory.

CONSOLIDATION OF MEMORY

A recently proposed model of consolidation sees the process as the interaction between two complementary learning and memory systems in the brain: The first is the chemically-based hippocampal system processing all new and on-going sensory input (which requires rapid processing and only short term retention of information). The second is the structurally-based cortical processing system in the association cortices holding our stores of past experience (which processes far slower requiring structural change, the formation of new synapses and probably changes in membrane structure). Although slower, the cortical system does provide long term retention of information.[28] It is the reason why we 'study' complex information by repeated inspection in order to learn it.

Transfer to long-term memory, as we all know, requires repetition, or having the same data presented repeatedly before it 'sinks in'. The sinking in process can be thought of as the time it takes to integrate the new information with our old memories, or, from the neurological perspective, as the time it takes to create changes in the synaptic connections in the memory association areas of the cortex. Thus, long-term memory is laid down slowly because it is based in actual changes in the structure of connections in these cortical areas. On each reinstatement, the cortical synapses change a little, and a number of reinstatements are necessary to complete the synaptic structure of a new memory.

The consolidation process is important for two reasons: First, it permits new information to be processed in short-term memory in the hippocampus, without the disruption of past memories which are held structurally in long-term memory. Secondly, it permits relevant information in short-term memory to be interleaved with previous memories of a similar type, making retrieval of the new and the related information more efficient.

All the evidence to date suggests that memories stored in long-term memory are codified into different classes, and that associated classes are stored together.[29] Such arrangement makes perfect sense in terms of the streamlining of information retrieval and the design ensures that similar information can be easily recalled to use as a reference in the processing of new information.

For instance, you know the word 'bed' means 'a place where you sleep.' But as you are reading, what happens if you come across the word 'cot?' The dictionary tells you that a cot is a 'portable, foldable bed'.

In the memory's frame of reference, 'cot' now links to the idea of 'bed' and as it is rehearsed, it is put in the same storage area. The two terms now help to define each other in an alignment which gives you the fantastic capacity to recall past information in order to give new information greater relevance.

It is a comparative function, which allows us to store data according to its similarities and distinctions. You now store 'cot', not only along with the concept of 'bed' but also with the recorded distinctions that a cot is 'a portable, foldable bed.' And so it appears that during the process of memory consolidation, new memories are stored directly in association with memories of a similar type.

Long-Term Memory. Long-term memory, also known as secondary memory, therefore appears to result from structural change in the neuronal membranes and their interconnections. Long-term memory is structurally encoded, perhaps as a change in the structure and number of dendrites and their synaptic connections.[30] Once that change has occurred, the memory is permanent because the neuronal arrangement containing its encodement will live in your brain as long as you are breathing.

Only information that is transferred into long-term memory can truly be said to have been learned. If information is not encoded in your long-term memory it cannot be retrieved and serve as a basis to modify your behaviour. After all, learning is about the retrieval of past experience referenced to current circumstance. Throughout your life you are therefore storing permanent memories of your relevant life experience.

Now, this is going to sound like a direct contradiction to the idea of the permanence of long-term memory, but the fact is, only about one percent of the information you have learned in you life is recallable without a trigger of some kind.

The other 99 percent is still in long-term memory but is just not consciously retrievable at the moment. Forgetting information stored in long-term memory is generally assumed to be the result of interference from later learning.[31] In a sense, the older memories are pushed into the back of the file drawer by adding new memories to the front. Unless a trigger stimulus causes you to pull the drawer all the way out, and look again at these old memories, we would say we have forgotten them.

Short-term memory is only a window to our immediate experience, a recall function that remains open for a minute, to maybe a week or two at most. The reason we get children to repeat their multiplication tables over and over again is to enable them to hold them in short-term memory long enough for transferal into long-term eidetic or image memory, where it is encoded as pictures. I learned my times tables more than 40 years ago and if I want to know the answer to 7×7, I literally look up into my visual memory which gives me the already encoded picture of the answer: 49. I do not have to do any mental calculation.

If I could not have transferred this information which was held in my auditory short-term memory, across and into my visual long-term memory, I could not have remembered my times tables. This is a common problem I see in children who come to me presenting with learning difficulties. They can laboriously learn their tables, have them down pat, but by the next day they just can't remember what they spent so much time and effort learning. While the data entered short-term memory, they never managed to get the information transferred into the brain areas storing that type of long-term memory.

WORKING MEMORY

Over the past three decades, research has alluded to another type of short-term memory that appears quite separate from the usual short-term memory involved in the laying down and retrieval of memory traces from the long-term memory. In their insightful book *Plans and the Structure of Behaviour*, written in the 1960s, Miller, Galanter and Pribham labelled this new type of short-term memory 'working memory' and considered it a temporary storage system for information used in connection with other, more complex tasks.[32]

Working memory can be thought of as a human-information processing system involved in the executive control of thinking and behaviour that also serves as a form of brief short-term memory. It can be on-line while other matters are being dealt with. It is a repository of conscious awareness where information not needed at present, but which will be required again shortly, is held. The facility is comparable to a mental scratchpad in which plans can be temporarily retained while they are being formed, transformed, or executed.

Working memory plays a vital role in our everyday lives. When engaged in conversation with a friend, working memory enables you to hold on to the beginning of the sentence while she gets to the end. It also provides us with the capacity to multi-task or to perform several different thoughts or actions all at the same time. We can look through our diary for an appointment time, talk on the telephone, and wave at a passing friend to get their attention to ask if they are free to go to the movies tonight.

Working memory also plays a vital role for authors. It permits us to hold many different pieces of information temporarily while working out how to put them together coherently. Working memory is where writers create and plan the outlines that when fleshed out became a completed chapter.

While the exact nature of working memory is not fully understood, several models have been proposed. In one model, working memory is seen as a single system constituting a mental workspace. This is comparable to a mental 'blackboard'.[33] The model I prefer sees working memory as a multi-component system that usually operates after access to long-term memory has taken place. It is quite separate from normal hippocampal-based short-term memory. In this system, the hippocampus plays a supporting role, while the central processing unit of working memory is operating in the dorsolateral frontal cortex, the area of cortex that is just above and between your eyes and ears.[34]

In the model I prefer, working memory is made up of three components that provide respectively: temporary verbal storage; temporary visuospatial storage; and a co-ordinating function or attentional control system. The attentional control system is termed the *central executive*, and is aided by slave systems, or buffers, responsible for temporary storage and manipulation of either visual material (the *visuospatial scratchpad*), or verbal material (the *phonological loop*) (see Fig. 4.3). The slave systems serve as 'working buffers' for visual and verbal information that has yet to be processed or is about to be recalled consciously.[35]

The verbal storage component, the phonological loop, acts as both a temporary verbal store and a rehearsal system. As you have conscious access to the contents of working memory, loss of information from this store can be prevented by silently repeating the information in your head. The visual component, the visuospatial scratchpad, is thought to be involved in visual imagery tasks and in temporary retention of visual and spatial information. It may include a companion system that retains movement sequences and may be used for visuospatial rehearsal.

The central executive is a limited-capacity attentional system that mediates between the verbal and visual components, and with knowledge that is stored in long-term memory. It is the central executive that is responsible for strategy selection and planning, and may even be said to 'contemplate' ways of using information in the phonological loop or visuospatial scratchpad.

Information can enter the verbal or visual subsystems, or both, either from direct sensory input currently being processed in the hippocampus, or, by recall from long-term memory.

Often, sensory input held in the hippocampus activates memory traces of related information in long-term memory, which then become available to the slave systems of working memory. Working memory appears to be particularly involved in the processing of novel information. By considering both verbal and visual aspects of a novel experience from sensory input, and by referral to long-term memory for any related or similar experience, the central executive can contemplate this information to decide what to do with it or how to make sense out of it.

For example, if the word 'horse' is heard, the sound representations of horse in your head create a sound trace of 'horse' in the phonological loop, which then permits you to rehearse or *speak* the word. On hearing the word, the visual and spatial properties of the word 'horse' become available to the visuospatial scratchpad, allowing you to temporarily *visualise* the word, which you could then write down.

General information about horses would then be available to the central executive, permitting an image of 'horse' to appear in working memory. The

138   A Revolutionary Way of Thinking

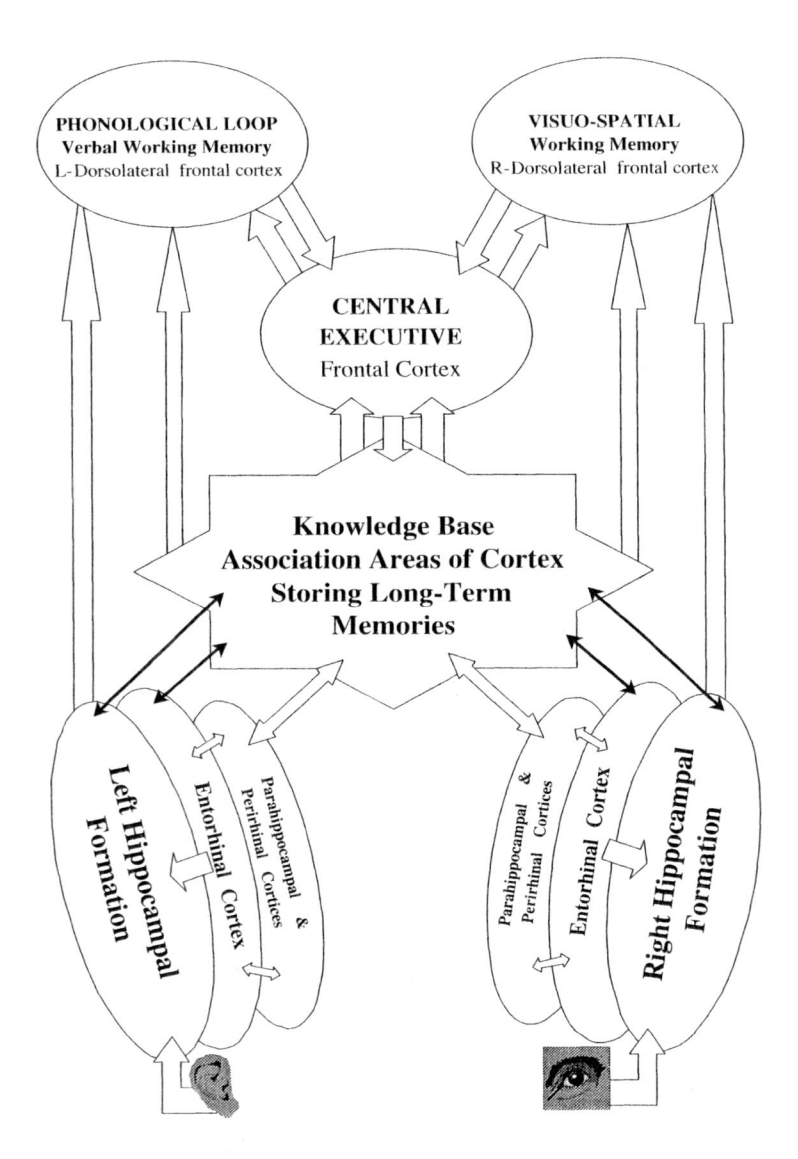

Figure 4.3. A Schematic View of Working Memory. Auditory and visual sensory experience processed in the hippocampal formation may enter the working buffers of verbal and visuospatial working memories of the dorsolateral frontal cortices. Likewise, long-term memories associated with these sensory experiences may also enter the working buffers directly from the association areas of the cortex. The central executive may then manipulate and contemplate this information to plan and execute various actions and behaviours.

central executive could then draw upon this information in both the verbal and visual loops to allow you to spell the word, break it into syllables, or rotate the image of the word in your head.

Thus, it appears that our access to various aspects of working memory is one of the ways by which we define ourselves. 'Oh, I'm no good at spelling' or 'I can easily visualise the finished chair that I am making'. It also appears to be the component of memory that begins to fade after the age of about 40. While the hippocampal-based declarative memories persist, and measures of hippocampal function, such as digit span, don't decay until late in life,[36] our dynamic, 'now-time' awareness of working memory slowly degrades. 'Where *did* I put my pen, I *know* I was just using it a second ago?'

EPISODIC MEMORY

Declarative memory comes in two major forms, semantic and episodic. Semantic or 'general knowledge' memory is the memory of words, the meaning of words, and objects and events recorded as encyclopaedic 'facts'.

Episodic memory is the subjective memory of objects and events put in the context of our personal experience and this includes our feelings of an episode or story from our life.[37] Episodic memories include everything, from the movie you saw last week, to getting your first two wheel bicycle at age six. Later in life it can be concerned with where you put your glasses?

You are reading and the doorbell rings. You take off your reading glasses and leave them on the desk as you go to see who is at the door. It's the mailman with a package that is being held for you at the post office. After returning from the post office, you go back inside and open the enclosed letter. 'But where are my reading glasses?' To find them you must then access your episodic memory to retrace your steps. 'Oh yes, I put them on the desk when I went to answer the door.'

Episodic memory is largely conscious, but it has the inherent problem of being selective in terms of what memories are retrievable. Fascinating experiments with human subjects have shown that virtually everything that has happened to us is held somewhere within our memory storage systems, but that much of this is not consciously retrievable. We seem to put a lot of memories into an archival area of memory with the result that memory retrieval is fragmentary.

Classic illustrations of this point come from the fields of neurosurgery and hypnosis. To treat cases of intractable epilepsy, Wilder Penfield and others developed techniques of cutting away a flap of bone from the roof of a patient's skull. He would then stimulate the exposed brain with electrodes to locate the diseased areas, and to spare important functions, such as speech, during the surgery. This stimulation of the cortex at times provoked remarkably detailed recollections of past experiences, or of events that had long since been forgotten.

One patient relived a scene from her childhood. Another watched in her mind a play she had not seen in years. Another patient was certain the doctors were playing a record of a song in the operating theater and she could not be convinced that there was really no phonograph in the room. The memory was not a memory to her, it was reality. Even more interesting, when the stimulation stopped, the song stopped, but when the stimulation began again, the record always went back to the beginning.

The attitude that an event is not a recollection, but is real, is a common one. Penfield even remarked, 'The patients have never looked upon the electrically stimulated response as a remembering. Instead, it is a hearing again and seeing again—a living through of past time'.[38]

Another example of this continuity of memory outside of conscious recall comes from the field of hypnosis. In a classic case, when a former bricklayer in his 80s was put under hypnosis he began to tell the experimenters about a particular wall he had built in his twenties as an apprentice bricklayer. Brick-by-brick he was able to describe the details and positioning of certain bricks and that some of the bricks were cracked, wrongly coloured or displayed notable bumps. As it happened, the wall was still standing, and when the researchers inspected it, they were able to verify that every brick was in place just as the man had described. Though he had laid millions of bricks since building that particular wall, and could not consciously even recall the wall, its exact detail had nevertheless been stored in his memory.[39]

While the above examples allude to the perfection and permanence of memory, how do we remember? And how accurate is our conscious explicit memory compared with these intact memories that are triggered outside of our consciousness?

MEMORIES ARE MADE OF THIS:

Replication or Recreation?

While our memories are experienced as a single unified event capturing the past event in full sensory display, much like watching a video playback, it is now known that each experience is not stored in its totality as a whole experience. Rather, each experience is fragmented into its sensory components and each component is stored separately in the various sensory association cortices which are widely scattered around the brain. (see Fig. 4.4.)

When an experience is laid down in our memory, each sensory component is distributed to the area of the cortex associated with processing this type of sensory data. In summary:

Visual Memory seems to be stored in the visual association areas in the occipital lobe, just in front of and surrounding the primary visual cortex.

Auditory Memory seems to be stored in the auditory association area in the superior lateral temporal lobes surrounding the primary auditory cortex.

Touch and Body Sensation Memory appear to be stored in the somesthetic association areas of the parietal lobes immediately behind the primary sensory cortex.

Taste Memory is stored in the gustatory association areas on the medial surface of the superior temporal lobes adjacent to the primary gustatory cortex in the posterior frontal lobes.

Olfactory Memory, or smells, are stored in the posterior and medial temporal lobes below the association areas for taste and near to the limbic centres that process smell.

Each of these sensory components is further partitioned into the elements making up that sense, and are stored in separate areas within each sensory association area. For instance, the visual component of the remembered event is partitioned into the colour, shape, spatial location and the actual static image, and each is stored in a different area of the visual association cortex. A remembered sound is likewise divided into the pitch, timbre, colour and loudness, which are stored in separate areas of the auditory association cortex.[40]

As we remember, these sensory components are reconstructed into the

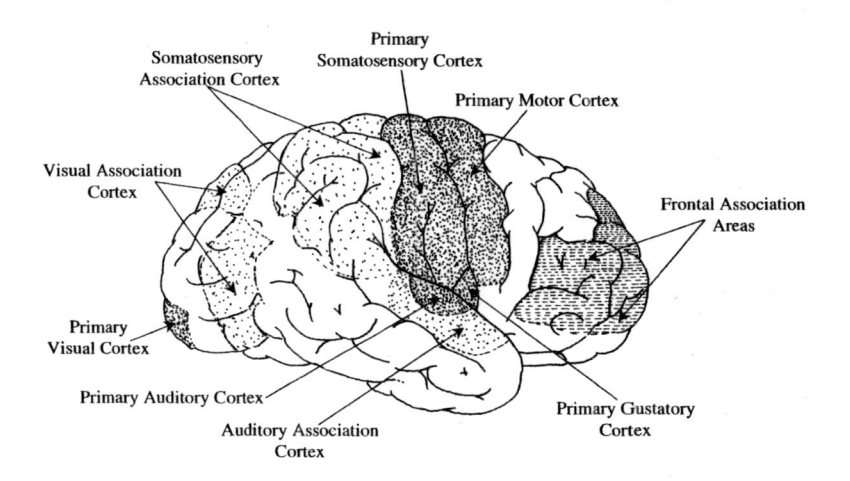

Figure 4.4. The Cortex—highlighting sensory association areas. The primary sensory cortices receive sensory data, which is then stored in the corresponding long-term memory association areas.

seamless experience of the on-coming car, the bonnet buckling in front of your eyes and the windscreen shattering. All against the background noises of the screeching brakes and crunching metal. Often, the smell of burning rubber and maybe even the taste of blood will fill out the horrible memory of a car crash.

Not only that, but what is stored appears to be little more than a summary sketch of the actual sensory experience. Upon being reactivated, it is reconstructed into our memory of the original experience.[41] Current evidence shows that our explicit memories result from a stimulus—whether external sensory input or internal mental input—which reactivates the various convergence zones such as the entorhinal cortex and hippocampus of the medial temporal lobes.

This activation then stimulates simultaneous and synchronous firing in the many anatomically separate and widely distributed neuronal networks in the association cortices, reconstructing the neurological pattern of the previous experience.[42] Thus there is no 'mind's eye' that records everything like a videotape, but rather, our memories are a present time interpretation and not an exact replication. They are a newly reconstructed version of the original event.

Although memory is experienced as a single seamless event, every element of each sensory component was reassembled in the convergence zone of that sensory cortex, and this reconstructed sensory component fused with the other senses involved in that memory in the major convergence zones of the medial temporal lobes. Finally, the reconstructed disparate parts emerge into our conscious awareness in our hippocampus and working memory as our memory of the event.

MEMORY RECONSTRUCTION:

Can It be Trusted?

A consequence of this reconstructed aspect of memory, is that our memories can sometimes be 'false'. Even 'flashbulb' memories that are made especially sharp because of the strong emotions associated with them—Where you were and what were you doing when President Kennedy was shot or the space shuttle Challenger exploded?— may not be totally accurate. While the flow of adrenalin does strengthen explicit memory,[43] the 'shock' of the situation may distract our attention from much else that is going on at the time.

If you are robbed at gun point, no doubt you will have detailed explicit memories of the experience. Yet, you may not remember what the robber looked like because your whole attention was on the size of the gun that was pushed into your face. Every detail of the gun may be indelibly etched into your memory, but the robber's face remains a blurred, incomplete image.

Likewise, because memories are reconstructions at the time of recall, the state of the brain at that time may significantly influence the reconstruction. (Remember that reconstruction is a dynamic synthesis of synchronous neuronal activity in many parts of the brain). Our mental state at the time of remembering, even our overall mood, may alter the timing and integration of neural events generating the memory. Also, since memories are reassembled from summary sketches of the original experience, it should not be surprising that our expectations and biases in the present moment may flesh out the sketch in a slightly different form than the original.[44]

Source Memory. The component which records where a memory originated, the so-called 'source memory', is particularly prone to error. To quote Daniel Schacter,[45] a Harvard University psychologist and memory researcher, 'One of the most vulnerable aspects of memory for an experience, is remembering the exact conditions in which the event occurred—remembering where it occurred and remembering whether it actually occurred rather than having merely heard about it.' Defects in source memory can create the common experience of recognising someone, but not being able to place where you know them from.

Once the source memory has faded, merely thinking or hearing repeatedly about a fictitious event can lay down memory fragments that may be hard to distinguish from reality, or that may be interwoven with real memories. An example comes from the trial of Carl Pettersson, accused of assassinating the prime minister of Sweden, Olof Palme. At the time of the shooting the prime minister and his wife had been walking home from a movie. Mrs Palme's memory of the event and her testimony were evaluated at different times after the murder. With the passage of time, her testimony became more and more detailed and vivid and it was argued by the defense that she had incorporated information from newspaper and television coverage into her memory.[46]

This tendency to lose the source memory along with the influence of expectation and association, have been shown to have a neurophysiological basis in a recent study of remembering and knowing. Volunteers were given sets of words that are related in meaning, such as 'sleep', 'tired', 'snooze', 'snore', and 'nap'. Thirty minutes later they were presented with a new list that contained some of the previous words as well as some new words related to the old words— 'drowsy' and 'bed'. They were also given some other quite unrelated words.

The subjects were then asked to note whether they actually remembered seeing the word, just knew the word was on the previous list although they could not actually recall seeing it, or, were not aware of having seen it?

While each subject recorded their results, their brainwaves were recorded by EEG and maps were drawn of this activity. Remembering and knowing produced different brainwave patterns, with knowing responses developing more quickly than remembering. More significantly, the subjective accounts closely matched the EEG patterns. Even when the subjects remembered 'seeing' a word they had not seen, their brains produced a remembering response. Thus, rather than matching accurate memories, the brainwaves matched what the volunteers 'believed' they had seen.[47]

The results of this study have been upheld in other psychological research which again used test lists of related words. The lists were read to the volunteer subjects. With each list they were given a related 'target' word but this was never spoken. For example, the list presented 'bed, rest, awake, tired, dream, snooze and blanket.' The unspoken target word was 'sleep'. The subjects were given four minutes to write down as many of the 'heard' words as they could. They were only to write the words they were sure they had heard. Guessing was not allowed.

On average, volunteers correctly recalled less than 40 percent of the words. More surprisingly, they also claimed to remember hearing 57 percent of the unspoken 'target' words.[48] In other studies where the lists were read in turn by male and female assistants, not only did the volunteers remember hearing the unspoken target words, they also recalled which experimenter supposedly said it.[49]

Such examples of faulty conscious recall on the one hand, and total recall triggered outside of consciousness on the other, allude to the fact that there are two types of memory retrieval processes: These have been called explicit and implicit memory.

REMEMBRANCE OF THINGS UNKNOWN:

Explicit and Implicit Memory.

The only type of memory studied for almost 200 years and intensively researched over the past 50 years, was declarative memory. The memory that could be explicitly recalled by conscious intent. A newcomer to the field of memory research is implicit memory, a term introduced only a decade ago.[50]

Declarative or explicit memory relies on conscious recollection of previous experience—explicit remembering. In contrast, implicit memory, also called nondeclarative memory, is information stored in memory that may be recalled and influence behaviour without conscious or deliberate recollection of the events that produced this memory.[51]

Explicit memory is conscious: consciously driven and consciously retrievable.

Psychologists have some favourite experiments that test explicit memory and these are termed free recall. Testers give a subject a list of 10 unrelated items or words that the subjects are to study for one minute or so. The list is then taken away and the person has to write down all the items they can recall at different time intervals following the study period. Most people get six or seven within minutes of reading the list. If they are asked to recall the items on the list a week later however, they will be down to naming maybe two or three, perhaps only one item. This loss of memory recall is known as memory decay.

Implicit memory is largely subconscious: with information subconsciously stored and retrieval generally 'triggered' by an event or object that has no conscious meaning.

A variation on the free recall experiment tests implicit memory: Subjects are given a list of words and as above, are asked to study it for a minute or so. Then, some weeks later they are shown a new list in which most of the letters of each word are blank. Taking the word 'mystery': The only information given will be '_ys_e_y'. Now many words could potentially fit this pattern but within seconds, the brain will solve the problem by seeing 'mystery' and the guess will be accurate almost 100 percent of the time. Further, if the test is performed even six months later, people retain an impressive amount of detail about the material that they had consciously forgotten. In fact, the test subjects reported they had no idea where the information came from.[52]

Implicit memory does not seem subject to the same type of decay that occurs with explicit memory. Given the right stimulus or trigger for recall, everything contained in implicit memory seems to be encoded and accessible whereas explicit memory relies more on conscious activation for retrieval and is prone to forgetting.

Implicit memory has also been demonstrated by presenting words to anaesthetised patients. Again, the patients do very well on triggered recall of the presented words, even though they were totally unconscious at the time of presentation. Such tests confirms that implicit memory is truly subconscious.[53]

Other research has also shown that explicit and implicit memory have quite separate neural substrates, and are carried out in separate brain systems. Explicit memory is dependent on the hippocampal system and its connections to the amygdala, hypothalamus and the cortical memory association areas. This hippocampal-cortical system then provides information to the working memory where we may contemplate and analyse it.

Implicit memory is dependent on different brain systems depending upon the type of implicit memory, but *not* on the hippocampal-cortical system. Indeed, one of the ways implicit memory was discovered was by the ability of people whose hippocampal system had been severely damaged to still demonstrate certain types of learning and memory.[54]

While the free recall tests show a type of implicit memory called priming which is demonstrated with words, other types of implicit memory include both motor skills memory and emotional conditioning. Motor skills memory, like typing and riding a bicycle, appear to reside in the basal ganglia and cerebellum, whereas conditioning of emotional responses depends on the amygdala.[55] Furthermore, new research suggests that the amygdala does not use working memory, which is perhaps the reason why it is so difficult to contemplate our emotions.[56]

Emotional memory appears to be largely subconscious in function, although not in effect. When a subconscious trigger stimulus activates memory associated with a particular emotion, you may then become conscious of the emotion, but not its source. This is much in the same way the subjects in the implicit word tests became aware of the correct words and yet were unaware of why they chose them.

It is this interplay between explicit conscious awareness of our emotions and often their implicit subconscious source that allows kinesiology to work so successfully. Kinesiology techniques give us the ability to access the subconscious areas of emotional memory that appear to be held intact. Often, people come to a kinesiology session aware of an issue, and during the course of the session the subconscious muscle response may reveal the emotions held in implicit memory that underlie this issue.

Once the implicit emotional context has been identified, it may then trigger explicit recall of the episodic memories associated with the original experience. The person undergoing kinesiology may become aware of something that has happened to them in the past, but of which they previously had no conscious recollection, or certainly no recent recollection.

Other times, the muscle response will reveal the underlying subconscious emotional memory, but there will be no explicit memories recalled. One of kinesiology's greatest strengths lies in its ability to access implicit emotional states underlying explicit issues in our lives. Even though it is out of our awareness, this implicit emotional conditioning from our past can significantly influence our consciousness of the present.

This is particularly true of subconscious emotional conditioning that occurred during early childhood. Because we did not have a logical, rational understanding of events that were occurring in our environment, and everything was new and didn't match any existing associations in our memory, much of what happened in early childhood was not encoded into conscious memory, but rather, appears to be stored in subconscious memory.

The inability to remember our experiences from early childhood, (roughly before the age of three), has been termed infantile amnesia. Freud was the first to recognise this phenomenon when he noted that a two year old child speaks easily and can handle quite complex mental situations, yet, the child appears to have no memory of what they said or what was said to them. Neither can they recall what they did or what was done to them during this period.[57]

In contrast, the same children can usually recall events that happened after about age three, especially if they were events with special significance, such as the cake they had for their fourth birthday. Every family has its favourite stories about what you said or did as a two year old, be it cute, clever or outrageous. Older members of the family can remember, even if you can't.

Recent studies provide a basis for these observations. Infantile amnesia appears to result from the prolonged period of maturation of the hippocampal system, which takes longer to myelinate and develop its full complement of synaptic connections with all the other brain areas than other brain regions. The hippocampal-cortical systems which encode conscious memory are therefore not fully developed until sometime between the ages of three and four, while the thalamic-amygdaloid system that encodes subconscious memory is apparently well developed at birth. Since the hippocampal-cortical systems are responsible for our consciously retrievable explicit memories and these systems are not fully developed until after the age of three, it is not surprising that we have so few consciously recallable memories that reach back into infancy.[58]

The catch to this is, however, that the amygdaloid-thalamic system was still recording the emotional content of experiences so that even things that you did not understand at the time, may have an emotional effect today. This is particularly true of the more subtle aspects of communication such as vocal tone, which carries most of the emotional content of speech. Because your subconscious understood these events in terms of reward or punishment, they were encoded in subconscious memory.

So many of the things that happened to you, especially as a very young child can still be influencing or colouring your adult behaviour because they have been encoded as implicit memory and are totally beyond your consciousness. Nevertheless, once elicited, these emotions can control our adult behaviour. How many adults have you witnessed acting irrationally, even childishly? No matter how rational one might become as an adult, you often find it difficult to change your irrational behaviour because the underlying source in your early childhood experience is outside of your consciousness.

Sometimes too, as a child, you misinterpreted what was happening. You punished yourself for something that wasn't necessarily your fault. This is common in children whose parents divorce. Even though they are not responsible for the split-up, the children often subconsciously blame themselves. Such subconscious association can have a profound impact on their adult relationships.

So while memory has all these different aspects in terms of its physiology and function, its ultimate end-product is the ability to modify or change our behaviour. As we have learned, we can only modify our conscious behaviour on the basis of memories that are available and accessible to our consciousness. So much more that is submerged in implicit memory can be brought right back on line with the right stimulus.

But why would the brain develop two apparently quite separate memory and learning systems, one conscious and explicit, but fraught with error, the other subconscious and implicit with generally excellent recall?

DUAL PERCEPTION-MEMORY SYSTEMS:

The Subconscious Control of Behaviour

Over the past decade research has revealed a startling fact. The brain has two perceptual and memory systems that provide the basis for learning. These two systems are normally seamlessly joined in our mental processing. One is cortical and creates the fine detail and nuance of our conscious experience. The other is subcortical and subconscious, providing only a coarse-grained view of our world.[59]

Though subconscious, this course-grained view is ever vigilant for 'threat and danger', and creates the subconscious emotional context of our lives. These two perceptual and memory systems are derived from parallel transmission of visual, auditory, and probably other sensory information to the brain.

They generate two different types of experience: One is via sensory input to the thalamus which is then relayed to the primary sensory cortex, interpreting that type of sensory information. Visual and auditory input go to the lateral and medial geniculate nuclei of the thalamus and are then relayed to the primary visual and auditory cortices, respectively. Similar pathways are probably followed by the other senses for conscious perception.

Visual and auditory information are then processed with reference to previous information of the same type held in association memory areas of the cortex, and intricate interpretation of the information is fully developed into conscious perceptions about our environment and about the objects and events in that environment.

The hippocampus appears to be instrumental in laying down memories about these events and objects, recording them as 'facts' that are then generally consciously accessible (at least for a time). The hippocampus also mediates the retrieval of these memories. This hippocampal-mediated declarative memory involves explicit, consciously accessible information about objects and their identity as well as spatial memory—the relationship of the object or event to its environment.

The hippocampus not only provides our moment-to-moment awareness of our sensory experiences, but in conjunction with past memories stored in long-term memory association areas of the cortices, also supplies the contents of our working memory. This allows us to contemplate both our current sensory experience and whatever this sensory experience may have triggered from long-term memory.

This contemplation may then allow us to come to a new understanding of the meaning of these experiences. For instance, the triggering of my feelings of hurt by yellow Fords eventually allowed me to reach a new understanding of the lessons in that relationship and then come to a long-term resolution of this particular episode in my life.

While an understanding of the dynamics of declarative memory has progressed rapidly over the past 50 years, the existence of the other perceptual-memory system has only begun to emerge over the past decade. These other systems are subcortically based, and the system controlling emotional conditioning appears to rely on the amygdala as its central processing unit for memory storage and retrieval.[60]

In the subcortical emotional conditioning system, sensory data is also relayed via the sensory thalamus, but directly to the amygdala—bypassing the multi-step cortical processing of conscious perception. Only a crude perception of the external world is presented to the amygdala, but because it involves only a few neural links, this perception is formed faster. For acoustic or sound stimuli, the amygdaloid processing is twice as fast as the cortical processing, and similar time differences are likely for the other senses.[61]

The coarse-grained perception which is presented to the amygdala is not used to understand our environment and the objects or events in it, but rather, to act as an 'early warning system' for potential threat and danger. The amygdala then lays down memory of these perceptions of threat or danger creating 'emotional memory', which is subcortical and subconscious as it has never involved any conscious areas of the brain.[62]

Current evidence suggests that this subcortical thalamic-amygdaloid system does not use working memory.[63] The implications are profound. While this system lays down and retrieves our emotional memories (often triggered by current sensory experience), we can not contemplate these emotional memories *directly*. We can only contemplate the cortical emotions and feelings generated by these memories. Thus, unlike less emotionally charged issues in my life which I could call forth into my working memory to analyse, come to understand, and thus quickly resolve, my inability to contemplate the emotional memories triggered by yellow Fords, meant that years went by before I could learn the lessons in this relationship and fully integrate them into my life's experience.

Thus, while the cortical conscious memory of the hippocampus-cortex system is declarative, with objects and events perceived only as cold 'facts', the amygdala-subcortical system generates 'emotions and feelings' about the objects and events crudely perceived.

These emotions and feelings are largely based on two factors: Firstly, are these objects or events 'threatening'? If they are, emotions based in fear are elicited and feelings of fear are experienced. Or, are these objects or events 'nurturing'? If they are supportive of my existence, endorphins appear to be released from the reward centres, creating positive, pleasant feelings and emotions.

The emotional memory generated by fear-based learning is stored and retrieved differently than the emotional memory created by pleasure-based learning. Current evidence suggests that fear-based emotional memory is stored and retrieved subcortically and is relatively permanent. Once that object or event has been subconsciously associated with fear, it is extremely hard to extinguish the behavioural response elicited from these fear-based memories.[64]

Witness phobias, which, although consciously irrational responses to 'neutral' stimuli, are extremely hard to extinguish. Somehow, these 'neutral' stimuli can activate an amygdala reaction and incorrectly assign it a potentially 'dangerous' label. They are stored in the fear-based emotional memory. Once established, this fear-based behaviour persists, even when the conscious mind 'knows' the behaviour to be totally irrational, and often quite consciously inconvenient. Imagine the frustration of not being able to use an elevator in a tall building or to fly in a plane?

As an example of how debilitating phobias can be, I had a secretary once who had an extreme fear of spiders. One day her mother, whom she had not seen in years, was arriving from Sri Lanka. But when my secretary went to get the car out of the garage, there was a small spider on the handle of the garage door. Her phobia was so extreme that she couldn't even use a broom to remove the spider. She was an hour and a half late picking her mother up because she had to wait for the spider to move of its own free will.

Pleasure-based memories, on the other hand, appear to be created subcortically, via output of the amygdala and the reward system. They are then stored cortically. When an animal has been conditioned to respond to a specific sensory stimulus to gain a reward, removal of the areas of the cortex storing this particular type of sensory memory, or the hippocampus, results in loss of the reward-based memory. In contrast, removal of the cortical areas storing memory of the stimulus that generated fear-based memory, does not affect this memory, or the behaviour it elicits. Effectively, fear-based emotional memory has little to do with cortical function and appears to exist entirely in the subconscious.[65]

The thalamic-amygdala pathways are, therefore, critical to survival, as they provide rapid response to potentially threatening, although not fully identified stimuli. Eliciting fear, or triggering fight or flight reactions in response to benign stimuli, is less costly than taking the time to consciously analyse and positively identify stimuli which may prove dangerous.

When the eyes see an object, as in Figure 4.5, the visual information takes two separate pathways, one subcortical and subconscious, and the other cortical leading to conscious perception. Visual information goes straight to the amygdala from the visual thalamus (A), which forms only a coarse-grained image based on rapid processing involving only a few neural links, and then immediately references subcortical memory of similar objects with special emphasis on potentially dangerous objects of similar shape.

The amygdala 'sees' a twisted object on the ground (B)—references 'snake'—danger, and sends signals to the hypothalamus to initiate the 'fight or flight' response. Signals are then sent to the adrenals (C) to release adrenalin increasing heart rate, blood pressure, and the power of muscle contraction, and you may jump back to avoid the object.

At the same time, visual information is also travelling back to the primary visual cortex via the optic tracts (A) and optic radiations (D) from the lateral geniculate nuclei of the visual thalamus. Once at the primary visual cortex, this information undergoes multi-step and multi-level processing involving

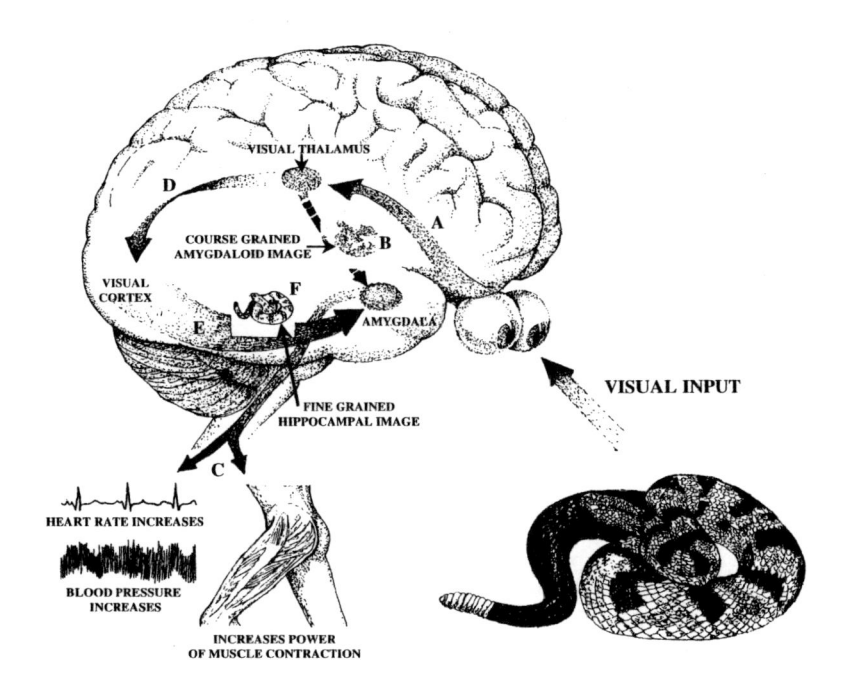

Figure 4.5. The Dual Visual and Memory Systems in the Brain.

many neural links (E), to form a fine-grained image of the object (F) which is then referred through the hippocampus to other cortical memory areas for final identification at the level of consciousness. Two outcomes are possible following this conscious image formation, which occurred well after the amygdaloid image had caused the 'fear' reaction. 1) the fine-grained image 'sees' a snake, in which case the 'fear' reaction and avoidance are continued. 2) the fine-grained image 'sees' a twisted bit of vine, in which case the amygdaloid 'fear' reaction is turned off and you walk calmly past the twisted vine, as your heart rate and blood pressure decrease once again to normal.

The tendency for the brain to err on the side of caution is also seen when two stimuli (objects or events) are presented simultaneously, one with fear-based aversion, and the other with pleasure-based reward. The subconscious fear-based memory wins out every time—the object is avoided and the behavioural response is one of fear, not pleasure.

A friend was swimming in the lovely warm waters of the Indian Ocean near Perth, when out of the corner of his eye he saw a shadowy shape approaching him at speed. His instant reaction and coarse-grained amygdaloid image was 'shark'—swim for your life! Upon reaching the safety of the boat, he looked back to analyse this stimulus with his fine-grained hippocampal-cortical system to find he had just fled a curious dolphin that had come over to play.

But why would the brain have evolved two perceptual-memory systems?

The answer is, probably to solve the evolutionary imperative—survive long enough to procreate and continue the species. The thalamic-amygdaloid early warning system has clear immediate survival value. It warns us of potential danger and implements the initial reactions to threat—releasing adrenalin and initiating the fight or flight responses. The catch is, to continue these energetically expensive fight or flight behaviors in the presence of innocuous stimuli may reduce long-term survival.

Thus there was an impetus to evolve a parallel perceptual memory system that creates a more detailed and accurate—if slower—perception of objects and events in our environment. To evaluate the actual degree of threat identified by the early warning system also has survival value. Analysis of the specifics of potentially threatening situations by the hippocampal-cortical system permits the development of alternative reactions to these circumstances in the future.

ACT FIRST AND LIVE:

Think about it Later
When man was on the savannah and there were lions about, survival for human beings was very much a day-to-day proposition. Man didn't often live

very long in those conditions and most died as a result of physical threat and trauma.

In prehistory, the hunter is out on the plain with his spear. Suddenly out of the corner of his eye he senses danger. He sees a form moving quickly towards him. The thalamic-amygdaloid system references 'lion'.

Run!

Adrenalin is released, pupils dilate and the hunter immediately goes into a flight response and races off. In his survival-oriented amygdaloid memory, the last experience he had of a large animal charging at him was resolved successfully when he managed to climb a tree and survive. So the only program he has operating in his brain is to climb a tree and escape. Spotting the nearest tree, our hunter redoubles his efforts and really goes for it.

On the way, he runs right past a rock outcrop that he also could have climbed to get to safety. But rock outcrops are not yet associated in his memory with the idea of safety, so he keeps running on towards the tree.

He runs, the lion chases and the man only just makes it. Jumping up into the lowest branches he starts climbing. Had the tree been five metres further on he would have been dinner.

Now he's up in the tree puffing and panting but safe. The lion walks around for a while, tries to jump up but gives it away and strides off. Our hunter continues sitting in the tree and as his adrenalin levels begin to drop he starts to think. Now, perceiving the environment more clearly with his hippocampal-cortical system, he says to himself: 'Look at that. I ran right past a rock outcrop. I could have been safe there but I almost died because I ran right past it'. Now in his memory he has the new association: rock outcrop, *or* tree. He has a new option for safety. He has broadened his survival options.

The human beings who thought first, 'Now where should I go to escape the lion? That outcrop or the tree?' generally left very few offspring. Similarly, those people who could not learn from their past mistakes didn't make it to the tree the next time. And they didn't leave many offspring.

But those who evolved a dual memory-learning system both survived in the short term and were given the greatest options for survival in the long term.

ASSOCIATION RESPONSES

Stimuli that activate the brain may come from on-going sensory experience or from a memory of sensory experience. Whether information comes from within (from the memory areas of the cortex), or from without (from an on-going sensory event) is of little concern to your brain. What is happening in the brain is, from the brain's perspective, 'happening now' and is capable of eliciting memories of reward and punishment. This means that a sensory experience retrieved from memory can be almost as strong a stimulus as an event happening around you, particularly if it is associated with a strong emotional memory.

In memory, it is the hippocampus that plays the role in recognising and categorising events and objects and the amygdala that remembers any emotional associations that colour that event or object.

As with my story of the yellow Ford, association of a declarative fact—a car—with powerful subconscious emotional memories of a broken heart, would elicit memories of my former girlfriend replete with all the things we used to do, and of my pain and hurt at losing her love. The same trigger stimulus would also elicit the physiological responses to my hurt; the feelings of heart ache and a churning stomach, almost as if it was happening anew or my girlfriend was in sight.

Once emotional memory is lodged in our subconscious amygdaloid circuits, a stimulus associated with the original circumstance may trigger these emotions and feelings to enter our consciousness, often with the same power and impact as the original event.

Seeing a car, smelling a perfume or hearing a piece of music can trigger a whole sequence of recognitions and associations in the brain. Music is an extremely powerful trigger, but the single most powerful trigger is smell. A familiar smell can provoke a powerful emotional experience of something you may not even have consciously noted at the time. People who have had bad experiences in hospital can become instantly fearful when they come across a strong antiseptic aroma. Another common smell trigger is food. Sometime in your life, you may have eaten a particular food that made you sick and from then on, it is likely that just the smell of the same food will trigger nausea.

The French novelist Marcel Proust provides a stunning example of this connection between smell and taste and recollection:

'One day in winter, on my return home, my mother . . . Offered me some tea . . . She sent for one of those squat, plump little cakes called 'petite Madeleines' . . . I raised to my lips the spoonful of tea in which I had soaked a morsel of the cake. No sooner had the warm liquid mixed with the crumbs touched my palate than a shudder ran through me and I stopped, intent upon the extraordinary thing that was happening to me. An exquisite pleasure had invaded my senses, something isolated, detached with no suggestion of its origin . . . Whence could it have come to me, this all-powerful joy?'

'I sensed it was connected with the tea and the cake . . . And suddenly the memory revealed itself. The taste was that of a little piece of Madeleine which on Sunday mornings at Combray . . . my aunt Leonie used to give me, dipping it first in her own cup of tea . . . And as soon as I recognised the taste of the piece of Madeleine soaked in her decoction of lime blossom, which my aunt used to give me, immediately the old grey house upon the street, where her room was, rose up like a stage set; ... and with the house, the town from morning to night and in all weathers ... So in that moment all the flowers in our garden and in Monsieur Swann's park. And the water lillies on the Vivone and the good folk of the village and their little dwellings and the Parish church and the whole of Combray and its surroundings, taking shape and solidity, sprang into being, town and gardens alike, from my cup of tea.'[66]

Proust went on to use this experience of the evocation of memory by tastes and aromas in his magnum opus, *Remembrance of Things Past*.

Smell is distinct from all the other sensory input because the olfactory pathways go directly into the limbic brain, bypassing the potential filtering that can occur in the thalamus.[67] The direct connection of the olfactory pathways to the amygdala and other subcortical centres involved with reward is often used in the psychology of selling.

If you want to sell a house, a good piece of advice is to bake bread and brew up fresh coffee just before potential buyers come in to inspect it. As soon as those aromas hit their nostrils, immediately the idea of 'home', 'family' and 'welcome' is elicited. Disreputable car dealers have also been known to spray leather upholstery scents on to the vinyl seats of cheap vehicles because there is an instant association of luxury and quality to the smell of leather. Your view of the car and your memory of the car as you drive away to consider its purchase can be coloured by the manipulation of a process that is beyond your conscious awareness.

It has also been established that people associate the scent of lemon with cleanliness, which is why so many cleaning products feature a lemon scent. The advertising industry is particularly skilled at playing on the mechanisms of memory in the way that it uses association responses to get their potential buyers to attach strong emotions of desire to objects. For instance, an agency might create an advertisement for a new model of green sports car and have it depicted with a very attractive person sitting at the wheel. Desire is thus associated with the idea of a green sports car and desire (or a potential reward) can be a very strong motivation for purchasing.

This process also explains the more recent innovation in the way bed linen is being advertised. In the past, these products were often promoted using images of housewives preening a new set of sheets. Since the advertisers started putting very well built young men between the sheets on the bed, sales have quadrupled. Why? Because women buy sheets and women often associate desire to well built young men.

The old Chinese jade merchants were masters at observing desire responses. They would show a customer many pieces of jade and take particular note of the ones that caused dilation in the pupils of the buyer's eyes.

Physiologically, dilation of the pupils is a sign of desire. The price of these pieces would instantly go up because they knew which piece the buyer truly desired.

More recently, seeking to find out what cover pictures would have the strongest selling potential, a women's magazine conducted an experiment around which pictures caused dilation in the pupils of the eyes of women readers. What they found was that the greatest dilation occurred when the women saw pictures of small babies. To the amygdala, babies elicit the nurturing response. This stands to reason because nurturing young children is the guarantee of the survival of the species.

These are classic association responses and association responses often include powerful emotional reactions that are subconscious. All it takes to activate a memory is the right trigger. Research with animals has further shown that even when an animal has been trained to override the memory of a negative event, the negative program will be reactivated under stress.[68] This is a survival-oriented arrangement because negative events potentially have far more impact on our survival than positive experiences.

MEMORY TRIGGERS

As we have now learned, there are two types of triggers: conscious and subconscious

A classic example of a conscious trigger is what can happen when you are driving along in your car listening to the radio. A song comes on that you haven't heard for years but the second you hear its first refrain, you will recall much of what was happening to you when you originally heard it. You can recall who you were with, what you were doing and how you were feeling. The song will trigger the return of a whole episode of events in your past life. Associated events have been triggered into conscious recall.

Music can elicit a whole cascade of memory, including smells, weather conditions, what you were seeing and how you were feeling. It all comes back as a package. You are conscious of what the trigger was for that recall—a song—but only a small percent of triggered memories can be accounted for consciously.

The rest are recalled from the subconscious implicit memory. Some other clue or stimulus that we are not consciously aware of will trigger the recall of associations from emotional memory. But what is triggered? Current research suggests that it is the amygdala which receives direct sensory inputs from the sensory thalamus, information about past sensory associations from the sensory association areas of the cortex, and information about the overall situation from the hippocampal formation. It appears that the amygdala is the adjudicator of these triggered responses. To quote Deloux in his fascinating recent book, *The Emotional Brain*, 'the amygdala is, in essence, involved in the appraisal of emotional meaning. It is where trigger stimuli do their triggering.'[69]

While smell is one of the strongest triggers, another is vocal tone. The timbre or loudness of a person's voice triggers within you memories of events associated with the same or similar vocal tones. Although consciously we generally pay little heed to vocal tone, it is a powerful trigger to elicit subconscious memories. As soon as you hear a particular earmark of tone it will stimulate your auditory memory to make associations.

When was the last time you heard a vocal tone like that? When you were five years old and your father was yelling at you for something you did wrong. Along with your association to your father will come all the emotional baggage of the event, so you can find yourself reacting to a new person in an old way. Their vocal tone, which happens to be very like your father's, may cause you to feel just as angry or hurt as you did when your father was actually yelling at you. Your amygdala will elicit the feelings of being angry or aggrieved. Yet you would be totally unaware of the source of these feelings arising from subconscious memory, and you are likely to ascribe them to the person who is talking to you now. ('He made me so mad!').

Why is vocal tone such a strong trigger? If you consider a child of two or three or even younger, you are dealing with a being who is by definition irrational. A young child does not have a strong vocabulary. Animals have no vocabulary, but they too know when they are in trouble by the tone in someone's voice. A dog knows it has done something wrong because its master's voice will be strident, commanding and loud. The dog knows immediately it is in trouble and its ears will go down, its tail will drop and it will try to slink away. The only clue was the tone in its owner's voice.

When I was a child I knew I was in big trouble if my mother said, 'Charles Theodore Krebs!', in a particular tone. I required no further explanation. And, as we have explained, even the thought of punishment elicits the response of a punishment circuit in the brain, so as soon as I heard that timbre, a negative association was instantly made. I was in deep trouble, and I would often start crying even before she spanked me because of the fear of pain.

There can be other more subtle triggers which recall similar events and produce almost irrational responses in us. The shape of someone's eyebrows, lips or nose. Television casting agents use this characteristic of memory when they are casting bad guys in drama productions. There are certain tapes in our subconscious memory that associate to stereotypes of goodies and baddies. In some shows you just need to catch sight of a villain to know he's the bad guy.

Much of what elicits memories, and much of memory itself, never returns to consciousness. What does enter our consciousness are the emotional associations.

So when your boss comes in and says, 'Where is that report! I need it for a meeting in 10 minutes!', and has the same vocal tone as your father had when he was yelling at you when you were five, you may instantly feel guilty or angry. You might even fly off the handle. Not because the boss's request was unreasonable but because he re-triggered your anger at your father. You are totally unconscious of the connection but you certainly feel what you feel, which is anger. And that anger is directed at the current source of the stimulus, which is your boss. 'The unreasonable bastard!'

Such triggers can also elicit depression, defeat or other types of negative emotional associations and again, this is where kinesiology is a powerful tool because it gives the ability to access the source of the subconscious reactions and to defuse their physiological and emotional content. With kinesiology muscle monitoring techniques I can tell if interaction with your boss creates stress, even if you believe consciously that you have a great relationship. The responses to muscle monitoring will tell me if there is any unfinished, unclear or negative subconscious agendas that have not been dealt with.

You may not be having any problems relating to your boss on a day-to-day basis but all that has to happen is for a particular trigger event to occur and the negative, unfinished business will be brought up again. Suddenly you might find yourself in an irrational fight. This is the definition of the psychological baggage that we all carry with us. And this is the baggage that kinesiology can defuse.

It also explains how kinesiology can have such a profound effect on learning. As we now know, learning is highly dependent on memory and if there are any unresolved or negative memories that are interfering with your ability to recall information, they can have an enormous impact on your capacity to learn.

However memory works, it provides the basis for learning. Learning has many of the same characteristics of memory—a multiple component parallel processing system that is widely distributed in the brain and dependent upon integration and synchronised firing patterns in these separate neural networks. And like memory, the conscious components of learning are heavily reliant upon subconscious processing. How you learn is the subject of our next chapter.

Chapter Five

THE MIRACLE OF LEARNING

LEARNING WHAT IS RELEVANT

Without memory, learning would be impossible. If we had no memory, we would repeat our mistakes (punishments) over and over again. Likewise, we would be unable to learn from our successes and accomplishments (rewards).

Reward and punishment provide the critical factor in learning. They are the motivation to learn, and learning does require conscious motivation. To hold information in our short-term memory long enough to transfer it to long-term memory requires the motivation to repeat the learning, as we must when we are learning our multiplication tables.

A significant aspect of learning is also provided by the relevance of the situation. It would be pointless to put all this energy into learning my times tables if I don't plan to use them. But if I intend to become proficient with maths then they certainly become relevant.

Learning can be relevant to our current interests so that we are sufficiently motivated to put effort into the task of rehearsing the information. Yet there are other circumstances in which rehearsal is not necessary for memory formation. This occurs when the emotional impact of the learning situation is so great that we can experience what is called 'one trial' learning. In such learning we only have to experience something once to have it lodged permanently in memory. It is usually associated with powerful emotional experiences—positive or negative.

For humans, interest, in itself, is often a motivation to learn. When you are truly captivated by a subject it can become an effortless exercise to pursue knowledge of it. In contrast, if you have little interest in a topic, find it difficult or just plain boring, it becomes almost impossible to learn. You just cannot sustain the motivation long enough to transfer the information from short-term memory to long-term memory.

Learning is an activity that requires conscious motivation, but there are a whole series of conscious and subconscious, cortical and sub-cortical functions also involved in the process of learning. So we are going to go back into the brain itself to look at the parts of the brain that are involved in learning.

THE PROCESS OF LEARNING

From the overview of the major brain structures and the workings of memory already presented, it is clear that both memory and learning do not involve a single, global hierarchical system in the brain. Rather, learning involves an interplay between many inter-linked sub-systems or modules.[1] Also, the timing and synchronisation of information flow between these sub-systems and modules appears to be critical to the success of learning.

For example, instead of the entire left hemisphere being involved in logic, we find that there are certain cortical columns in the left hemisphere that come into play during certain types of logic processing. They become a module interconnected to many other cortical and subcortical areas on both sides of the brain.

Information is relayed to the hippocampus and amygdala. These then send the impulses back into the association areas for reference, and forward again into the cortex. It is at this point that we may become conscious of the answer or result. In simpler terms, a number of processing units are interconnected and involved in any one type of processing and these are further inter-linked to other areas of processing which perform other processing functions, and so on.

Complex? Yes, but it all happens in a split second.

To illustrate: Adding one plus one is a task that brings into play the Logic cortical processing unit involved in symbolic reasoning. These functions are consciously activated by the thought 'I want to add one plus one'. This command feeds the request down into the subconscious areas of the amygdala and hippocampus via projection fibres and also, via the association fibres, to information stored in the cortical association areas.

The request is maintained in our conscious awareness in the left hippocampal formation, while the cortical association areas storing numbers, are activated and the numbers are fed into the phonological loop of working memory. Here we become conscious of the numbers as words.

At the same time, activation of the right hippocampal formation feeds this information into the visuo-spatial scratchpad of working memory, where we become conscious of the images of the numbers. Other areas of our brain, predominantly in the frontal cortices, then manipulate this information in working memory to form the conscious perception of the answer as thought, and then as speech. The expressed answer: 'One plus one equals two'.

If in the past you've experienced tremendous problems adding even simple numbers, such a command may be perceived as a punishment and the process will become very difficult. Seeing 'punishment', your amygdala, operating at the subconscious level, will activate avoidance behaviours. In an attempt to justify the avoidance, your conscious, rational mind will virtually tell you that you are 'too stupid', or that 'maths is boring, and when would you ever use it anyway?' This is the path to future failure.

On the other hand, if you've been successful in addition and get the correct answers, the amygdala perceives a potential 'reward' and will not only allow you to do maths easily but may seek a more difficult task for an even bigger reward.

You can see how brain areas are constantly interrelating through complex integrative pathways, which provide for synchronised and integrated activity. All the systems must integrate well in order for you to produce a conscious outcome: the answer. It is only when you can consciously retrieve what you have learned that you can say you have really learned it.

BRAIN DOMINANCE:
The Right and Left Hemispheres

Since the late 1800s Broca's and Wernicke's Areas have been known to operate in concert. The brain areas involved in the ability to organise thoughts and think consciously (Wernicke's Area), and the brain areas involved in expressing those thoughts as speech (Broca's Area), are usually located in the left side of most people's brains.

In older neuropsychological literature, the hemisphere housing these two speech centres was termed the 'dominant hemisphere' and the majority of people were said to have their speech centres in the left hemisphere.[2] More recent evidence indicates that women tend to have Broca's Areas in both hemispheres. It is not yet known why this is so, but it appears that due to this arrangement, women can suffer a greater degree of brain damage before they demonstrate significant speech problems.[3]

Nevertheless, more than 95 percent of men and women tend to have Wernicke's Areas (thoughts into words) in the left hemisphere. The rest have both speech centres in the right hemisphere or, can control speech from either hemisphere.[4]

It has been hypothesised that in many cases where Wernicke's area is found to be located in the right hemisphere, the arrangement may be the result of brain damage that occurred during foetal development.[5] That the brain can reassign such important functions during development exemplifies its extraordinary plasticity and adaptation. (Incidentally, people with their speech centres in the right hemisphere are predominately left-handed and fifteen percent of left handers have speech in their right hemisphere. Another fifteen percent have speech in both hemispheres compared with less than five percent of right handers having speech in the right side.[6])

While Wernicke's area in the left hemisphere does appear to be the centre for comprehension and thinking, the homologous, or same area in the right hemisphere, makes its own unique contribution to thought and speech. As the left Wernicke's Area selects our words, the right Wernicke's Area contributes to how we feel about the words, and controls the vocal tone with which the words are expressed.[7]

Therefore, while the text books make declarative statements about the location of the speech centres, evidence shows that in reality, things are not so clear cut.

The confusion may result from the fact that the original studies were conducted on right-handed men, who are more lateralised than women and left-handed men. Secondly, until recently we could not image where in the brain a person was doing their thinking or speaking, only that they were doing it. With the advent of real-time brain imaging techniques such as Positron Emission Tomography (PET) and functional Magnetic Imaging (fMRI) scans, the actual areas of the brain involved in various mental functions can be observed.

Multilingual people can show some interesting variations from the normal left dominant Wernicke's Area for speech. I once worked with a Japanese-American woman who was a simultaneous translator. She was left hemisphere dominant for English and right hemisphere dominant for Japanese. Perhaps one of the reasons why she could translate simultaneously was that she could literally be listening to the end of a sentence in English while she was already beginning to speak it in Japanese.

I also know of a trilingual left-handed psychiatrist who was born in Russia, but raised in Australia, so he spoke both Russian and English fluently as a child. Later in life he also learned French. When half his brain was experimentally anaesthetised in what is called a Wada's test, he could only speak some of the languages, and the languages that remained depended upon which hemisphere was anaesthetised. When the left hemisphere was anaesthetised, he could speak only Russian and English. When the right hemisphere was anaesthetised he could speak only French.

Despite these fascinating findings it is easy to understand how, for many years, the right hemisphere was known as the 'silent hemisphere'. It did not appear to contribute to overt functions, such as speech.[8] Now it is understood that the right hemisphere is really doing a great deal.

REDEFINING THE TERMS

In the literature of kinesiology, a vitally important distinction is made in the use of the term 'brain dominance'. While in the neuropsychological literature the term refers only to the location of the speech centres (particularly Wernicke's Area), in kinesiology the term defines *the area of the brain which plays the dominant or lead role in mental processing.*

In kinesiological terms you can be 'right brain or hemisphere dominant' or 'left brain or hemisphere dominant' depending on the type of mental processing you are doing at the time:[9]

When doing a predominantly logical, linear, analytical task, most people activate cortical columns of their left 'Logic' hemisphere. Likewise, when most people are performing creative, or visuo-spatial tasks they would be activating cortical columns of their right 'Gestalt' hemisphere.

Inductive reasoning, based on global, simultaneous processing, which we term 'intuition', appears, in most people, to rely chiefly on the right hemisphere lead functions. Conversely, deductive reasoning, based on the linear, analytical processing of 'facts' appears to be initiated by lead functions that take place in the left hemisphere

'Inductive' refers to the process of looking at the whole of a situation, appreciating the overall pattern and not so much the pieces that make up that pattern. This process was named after the German word 'Gestalt' which means 'pattern' or 'form'. Generally, the functioning of the right hemisphere is intuitive and non-rational.

Deductive or logical reasoning is used to analyse the relationship of the pieces that make up the whole, a process that is inherently rational and analytic.

Some tasks, like remembering someone's face, are predominantly Gestalt. Some tasks, such as solving a maths equation, inherently use Logic functions. Ideally, you should have access to whichever mode is more efficient to tackle the task at hand. More ideally still, you should be able to integrate the functions of both hemispheres because whole brain processing leads to a higher level of thinking and understanding than either of its two parts.

The brain seems to run by a program that says, 'Do it the most efficient way possible'. In all of its functions, the brain seeks optimum efficiency. The line of least resistance. If one particular function is not accessible, the brain will automatically go on to the next most efficient process for doing that particular task. If that second process is not available, it will go to the third, the fourth, the fifth most efficient and so on. Because each alternative process is less efficient, it is inherently more stressful. The brain will keep searching for an appropriate processing method, until eventually, the activity may become so subconsciously or consciously stressful that the person will choose to give up trying to do the task altogether.

It is very much like water running down a hill. Running water takes the most direct possible route. But if you block the water flow, the water will find the next most direct route. If you block that, it will move towards the next most direct line.

Each new block gives the water a longer journey to the bottom, and too many blocks means the water might be absorbed before it gets down the hill. This is exactly how the mind operates. If you ask your brain to do a task but there is a block, then it will then take the next best route, or the next, or the next to accomplish the task requested.

We all recognise this situation. Whenever we have difficulty doing something, we become aware of the mental stress that is required to do it. This mental stress will often cause us to avoid doing that task.

Where does that most difficult task you have to do today go on your list of daily activities? At the top? No. At the bottom and somehow, you never quite get to it, at least not today.

CONCEPTS OF LOGIC AND GESTALT

I have said that Gestalt processing and its basis in intuitive knowing is, by definition, non-rational. That should not be taken to mean that it is inferior or less correct than logical, rational, deductive reasoning. The only distinction is the avenue or pathway taken to arrive at the correct result.

Since much of our Gestalt processing takes place outside of our conscious awareness, it may indeed use rational processes to generate the answer that comes to us as an intuition, and is hence non-rational rather than irrational in a strict philosophical sense. But for the person experiencing the intuition, what they intuit can appear irrational because they have no idea how they generated the information.

In contrast, Logic processing is dominated by our conscious manipulation of information following a formal set of logical rules. It appears entirely rational. You are not only aware of how you got the answer, but you can rationally explain the process. The major difference then between Logic and Gestalt processing, may not be in the underlying processing, since both rely heavily upon the same subconscious neural substrates, but rather on our conscious awareness of that processing.

Historically in the western world, there has been a tendency to revere rational thought and to somehow diminish reasoning based on intuition or Gestalt processes. From the time of the ancient Greeks we have maintained the notion that logical, analytical reasoning is somehow superior to intuitive reasoning, which has been more often associated with superstition. Indeed, one of the most insulting things you can say to anyone in the West is, 'That's irrational!' Nothing could be further from the truth because history shows time and again that many ideas that seemed perfectly rational can turn out to be totally wrong in the light of new facts.

For thousands of years it was assumed that the earth was flat, rather like a plate. It was further believed that the earth was the centre of the universe with the planets, stars and the sun orbiting around it. Based on the facts available at the time, both assumptions were logical. As more facts came to light, however, both assumptions proved to be wrong.

Yet it had seemed so logical. After all, when people stood on the top of a mountain and looked around, apart from undulations of landscape, the earth did indeed appear to be flat. When they looked out over the ocean it even appeared to have an edge. It was not obvious to the person standing on the earth that the ground beneath was actually spinning at 1600 km per hour, and that the whole earth was hurtling through space at even greater speed. To the early observers it was sheer commonsense that the earth was motionless, and that the sun raced across the daytime sky and the stars transited the nighttime sky.

In the late 1400s, Columbus bravely sailed over the horizon and never came to the edge. Soon after, many others were circumnavigating the earth in a great frenzy of discovery.

In 1543, Copernicus began working with the newly invented telescope and made accurate observations of the heavens. No matter how he analysed his observations, they did not work if the earth remained at the centre of the universe. The only way he could logically explain his findings required a new way of looking at the universe. It could only work if the sun was a star, like the other stars in heaven, and was orbited by a series of planets. Copernicus had no choice but to throw out the old model and present a new one based on the new facts.

The major strength of Logic is that it allows us to construct detailed models of the world that have predictive value. Logical models make it possible to deduce what will happen next. The major drawback of Logic, however, is that the model is always based on the facts as they are known right now. As new facts accumulate, what is logical today may become illogical tomorrow. Ultimately, history will say, today's model will prove to be wrong in the long-term.

Nevertheless, in the short-term, these predictive models are very useful because they help us to construct a way of thinking about the world in which we live. Most of western science is the product of fact-based, deductive reasoning and it has certainly brought us many phenomenal advances in telecommunications, nutrition, travel, medicine and computing.

Consider that it was only a century ago that physicians were attempting to heal people by bleeding them; by applying leeches to their skin. A doctor of today looks at this practice and considers it irrational. But the physicians of yesteryear were not stupid; they were highly intelligent, caring people who happened to be following a model of health different to the one we follow today.

Doctors of that time saw the health of the body as being determined by the balance of the four bodily fluids, or 'humours': blood, lymph, bile and cerebrospinal fluid. Of the four fluids blood was the most accessible. So when a person was ill, the most logical treatment was to bleed them to re-balance their humours.[10] (By the 16th century the Latin term 'humour' had been modified to denote an unbalanced mental condition as mood or a folly, and became a subject for writers of comedy).

It is also interesting to note that recent western medical research has shown that the removal of blood indeed does stimulate haemopoeisis, and increasing the production of new red blood cells can be a significant benefit in many disease conditions.[11] So these physicians of old often had positive effect, but not for the reasons their model predicted. On the other hand, there are many other disease conditions in which bleeding was a death sentence. In fact two American Presidents died as a result of this practice.

Our late 20th century medical model is based on biochemistry and biomechanics—the Newtonian view of a rational material world. The basic assumption in this model is that man is nothing but a biochemical/biomechanical machine, however sophisticated. If there is sickness or disease, clearly the biochemistry has been upset and the proper treatment is to adjust this chemistry by prescribing the intake of chemicals—drugs. Or, the person has a mechanical problem (such as a broken arm) and the proper treatment is to realign the bones mechanically so that they knit together again. Fifty years from now the doctors may view some of these procedures to be as irrational as bleeding by application of leeches.

As it is based on known facts Logic has a use-by date. As new facts come along, so our understanding changes.

Logical analysis also depends upon the development of premises or hypotheses based on assessment of the known facts. Sometimes these hypotheses are wrong, and the solution is to be found in a new hypothesis based on a premise that was intuitively derived.

These two types of reason complement each other. In a sense, the expressive Yang of Logic needs to be balanced by the hidden Yin of Gestalt. Not only that, but the Yin, or intuitively derived Gestalt premise may be transformed into a Yang or logically supported theory.

Where Logic is limited by paradigm-dependent facts, Gestalt is only limited by imagination. Gestalt can jump beyond present evidence because it can conceptualise what does not now exist and what has never existed. It can look at the same old facts and put them together in an entirely new way, allowing a leap of insight. From looking at the whole, Gestalt can divine a sense of knowing. It may not be provable at the moment, it's just something you know to be true.

When Einstein came up with the Theory of Relativity in 1905, it was based solely on his intuitive experiments. He knew it to be true even before he could prove it mathematically. He could then use his deductive reasoning to provide a logical construct for his intuitive concept. And while his model was valid mathematically it was several decades before the instrumentation was developed that could test it. So far, all tests on his theories have proven them to be valid. This is truly how science progresses.

Thomas Kuhn, a professor in the Faculty of Science at Harvard University, proposed a new theory about the progress of science in a book he wrote in 1962. In *The Structure of Scientific Revolutions*, Kuhn proposed that science has advanced through a series of accumulative, consolidative phases until, at a critical point in that accumulation, a Gestalt thinker comes along, makes an insight and moves scientific thought to a whole new level, a whole new conceptual understanding of reality (see Fig. 5.1). This is otherwise known as a paradigm shift.[12]

What Kuhn showed was that science actually proceeds through an interplay—or dance if you like—between Logical reasoning and Gestalt conceptualisations. He showed how science accumulates facts to back up

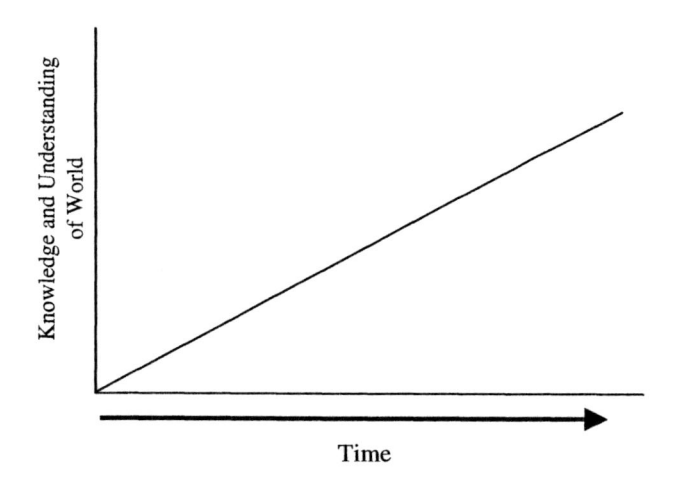

Figure 5.1a Traditional Model of the Progress of science and understanding of our world. Scientific investigation leads to the gradual accumulation of knowledge over time creating a fuller understanding of our world.

existing models of thought, but that every so often a fact arises that doesn't fit with the current model. This unworkable fact is put under the carpet, so to speak. Eventually however, a scientist trips over the lump, throws back the carpet to take a look at what's underneath and, based on what he or she finds, is able to make a conceptual leap to a new paradigm. All the data that had no place in the old model can sometimes add up to a revolutionary new model in the mind of a creative thinker, explaining not only the information in the old paradigm but also encompassing those facts that previously didn't fit.

When the new model is being put in place there will be a lot of activity to investigate it and to back it up with a whole series of logical, sequential

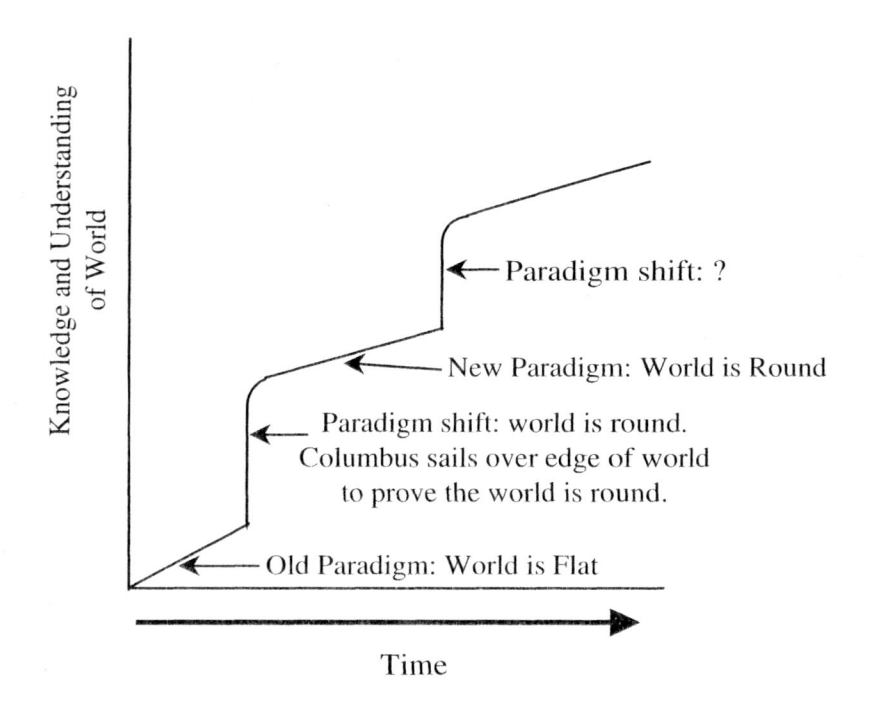

Figure 5.1b Kuhn's model of Paradigm Shifts or Scientific Revolutions. In this model, investigation leads to a gradual accumulation of knowledge about a particular paradigm or world view. Slowly observations accumulate that do not fit the current paradigm. An original thinker may incorporate these observations into a new paradigm leading to a revolution in the way scientists view the world. Then once again scientists set about gradually accumulating knowledge about the new paradigm. New observations accumulate that do not fit, and this process is repeated.

facts and scientific studies. But what happens as those facts are being put in place? New facts arise that don't fit. Back they go under the carpet, until a critical mass is again achieved and someone else trips over all this unaccountable knowledge that they can then use to create a new world view.

All scientific revolutions have followed this pattern that shows the wonderful interplay that is possible between Logic and Gestalt processing and how we make use of these marvellous tools in application to our human understanding of our remarkable world.

Whole brain thinking, which is when both hemispheres come into play, very often leads to a process that is greater than either could manage alone. What is inherent (Yin), or Gestalt, must be made manifest (Yang), or expressed, and expression is a Logic function.

MODELS OF LEARNING BASED ON GESTALT AND LOGIC

As I have alluded, for the past 20 years or so the Right Brain-Left Brain model of learning has popularised the notion of 'right brain' designating the right cerebral cortex, and 'left brain' referring to the left cerebral cortex.[13]

While Gestalt functions do appear to predominate in the right hemisphere and Logic functions appear to dominate in the left hemisphere, I argue that this model oversimplifies to an enormous degree the complexity of the many cortical subsystems—many of which are located in *both* cerebral hemispheres. Further, the prevailing theory totally ignores the subcortical processes that are, in fact, major centres of our mental processing. It is the subconscious that *does* most of the actual processing but it is the conscious areas of the cortex that *direct* what is processed.

It is a controversial view because I believe that a specific hemisphere does not entirely dominate either Gestalt of Logic processing. Rather, what they do is provide the lead, or the conscious intent that activate a number of other cortical and subcortical areas to perform the essential processing.

An analogy of this process is what happens when you decide to turn on a light. This is a conscious mental decision. As soon as you flick the switch, a whole cascade of other events occur. Electrons begin to flow invisibly through wires, junction boxes, the light fixture itself and into the bulb. All of this occurs outside your conscious awareness. All you are aware of is that the light has come on. This is an electrical model, but it is very similar to what happens in the brain. In the brain, you make a conscious request to do something—whether mental or physical—and this conscious input from a particular cortical lead function creates a subconscious flow that results in the processing of that request. The end result is conscious awareness of the outcome.

The essential point of the theory is that the conscious cortical lead functions in each hemisphere merely provide the entry point. And the cortex can only provide a lead if the point of entry is intact or accessible. If the lead function or entry point has been damaged in some way then we have a situation very similar to what happens when you damage the keyboard of your computer. The computer still works, all the processing is still available, but you cannot consciously access the processing capabilities of the machine because you have no way of talking to the computer. When this happens in the brain, in a sense, you become unplugged from the processing units required to do that task.

The reason for so carefully outlining this theory is that it has relevance to the rest of the information in this book. From here on when we talk about a Logic function or a Gestalt function we are referring to the *lead process* that is involved.

Watch how it works: Perhaps you see something in a store. It is advertised as being one-third less than its usual retail price. That makes it very attractive. You now have a motivation to consciously activate a series of Logic functions that allow you to calculate the price. You may then activate another lead function with a request to make the comparison of the amount of money you have in your purse with the sale price. You can now decide whether you can afford the item—a conscious decision based on answers processed largely in the subconscious.

Look at conscious intent as the lead into the biocomputer of the subconscious mind. The subconscious units then do their best to accomplish that conscious intent. Therefore the conscious mind is not determining *how* the brain should process merely *what* it should process.

While conscious processing is free-form, subconscious processing is dictated much more by formal rules. Using a computer analogy, you, the operator, are the consciousness. But once you strike the keys to bring up a particular file, the computer follows a specific pathway, and if it is a well-written program, it will be the most efficient and direct pathway to bring the file out of memory and into your consciousness on the screen.

If however, you make the same request to retrieve that same file and you get an error message, 'no matching file found', you then have to work out a new pathway into that file because the most expedient way is blocked. This may take some time and effort. Depending upon how important the retrieval of that file is to you, you may or may not choose to invest that time and effort.

Every time the route gets longer it becomes less and less efficient and takes longer to do. To the mind that translates into stress and the more stressful it gets, the more resistance there is in the brain to performing that process. If the task is associated with less efficiency and hence more stress, then the person will be less inclined to do it because it takes so much mental effort.

Ideally, the brain is set up so that all areas of Gestalt and Logic processing are accessible, and so that all the integration routes that connect them are totally clear. With this perfect set-up, all types of learning will be easy. Any blocks will make the process less efficient and more stressful.

BLOCKS IN MENTAL PROCESSING:
Organic Blocks/Functional Blocks

People who find learning joyful and easy have very few blocks in their mental processing so anything they put their conscious intent into will be successful. (They may still have some blocks to specific functions, but not in essential academic areas). A survey of 1600 people in Britain who have achieved fame in various professions revealed that some 85% of scientists were students who really enjoyed their schooldays.[14] These people were able to fully utilise the very purpose for which their brains were designed—learning.

As a child I too loved learning but I noticed there were a lot of other children who were having difficulties with spelling and understanding the simplest arithmetic. I used to wonder why. When I talked to those children they didn't seem to be different from me, or stupid. They were as creative as me but they had trouble with particular tasks that were easy for me. I couldn't understand it. Now I do.

Blocks to mental processing take two forms: organic or physical blocks, and functional blocks.

Organic or physical blocks can result from a variety of causes. One is that during the development of the brain, at between four to six weeks of gestation, the foetal brain is a neural tube that closes from the front to the back. When the tube doesn't completely close it can manifest as Spina Bifida. In the normal developmental process, the neurons that will form the grey matter on the outside of the adult brain are at this point on the inside of the foetal brain. An extraordinary process called neuronal migration then occurs.[15]

In neuronal migration, the nine billion or so neurons lying in the centre of the developing brain migrate to take their place in the cerebral cortex. It is a marvel that these neurons end up lying next to the neurons that in future they will need to co-operate with. What is more amazing still is how often this process occurs correctly. On occasion, however, it goes awry and neurons end up in the wrong place, leading to future functional problems. It is the neuronal migration phase that is often interfered with by excessive alcohol intake by newly pregnant mothers which can lead to a condition of partial mental retardation called foetal-alcohol syndrome.[16]

Another major cause of organic or physical blocks is micro-bleeding in various areas of the brain, due perhaps to a difficult or too-rapid birth. This micro-bleeding is the breaking of very small blood vessels in certain areas of the brain and it can lead to oxygen starvation of the cells in this area. Hypoxia (or a lack of oxygen), can kill off brain cells, creating dysfunctional areas of brain tissue. These areas can vary from very small to reasonably large, with corresponding levels of dysfunction.[17]

Two factors determine the nature and extent of brain damage resulting from hypoxic episodes: at what age and exactly where it occurred in the brain. Much of the cerebral cortex is quite plastic and one area can easily take over for another area that is damaged, but this plasticity decreases with age. Part of this plasticity of brain function before the age of eight appears to result from the active myelination and elaboration of various nerve pathways that is still occurring. After this age, the neural networks undergo pruning and sculpting to increase efficiency, but with a concomitant decrease in plasticity.[18]

Secondly, there are parts of the brain, particularly old brain areas such as the hippocampus, that perform critical functions which cannot be performed by any other brain area. When these areas are damaged, dysfunction almost always results, with the degree of dysfunctional paralleling the degree of damage.

The other common cause of physical or organic blocks is a blow to the head at any time in life. Such events may also cause micro-bleeding with concomitant dysfunction. Again if this damage occurs early in childhood, generally before age eight, and particularly if it occurs in the first few years when the brain is most actively myelinating pathways and developing new circuits, the function of the damaged areas may be completely taken over by other brain areas. If, on the other hand, the damage occurs later in life, the same initial degree of damage may produce more far-reaching and long lasting effects.

Functional blocks are far more common and appear to be caused by emotional stress. For some reason, emotional stress can cause processing modules to go off-line in our biocomputer. Although the structures remain intact, they are not available for use. An extreme example of this from psychiatry are cases of hysterical paralysis, when a person may become totally paralysed, yet have absolutely no detectable organic dysfunction. Episodes of hysterical paralysis may follow emotionally traumatic events, and then just as suddenly be resolved with full return of movement.[19]

From my perspective, functional blocks are the most common cause of learning problems in children and adults. By comparing the results of standard psychological tests used to assess learning disabilities, with access to specific brain functions and integrative pathways (such as the corpus callosum) which we can determine by specific kinesiology tests, we have found a very high correlation between poor access to specific brain functions and poor performance on the standardised tests. This will be discussed in greater depth in Chapter 9.

Because it prevents the effective integration of Gestalt and Logic functions so essential in academic pursuits, 'blocked' flow across the corpus callosum is found in almost every case of learning difficulties. And blocked flow across the corpus callosum is usually most strongly correlated with the poor development of Logic lead functions. In rarer cases, poor development of Gestalt lead functions may also be associated with 'blocked' flow across this vital integrative pathway.

The other major factor is blocks to access of key lead functions required to perform specific tasks. Again, poor access to critical lead functions, assessed using kinesiology, correlates highly with observed learning problems. Whenever there is an area of learning dysfunction, we can measure corresponding stress in accessing the lead functions associated with this area of disability.

For instance, children generally find spelling difficult if they are unable to create visual images in their mind. The child's brain will automatically look for the next most efficient process and switch into auditory processing in an attempt to spell. The spelling will tend to be phonetic, putting letters together to sound like the word. But, unlike many other languages, English does not follow such logical rules and words often do not look like they sound. Imagine someone trying to guess the spelling of 'phonetic' or 'write'.

What does the brain do to spell when it cannot create long-term images of words?

It does the very best it can, which is to attempt to put letters together to sound like the word sounds. Phonetic spelling is, almost universally, the type of spelling attempted by poor spellers because it is the best the brain can do.

Many children know how to spell, but they cannot do so because they do not access a critical brain function, or can not integrate the functions that they do access. This is true for all of us at some time or in some situation. There are blind spots in our mental abilities and we just accept them: 'That's us'. We don't understand that we may not have to be like this as many of these blocks are functional and can be removed.

In the 1960s, dyslexia was believed to result from an organic lesion or scar in the corpus callosum, the major integrating pathway in the brain. When autopsies were performed on people who had been dyslexic throughout their lives, however, there was often no evidence of any physical lesion. Since these dyslexics functioned as if there was a physical lesion, there must have been something blocking the flow.

One of kinesiology's seminal thinkers, Dr Paul Dennison is a case in point. Profoundly disabled by dyslexia throughout the early part of his life, Dennison presented as if he had impenetrable blocks in his mental processing. After Applied Kinesiology treatment, he demonstrated remarkable improvement in his learning ability to such an extent that he was able to successfully complete his doctorate. Clearly, the blocks were functional and not organic.

When the block is in an important academic area, such as reading, spelling or maths it reflects on other aspects of ourselves, such as our self-confidence and self-esteem. We perceive ourselves as dumb or just hopeless in some area of function, outcomes we will discuss in later chapters.

Essentially, all specific learning difficulties result either from lack of access to specific brain functions, or the inability to efficiently integrate those functions that we do access. Many functions, like reading and spelling, require the use of both Logic and Gestalt lead functions simultaneously and in highly integrated patterns. If you can't integrate these functions, even though you can access them, you simply cannot read or spell effectively. This lack of access to specific lead functions and/or lack of integration of these functions, I call loss of brain integration which is the underlying cause of the vast majority of learning disabilities.

GESTALT AND LOGIC LEAD FUNCTIONS

Both sides of the brain are constantly interacting and the way we learn is the result of the degree of integration in the lead functions of both cerebral hemispheres.

Each hemisphere provides the entry point to an integrated module of cortical and subcortical function, involving the relaying of sensory information to both cortical and subcortical areas and the laying down of new memories that may then be consciously recalled.

Each lead function contributes its own special capacity to all of our thought processes.[20] Certain tasks require certain lead functions. Other tasks require other functions, but all are using the same central processing units, located in our subconscious mind. We just use different combinations of the existing modules or arrange them in a new order— multi-tasking—to do different types of processing.

The human biocomputer is indeed very well designed.

To highlight my proposition I quote Levy and his explanation of the role of the right brain and left brain in reading. Instead of using his terms 'right brain', 'left brain', I have substituted 'Gestalt lead functions' and 'Logic lead functions':

'When a person reads a story, the Gestalt lead functions may play a special role in decoding the visual information; making an integrated story structure, appreciating humour and emotional content, deriving meaning from past associations and understanding metaphor.

'At the same time the Logic lead functions are playing a special role in understanding syntax, transforming written words into their phonetic representations and deriving meaning from complex relationships.'[21]

Reading is a task that clearly requires Logic and Gestalt lead functions to work well together. To orchestrate this highly complex integration of a large number of both Gestalt and Logic functions, and to synchronise these functions with many subconscious cortical and subcortical modules, an awesome degree of automatic organisation and coordination is essential.

In the next chapter we examine what happens when this automatic brain integration is compromised, or various processing modules are either not accessible, or only accessed poorly.

Chapter Six

MAJOR PATTERNS OF DYSFUNCTION

LEARNING DIFFICULTIES:

MAJOR TYPES OF LOGIC AND GESTALT FUNCTION

If you look at Figure 6.1 you will see that Logic lead functions are typically found in the left hemisphere and tend to be linear and sequential, involved with proof, facts, detail, order and consistency. In contrast, the Gestalt lead functions are typically in the right hemisphere and are simultaneous and global, involved with spatial awareness, creativity, visualisation, and beliefs.

One of the primary Logic lead functions is to construct internal visual images for instance of letters, forming words. It is therefore involved in spelling and learning new words. If we spread a set of alphabet blocks out on a table and then ask a child named John to spell his name, he will look around the table until he finds the 'J' block. Then he will look until he finds the 'O' block, then the 'H' and the 'N' and will arrange them to construct a physical, visual image of the word John.

This is exactly what happens in the visual construction process of the Logic hemisphere, except instead of moving physical blocks around, it is instead moving symbolic letters around in your mind's eye.

Once the visual image has been constructed from its pieces then, in a sense, a 'picture' is taken which is transferred to the Gestalt hemisphere where visual memory is located. Visual memory is where we store eidetic information or images, which can then be recalled into active memory. While we talk of these as visual images and perceive them as pictures, if you will remember from Chapter 4, visual memories are not actually static images like a snapshot, but rather reconstructions based on a record of the neural activity stored in the sensory cortices. Reactivation within the visual 'convergence zone' by the act of conscious recall causes ensembles of neurons storing the pattern to reconstruct the image in our mind's eye.[1]

When you go to spell a word, you activate your eidetic memory of the image that you created perhaps years ago, and that image suddenly appears in you mind's eye. To spell the word you then merely read off the letters in the order in which you see them. Likewise, if you have written a word, and are not sure if it is spelled correctly, you will often find yourself looking up into your head and then saying' Oh yes, it is e-i and not i-e' as you successfully reference the image in your mind.

If we consider reading, we find that reading begins with a Gestalt lead function—the interpretation of or decoding of symbols; the recognition of the individual letters, which are grouped as words. The decoded words are then sent to Logic lead functions to have meaning assigned to them in a process called 'meaning assignment'. Therefore, reading comprehension is based not only on the ability to decode symbols and to know what the word is, but more importantly the assignment of meaning to the decoded symbol.[2] Reading is after all the process of extracting meaning from written language.

When we are printing, the process is largely a Logic function because in printing you write one letter or symbol at a time in a linear sequence. If you change your writing mode to cursive script, or connected writing, then you switch to a Gestalt lead function because spatial flow is involved. Cursive writing is one continuous function rather than a series of individual actions requiring continuous spatial awareness.

Language, as you can see in Figure 6.1, is located in the left hemisphere in most people's brains.[3] The language that we are defining here is speech or verbal communication. It is the ability to assign meaning to words, to edit your thoughts and to say them. It also governs written language and applies the rules of grammar or syntax.

But there is also the language of the Gestalt—a language that is largely non-verbal. It takes the form of utterances, 'Uh! Uh!', and use of body movement. A two-year-old doesn't speak very well, but will make guttural sounds and point to indicate what it wants. The child is using two forms of Gestalt language: gesture and guttural utterance.

Many races are known for their Gestalt language. There is an old saying that if you tie the hands of southern Europeans they will not be able to speak because to them, much of the communication, or certainly the emphasis of what they are saying, is provided by hand gestures.

If, when speaking with such a person, you heard only the words he was speaking, you would miss a great deal of information and meaning because so much is conveyed by the way he holds his eyes, animates his facial muscles and moves his hands. Gestures enhance our communication to a great degree so much of the information we put across about ourselves is actually

178 *A Revolutionary Way of Thinking*

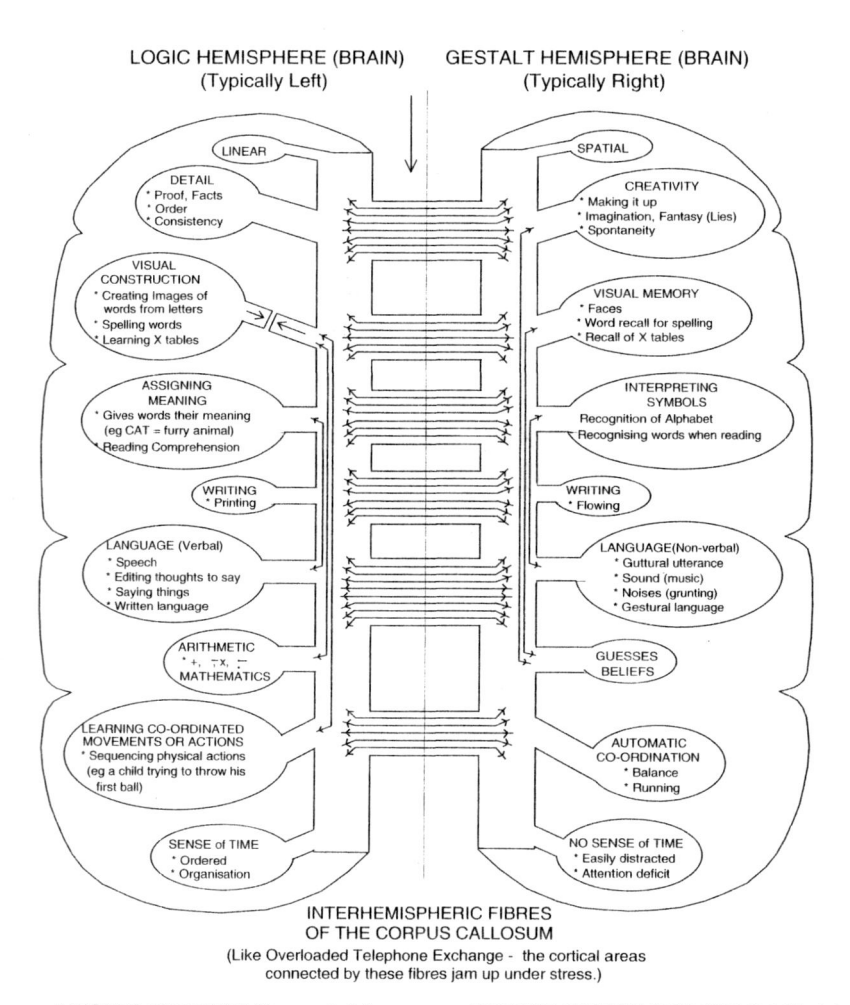

LOGIC HEMISPHERE (BRAIN) (Typically Left)   **GESTALT HEMISPHERE (BRAIN)** (Typically Right)

- LINEAR
- DETAIL
  * Proof, Facts
  * Order
  * Consistency
- VISUAL CONSTRUCTION
  * Creating Images of words from letters
  * Spelling words
  * Learning X tables
- ASSIGNING MEANING
  * Gives words their meaning (eg CAT = furry animal)
  * Reading Comprehension
- WRITING
  * Printing
- LANGUAGE (Verbal)
  * Speech
  * Editing thoughts to say
  * Saying things
  * Written language
- ARITHMETIC
  * +, −×, −
  * MATHEMATICS
- LEARNING CO-ORDINATED MOVEMENTS OR ACTIONS
  * Sequencing physical actions (eg a child trying to throw his first ball)
- SENSE of TIME
  * Ordered
  * Organisation

- SPATIAL
- CREATIVITY
  * Making it up
  * Imagination, Fantasy (Lies)
  * Spontaneity
- VISUAL MEMORY
  * Faces
  * Word recall for spelling
  * Recall of X tables
- INTERPRETING SYMBOLS
  * Recognition of Alphabet
  * Recognising words when reading
- WRITING
  * Flowing
- LANGUAGE (Non-verbal)
  * Guttural utterance
  * Sound (music)
  * Noises (grunting)
  * Gestural language
- GUESSES BELIEFS
- AUTOMATIC CO-ORDINATION
  * Balance
  * Running
- NO SENSE of TIME
  * Easily distracted
  * Attention deficit

INTERHEMISPHERIC FIBRES OF THE CORPUS CALLOSUM
(Like Overloaded Telephone Exchange - the cortical areas connected by these fibres jam up under stress.)

* WORKS BIT BY BIT (Sequentially)   * WORKS SIMULTANEOUSLY (Intuitively)
* TIME ORIENTED (Organisational)   * NO SENSE OF TIME (Only-Now/Not Now)

Figure 6.1. Essential Lead Functions. This is a diagrammatic sketch of some of the major Gestalt and Logic lead functions and the role they play in our mental processing.

communicated by body language. It has been estimated that body language accounts for more than 60 percent of total communication between people. Only about 7% is actually carried in the words.[4]

The other type of Gestalt language is colour, form and vocal tone, which again provides emotional emphasis to what is being communicated verbally. Research has shown that about a third of the information content in speech is from tone and inflection of the voice.[5] Damage to the right temporal cortex in the analogous area to Wernicke's Area on the left, impairs people's ability to give affect to their speech by changing vocal tone and inflection. Instead, they tend to have flat intonation and little prosody or vocal intonation to give meaning to the words and sentences they say.[6]

To show how much vocal tone adds to the meaning of what we say, consider what happened to a woman who suffered damage to this area. While the damage left her reasoning and her speech totally intact, she could no longer enhance the meaning of what she said by vocal colour and intonation, nor could she appreciate the intonation in the speech of others. She was, at the time, a high school teacher and was forced to give up her career because she could no longer engage the interest of her students. Neither could she control their behaviour because she could not put emotional emphasis into her statements. She knew that to have effective control of the class she occasionally needed to use an angry, commanding tone, but she could no longer do so.

In the realm of numbers, Logic governs. There are particular Logic functions involved in symbolic reasoning of which the simplest form is arithmetic: adding, subtracting, multiplying and dividing.[7] Writing 'one plus two' means making use of mental symbols to represent concrete realities, like one pencil and two pencils.

If you move to higher levels of abstract conceptualisation you get mathematics: 'X plus X equals Y'. No number of Xs can ever equal a Y concretely, but if they are standing for abstract proportionality, they constitute a very valid statement. Abstraction and abstract functions can only be appreciated via the entry point of access to Logic lead functions.

On the other hand, Gestalt lead functions allow us to draw on the overall situation, pattern or picture, and guess what the answer might be. If you get the overall idea you often develop a belief based on your feeling or hunch about the situation which is often correct.

As you can see in the Figure 6.1, when we move to the operations of the physical body, learning to develop a coordinated action relies initially upon Logic lead functions to organise and plan a motor sequence in conjunction with the subconscious caudate nucleus and cerebellum. It is Logic led.

You first have to learn a sequence of individual physical movements to perform a whole action smoothly. You know what it is you want to do, this conscious desire then activates Logic lead functions that initiate the frontal cortex-caudate nucleus conversation that eventually results in a successful motor program to perform a physical action. This process is graphically illustrated if you watch a very young child attempting to pour milk out of a carton and into a glass. You can almost see the brain sequencing the movement: ('Grab the carton. Put it above the glass. Tip . . . tip. Whoops! Now bring the carton back.')

As discussed in Chapter 3, the motor sequences to perform the desired action result from the interplay between the Logic lead functions, frontal lobe motor areas, and the head of the caudate nucleus. But once the sequence for this motor function has been transferred to subconscious parts of the brain (basal ganglia and cerebellum) they now appear to be run by Gestalt lead functions which simply activate the subconscious 'Pour a glass of milk program' and this then becomes a single, integrated movement.

The Gestalt brain also controls the body's spatial awareness and this perhaps explains why people who are Gestalt-dominant in processing are often athletically gifted because they have a great sense of their body orientation in space.

Another important area of Logic is a sense of time. Logic provides us with the ability to perceive the linear sequence of time passing: one minute, 10 minutes, 60 minutes, two hours. This function resides in the same part of the brain that allows you to order your actions and to organise.

By contrast, the Gestalt hemisphere has no sense of time. Gestalt-dominant people will tend to have poor attention to detail and they can sometimes suffer Attention Deficit Disorder. Why? Because to be ordered and sequential in your functions you have to concentrate, and concentration is a matter of paying attention over time. If you have no sense of time, how can you pay attention over it? Without a linear time sense to give you a reference point for your activity, you tend to jump from one activity to another, to be easily distracted and have great difficulty in holding your attention on any particular task for any length of time.

In overview, you can see how you have a set of Logic lead functions that are in most people predominately located in the left hemisphere. Logic lead functions basically work in bits, they are sequential, linear and analytic. They are also time-oriented, which means they are ordered and organisational.

By contrast, Gestalt lead functions work simultaneously, allowing us to intuit or 'know' things. There is no time in the conventional linear sense, there is only Now! or Not Now!

If ever you've experienced a two-year-old child, you are looking at the Gestalt processing in action. If you tell a two-year-old he can have a treat in half an hour he will probably react as though he's been told he will never get it. When you are two 'Not now' and 'never' mean essentially the same thing. Children this age are not capable of reasoning, of understanding that they will get the cookie, but in a few minutes. Later is not a real time to someone who is living totally in the NOW.

That's why, when you go on a trip with children, before you've even backed out of the driveway, you have the kids asking, 'Are we there yet?' There is no sense of time. To them there is only now, now, now. (We're told that you can get back to a more subtle form of this understanding when you become a Zen master.)

Another feature to take note of in Figure 6.1 is that the Logic and Gestalt lead functions are wired together for integrated function. This wiring takes the form of the neuropathways crossing through the corpus callosum, which is the major interchange for the communication of information between the two sides of the brain.

In the examples above, of spelling (creating images on one side and storing them on the other) and reading (decoding symbols on one side and assigning meaning on the other), it becomes clear that the commissural fibres passing through the corpus callosum are the centres of integration for many cortical functions.

So although it is essential to access relevant lead functions, both Gestalt and Logic, it is equally important to have clear communication between them. But what happens when you have problems in accessing those functions or their interconnections?

PATTERNS OF DYSFUNCTION

The explanation that follows is based on models of learning from the literature and on my clinical experience. I am talking more about lack of or poor access to specific cortical lead functions essential for certain types of learning and thinking. If any of these cortical lead functions is functionally 'blocked', types of thinking and behaviours dependent upon access to that function are just not available.

My model is also concerned with the integration of different functions at many levels within the brain, from the integration of Gestalt and Logic lead functions initiated by conscious intent, to the integration of the many basal subconscious functions carrying out the intended processing requested by the lead functions. This multi-level integration of the functions of many disparate areas in the brain, both conscious and subconscious, I term 'brain integration', a concept I will develop in more detail in the next chapter.

In this model, problems with learning, either in general or in particular areas, appear to originate from one or more of five major sources:

- A failure to access or poor access to specific Gestalt or Logic lead functions. Access to these functions is blocked.
- The pathways across the corpus callosum and other commissure fibres are blocked preventing effective integration.
- Access to specific subcortical processing modules is blocked.
- The integrative pathways connecting the subcortical pathways are blocked.
- The integrative pathways linking the cortical and subcortical processing modules are blocked.

By 'blocked' I mean that access to these processing centres or their integrative pathways is not available, the nature of this block is discussed below and in the next chapter. Whatever the causes, all the blocks will result in some type of learning dysfunction. In the context of learning difficulties, I find the most common pattern is Gestalt dominance in mental processing due to blocked flow across the corpus callosum. Because our Gestalt functions are well developed from birth, if the flow of information across the corpus callosum is blocked at an early age it appears to inhibit the development of Logic functions. In its extreme expression, Gestalt dominance in mental processing is currently recognised as Attention Deficit Disorder.

Normally, there is a complementary relationship between Logic and Gestalt with one balancing the other. But what happens when, for some reason or other, you lose that balance? What happens when you can access Gestalt functions well but have only limited or poor access to Logic functions? This lack of balance results in the expression of quite consistent patterns of behaviour.

GESTALT DOMINANCE IN MENTAL PROCESSING

Behavioural Symptoms

- A tendency to be impulsive.
- Little appreciation of cause and effect. There is rarely a thought about what will happen as a result of impulsive actions—you feel the impulse, you do it.
- Difficulty in budgeting time. This will mean that organisational skills are poor and projects are often left incomplete.
- Difficulty in concentrating. Concentration is merely paying attention over time. Difficulty in spelling. Generally spelling is phonetic; putting letters together so that they sound like the word.
- Difficulty with mathematics. Often difficulty remembering multiplication tables and usually, in understanding abstract mathematical concepts, starting with the concept of fractions.

- Reading may be fluent, but reading comprehension is usually poor. Symbols may be interpreted easily (Gestalt), but there is difficulty in assigning meaning to the words interpreted (Logic).
- Often well coordinated, even gifted athletically, because Gestalt functions control body awareness and orientation in space.

Reading comprehension gives a very good illustration of the problems of Gestalt dominance in mental processing. Problems with reading comprehension are generally expressed in three forms with people demonstrating Gestalt dominance:

1. Reading may be fluent but there is often poor comprehension of what is read. While the child can decipher each word in sequence, word-word-word, the part of the brain that assigns meaning to the words may be off-line. Remember, each visual image of a word is only held in the sensory store for a fraction of a second, and if no meaning or relevance has been assigned to it, it will be dumped or immediately over-written by the next word.

   So by the end of the reading very little of the story content has reached short-term memory. This type of child is merely functioning as a word processor. Ask them what they read and they will have little or no idea. 'A boy did something.' Since reading is extracting meaning from written language, these children are not reading in the true sense at all.
2. The child can only assign meaning to a portion of a sentence or paragraph. By the end of the paragraph, the stress of attempting to keep the rate of assigning meaning synchronised with symbol decoding will often result in the omission of meaning. For the rest of that sentence, or the next few sentences, the child will then be word processing, merely reading word, word, word but assigning no meaning. This child may be left with a patchy idea of the storyline but very few actual details.
3. The child, armed with a highly creative Gestalt mind, will commonly fill in the details between the few words they have actually managed to comprehend when reading. This means that the story they remember, though interesting, may have very little to do with the story they actually read.

I had a young boy who was given a story to read in which the old unit of Australian money, a penny, was used. When he told me what the story was about, it had been transformed into a story about a girl named (you guessed it!) Penny.

It is often assumed that these children read well. So when they fail to answer questions about what they have read, or give answers that are way off the mark, they are presumed to not be paying attention or not concentrating.

This poor reading comprehension often spills over to create problems in other areas. These children often do well as long as maths problems are presented numerically, but suddenly they can't seem to do the same problem when it is presented as a word problem. They don't have problems with maths, but with comprehending the question they were being asked.

These children often avoid reading or state, 'I hate reading' because for them reading is largely a pointless process. If you put considerable effort into reading but remembered almost nothing, why bother?

Another common behavioural characteristic of these children is that they have highly creative minds, which can be used in two ways. The introvert will tend to look out the window and create their own daydream world. The extrovert who cannot get positive attention for what they know, will use their creativity to entertain other class members becoming the classic class clown.

Because Gestalt-dominant children cannot rationalise, but are intuitively sensitive to people around them, they often tend to take things very personally and are easily hurt or bullied. Such children are often described as overly sensitive and emotionally immature.

LOGIC DOMINANCE IN MENTAL PROCESSING

Those people who have Logic dominance and poor access to Gestalt processing represent only a small percentage of those with learning difficulties. Among the most extreme members of this group are the true dyslexics. Other people displaying dyslexia may not be simply Logic dominant, but suffer from neurological processing problems in their visual or phonological systems.

Behavioural Symptoms

- Also cannot spell, or do so almost entirely phonetically by putting letters together so they sound like the word.
- Have great difficulty reading, usually stumbling over words, misreading words or unable to sound the words out effectively. However comprehension of what is read is often excellent. Again, some of these types of reading problems may be based in visual perceptual or phonological problems quite apart from blocked access to Gestalt lead functions.
- Display dysrhythmia or an inability to clap in time to a tune.
- Physically uncoordinated or clumsy.

One of the first children I worked with in this field was a young boy, Lex, who was unbelievably clumsy. His mother said that when Lex walked across a room he would trip on his feet, your feet or the leg of the table. Lex had very poor access to Gestalt functions, which take care of the body moving in space, but was excellent at maths. Quite literally, unless he was thinking about moving his feet while he walked, his feet went everywhere. Walking, which is normally a semi-automatic Gestalt-led function, was certainly not automatic for him.

There was another little girl, Sally, who at age seven had an IQ of 160 but who was considered retarded because she was totally Logic-dominant. Her mother explained how affronting it was to have a young child argue with her and win through sheer force of logic. But this same child had to be taught commonsense things that other children seem to pick up naturally. Logic-dominant people are attracted to fields where they can work with mathematics, computing or physics because it is so easy for them. They are the classic 'nutty professors' who had difficulty learning to tie their shoes, can't replace a light bulb or use a screwdriver.

LIMITED ACCESS TO GESTALT AND LOGIC IN MENTAL PROCESSING

The second most common type of learning difficulty results from limited access to both Logic and Gestalt processing. This results in serious learning problems. When you have limited access to Gestalt but good access to Logic, or vice versa, it is possible to compensate to varying degrees by compensating with the functions you can access. In fact, the more innately bright you are, the better you compensate. But if you have deficits in both the Logic and Gestalt processing your ability to compensate is severely compromised. How can you compensate a deficit with a deficit?

Behavioural Symptoms

- Language development is often extremely delayed for age.
- Reading is very delayed for age. There is often difficulty even recognising very simple words, or word recognition is a struggle. The words recognised are often forgotten almost instantly.
- Spelling is very delayed for age. Often words of more than three or four letters are impossible.
- There is difficulty in understanding numbers, even basic numeracy and arithmetic. There are often problems in learning to count, telling time or even knowing the days of the week.
- There is no concentration or focus. They are 'away with the fairies'.
- They often appear confused, lazy or just mentally slow, and seem apathetic, lethargic or display no zest for life.

In the extreme form, these people are often functionally illiterate and look blankly at a very confusing external world. Their tendency is to withdraw into themselves where they live in their own little world. Many children with these problems won't go much beyond primary school because learning is just so difficult for them. Others, with these problems to a less extreme degree may be able to get through school but only after a heroic struggle.

In every school, in every class, there are a few kids who have a kind of slowness about them. They are slow because their mental processing is so confused that there is a much greater time delay in doing most tasks. They may be able to get the right answer but it takes them far longer than anyone else in the class.

A woman I worked with who had this limited access to both Gestalt and Logic processing reported that she had always felt there was an extra step in everything she did mentally. In a way she was right because indeed everything she did required double-processing.

POOR INTEGRATION OF GESTALT AND LOGIC IN MENTAL PROCESSING

Representing less than one or two percent of the population, this last group is the least common pattern of learning difficulties. These individuals are fortunate to have good access to both Gestalt and Logic lead functions but the misfortune not to be able to integrate them because of poor access across the corpus callosum. This means that the two hemispheres cannot effectively talk to each other and integrate their activities.

Behavioural Symptoms

- Reading is very difficult. Often it is so stressful that reading will only be attempted for a few minutes or avoided altogether.
- Spelling is totally phonetic.
- There is difficulty with higher mathematics (algebra or above) even though numeracy, arithmetic and basic mathematics may have been perfect.

For such people, school is often a frustrating experience because so many essential academic functions, such as spelling and reading, require good integration. Learning becomes very stressful and the individuals who suffer it can become very frustrated and angry. They are intelligent, and they know it, but cannot do so many fundamental tasks that they are often presumed to be stupid.

I once worked with Ron, a 42-year-old American who was a classic example of poor integration. He was innately bright with good access to Logic and Gestalt but with almost no communication occurring between them. Ron had never learned to read and he only spelled phonetically.

When he was 14 and a big, athletically well-developed youth, a teacher admonished him in front of the class by saying, 'Ron, you're so stupid, I don't know why you are here. You are wasting your time, my time and the school's time.' Any other child might have stormed out of the school, never to return, but Ron took it as a personal challenge. He became absolutely determined to finish high school even though he couldn't read.

He managed this seemingly impossible task by getting friends to commit their class notes to tape (he had good auditory comprehension and recall), and by cleverly cross-examining teachers during tests. When it came to written exams he would look through the questions and manage to recognise some words. Then he would ask his teacher a question about the question and from the answer, would then guess what the question might be. He already knew the answer because he had studied, he just couldn't read the question. By this and many other ingenious methods, he was somehow able to graduate from high school, and in the manner of the athletically gifted, he was given a football scholarship to university.

After six months of continually failing exams and of it becoming increasingly apparent to his tutors that he was illiterate, he flunked out. At 19, he was a very angry, very frustrated young man. He bought a Harley Davidson, joined a gang and took to the road for the next 10 years. And on many Saturday nights he found himself fighting in a bar to vent his internal rage.

The only difference between Ron and many prisoners is the fact that he did not happen to kill or permanently maim someone in one of these Saturday night brawls. If he had, he would probably still be behind bars. One of the only commonalities that has been found among prisoners who commit violent crimes is that they are almost all functionally illiterate.[8]

One day, he happened across an old school friend and they got talking. The friend was pursuing personal growth and seeking spiritual answers. Ron was fascinated. He desperately wanted to know more, but found that most of the answers were written in books. He needed to be able to read. He traded in his colours, built a landscaping business that became quite successful because it relied on his innate creativity and, he married, as it happens, to a primary school teacher.

With the motivation of wanting to read esoteric books, over the next two years Ron learned how to read. He succeeded only by force of will. To read he would willfully jam the functions of his Logic and Gestalt together. At the end of about 10 minutes of reading, however, his eyes would be streaming, his stomach churning and he'd have to stop. Half an hour later he'd start reading again, forcing himself to succeed, albeit in short bursts.

After a couple of hours of treatment which opened the flow through his corpus callosum, and defused his negative attitude toward reading, Ron was able to read effortlessly for hours. He still does so to this day.

Extremely motivated individuals like Ron are very rare. He was motivated enough to overcome the stress involved in surmounting the barriers to knowledge. For most people, when the stress gets high enough they just avoid tasks.

I had another adult patient, a 32-year-old woman who could read very fluently—in fact too fast, but could remember virtually nothing of what she read. She was just word processing, not reading. She could write, but in terms of reading, was functionally illiterate. Her bright personality had been sufficient to allow her to get on in the world and she worked at many jobs including being a waitress. In order to explain the menu to her customers, at the beginning of each day she would go to the chef and have him explain each dish to her and show her which one it was on the menu. When people ordered she would have them point to the dish on the menu and in this way she could tell what they were ordering.

She was eventually offered the position of maitre d' of the restaurant. Yet because she felt she couldn't do a job that required greater literacy, she left the restaurant. Instead of being confronted with what was difficult for her, she avoided it altogether. This was not the first time she had opted out of the stress loop.

THE STRESS LOOP

Lack of integration of brain functions, or lack of access to specific lead functions, results in stress in doing certain tasks. Because of the stress, you avoid the task.

Particularly when you are a child in school, there are certain tasks that may be difficult such as reading, spelling or maths. You try to avoid doing them. Your teachers and parents however, recognising the importance of these subjects, will often force you to attempt them.

You keep being told, 'Try harder; pay attention' and 'Don't be so lazy. Do your homework!' As a last resort they will try punishment but punishment only generates more stress because you genuinely can't do it or can do it only with enormous effort. More avoidance and thus, more stress.

The stress actually creates a greater loss of brain integration, and so the loop goes around and around until an individual develops such avoidance behaviours they are regarded as misbehaving or withdrawing deliberately. Children in this loop are often labelled troublemakers, daydreamers or class clowns (see Fig. 6.2).

But people's behaviour always tells you the truth. It's just a matter of being

The Stress Avoidance Cycle
generated by Loss of Brain Integration

Lack of access to specific brain functions or the inability to effectively integrate these functions.

Increasing anger, frustration, stress leading to further .....

Difficulty performing tasks generating a degree of *stress*

Resulting in Punishment. Extra work. Being singled out. Labelled a behaviour problem. ***Punishment***

Avoidance behaviours I hate... I won't do .. I'm angry.... I'm dumb ... I'm distracted..*stress*

Misinterpreted as misbehaviour Not doing as you are told. Not concentrating. Not listening. ***Punishment***

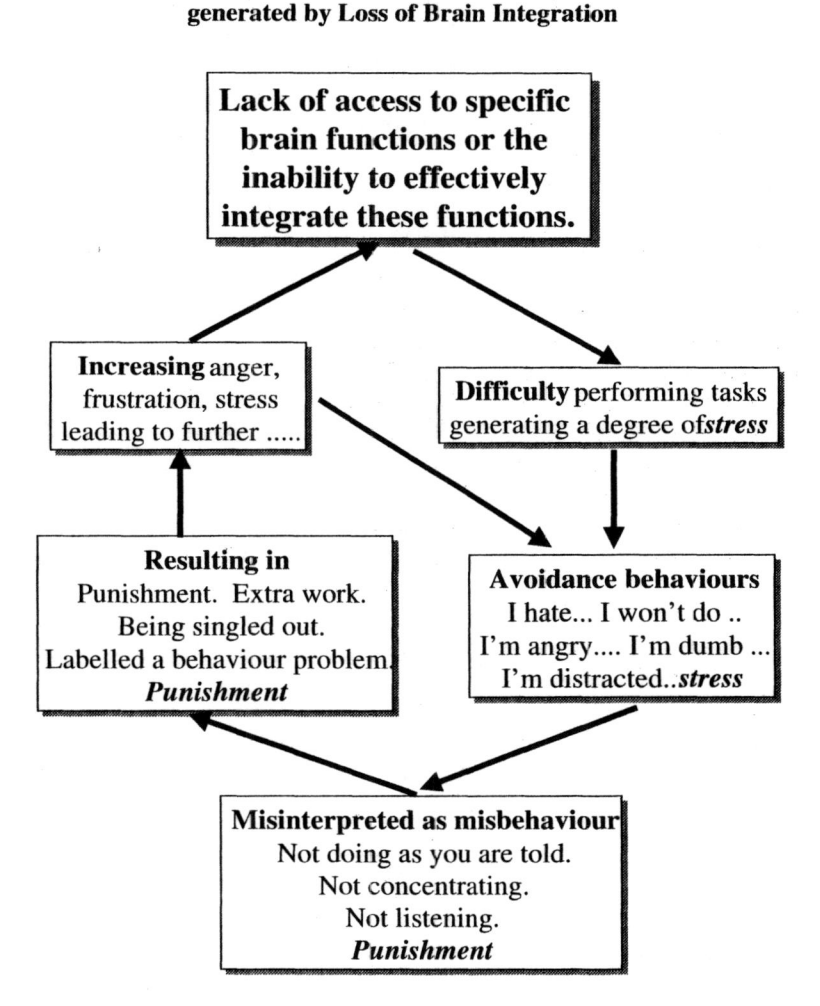

Figure 6.2 The Stress-Avoidance Cycle. Whenever there is lack of access to specific brain functions or the ability to integrate these functions this initiates the avoidance of tasks dependent on these brain functions. This is often misinterpreted as misbehaviour.

able to understand what the behaviour is really telling you. From a conventional perspective, a child not doing what he is asked is believed to be purposely misbehaving and therefore, the proper response is to encourage them to do that which they are avoiding, and if this doesn't work, to punish them.

Yet if the child could learn to spell, they would spell. Any child that can read and comprehend easily, enjoys reading as there is always something interesting to read about. They do not avoid it. What is not understood is that these children often do know *how* to spell but they just lack access to the essential functions needed *to* spell.

When young people say that they hate maths or English, what I understand them to be really saying is 'I cannot do this task easily,' or, 'I can only do this task with a great deal of emotional and mental stress and if I can, I will avoid it.' If you think about it, it is perfectly rational to avoid something that both tortures you and gives you very little in return for the effort.

Avoidance behaviour is largely misinterpreted in our society as misbehaviour, plain and simple. But if we understand what their behaviour is actually telling us we could then have compassion for them having to attempt that which is very difficult.

I find that most people with learning problems are innately very clever. In my clinic we have worked with thousands of so-called poor learners and constantly find that the highest percentage are not stupid or slow, they just lack access to functions that allow them to express their intelligence. In fact, the majority are highly intelligent as demonstrated by their ability to understand concepts and solve practical problems, they just find it difficult to perform basic academic functions like reading and spelling.

All of us have a sense of our own innate intelligence. If you have a sense that you are intelligent but cannot perform simple tasks that most of your peers can master easily, you start feeling stupid, and find yourself constantly failing. And every time you fail you become more firmly entrenched in a downward spiral of loss of self-esteem and self-confidence which, of course, constitutes more stress—more loss of integrated brain function—leading to more failure.

Brain integration is very fragile, in the sense that it is largely determined by your stress levels. Even the most well integrated person, given enough stress of a specific type, will lose integration and become temporarily dysfunctional. One of the major differences between people is the type of stress and the extent of stress required to cause loss of brain integration.

In a sense, we are all dyslexics, or learning disabled under certain circumstances.

People who already suffer poor access or poor integration, are already in a state of partial loss of brain integration and hence need very little extra stress to become totally dysfunctional. This may occur largely in one area of function. For example, they will look at a maths equation and won't even know where to begin. They will state: 'I'm hopeless at maths', not recognising that they have merely lost integrated brain function in that particular sphere. They have not lost their intelligence.

Here's a common experience: If I ask you someone's name and you can't remember immediately, I agitate you: 'Come on, come on, I'm in a hurry. I need the name right now!' You now have almost no chance of recalling the information under such pressure because it has just increased your loss of brain integration. What you really need is to relax to allow your brain to re-integrate, to come back together again. In fact, you'll probably find yourself minutes or hours later suddenly recalling, 'Jenny!' This occurs because trying only creates stress that exacerbates loss of integrated brain function.

The opposite of the downward spiral is what happens when someone has been reconnected to their integrated brain functions. They attempt a new task, and now being able to bring fully integrated brain functions to the task, perform it with ease. Tasks now begin to have positive outcomes. And as success is reward and stimulates release of dopamine into the reward centres of the brain, you will now look forward to the next challenge. If you once again maintain integrated brain function you will be successful again: further reward. You become more and more confident of your ability to succeed and this is the essence of self-confidence.

Self confidence is a common outcome of integrated brain function. I will elaborate on this ephemeral thing called brain integration in the next chapter.

Chapter Seven

THE NATURE OF BRAIN INTEGRATION

BRAIN INTEGRATION AND PERFORMANCE

Now that we understand the basic structure and function of the brain and have a model of learning based upon the integration of Gestalt and Logic lead functions, it is timely to consider what brain integration is and how it affects our performance.

Because I am proposing a new concept of brain integration, I first must define exactly what I mean by this term. Brain integration is the state of having access to all relevant Gestalt and Logic lead functions, the subconscious processing centres and the pathways to integrate these processing modules. In this state, you are in optimal learning mode. Every function you need to perform any type of learning is accessible and you can easily integrate all relevant functions to perform these tasks.

In the state of complete brain integration there is virtually nothing the brain finds difficult to learn. Yet only a very small minority of people (probably less than two to three percent) have managed to survive childhood with most of these functions intact.

Being one of the lucky ones, I always found learning fun when I was at school, particularly at high school when I got into more challenging academic areas. My big problem was boredom. I understood too quickly and there was often nothing to occupy my mind. The result was that I got into trouble because I had a creative mind that wasn't being fully occupied in class, so I entertained it with things which resulted in me visiting the principal's office.

By the same token, I used to spend three hours a night doing my homework. My mother never once had to tell me, 'Charles, go do your homework!' I found homework so enjoyable I could hardly wait to sit at the desk. It was challenging and difficult at times, and I had to put in effort, but because I was successful, it was enjoyable and rewarding.

Integration allowing ease of learning and mastering tasks is actually the birthright of all human beings. It is not always what happens. To understand why, we need to look at the nature of brain integration.

THE CHOREOGRAPHY OF THOUGHT

Nature designed the brain as a fully integrated functioning unit in which many separate parts (carrying out various functions) were designed to work seamlessly together. The key to this ideal functioning is to maintain a level of stress which will not interrupt this process. Once stress exceeds a certain threshold various functions may be compromised, or the integration of these functions may be lost.

But what is the inherent nature of this integration that can be so easily compromised?

Conventional neurological theory presents a view of the brain as a mass of neuronal connections, and it is believed that it is via these neurons (wires) and their connections (junction boxes) that mental processing occurs. In such a model it might be difficult to understand how the connections could break down when subject to a specific stress and then suddenly be regained when the stress is removed.

Recent neurological research, however, has suggested that this picture is a very limited view of the actual processes involved in thought and other types of higher mental processing. The new view of the brain suggests that much of the integration of functions occurs not by information flowing to a particular area that then integrates this information, but rather, that it is the *synchronisation* and timing of processing occurring in widely distributed subsystems in many different areas, at the same time, that constitutes integrated brain function.[1]

Using the analogy of a railway system, the old view was that there were a lot of stations connected directly by tracks. Trains could not leave the tracks and could only change direction at the shunting yard in the station. It was a fixed, linear system in which it was assumed that for processing to occur, information needed only to reach its destination, like a train pulling into a station.

The rails are still there in the new theory, but now the trains also communicate by radio, as well. Some of the information coming into the station is also carried by vehicles other than trains: cars, bicycles and trucks—all travelling at different speeds on different routes, and some are not limited to the tracks.

For example, for just one mental process to occur, it requires not only the timely arrival of information carried in a number of trains to converge on the same station at the same time, but also radio transmissions about the information being carried on other trains, running on other tracks and entering other stations, which must also arrive right on time. But still, only part of the necessary information has reached the Grand Central Processing Station. Other essential information must also arrive via other vehicular traffic. Only then can the information be integrated to perform one sometimes quite simple function. This is what it takes to add one plus one.

A further potential difficulty in this highly complex system is that the trains only remain in the station with their information for a fraction of a second. In that short time, all the other vehicular information must arrive, and the correct radiowave transmissions be received for well-integrated processing to occur.

So clearly, the nature of brain integration is timing and synchronisation of neural events. Loss of timing results in a massive traffic snarl in which little information gets through. Any information that does move is often meaningless because it does not seem to be related to anything else.

In short, this is what happens when you try a mental process that you find particularly difficult. If you have difficulty understanding maths, the loss of synchronised arrival causes an information jam in the processing modules that are involved with doing maths. You just do not have the right information coming together at the right time to allow you to comprehend and solve that type of mathematical problem. It does not compute.

From a neurological point of view, it has been recognised for a long time that the brain is a mass of some one hundred billion neurons, each of which has one thousand to as many as one hundred thousand other connections. And these are just the trains and the stations! Nerve impulse conduction in any one neuron also generates electrical and electromagnetic fields (like the radiowaves in our analogy), that broadcast information to other neurons about their activity. These can be recorded electrically as EEG patterns.

More recently, it has been shown that considerable information flow in the brain is actually not carried by neuronal connections at all. Rather it is carried by volume transmission.[2] Volume transmission is the information carried by various chemicals both within and between the neurons and at different rates of speed—all those bicycles, cars and trucks that aren't running on the railway lines.

Antonio Damasio, a leading American neurologist, proposed that thought and mental processing is the result of synchronised neural, electrical and chemical activity generating higher-order information flow within the brain. There seem to be what he describes as 'convergence zones', where information from different areas comes together to create another level of mental processing, one that borders on what we might term 'thought'.[3]

The synchronous firing of neurons in many separate brain areas to create conscious thought appears to be dependent upon some type of 'time binding' requiring powerful and effective mechanisms of attention and working memory. This time binding of disparate inputs to the various convergence zones appears to rely upon the global attention and working memory areas of the prefrontal cortices and their connections to the various limbic structures such as the anterior cingulate, amygdalae and hippocampi.[4]

The timing and synchronisation of neural activity in these diverse brain regions, both cortical and subcortical, must be maintained to produce coherent 'thought'. Because our thinking is dependent upon this integration of separate processes into meaningful combinations, any mis-timing or loss of synchronisation between these processes can result in learning disorders. To quote Damasio 'any malfunction of the timing mechanism would be likely to create spurious integration or disintegration'.[5]

From this new perspective, therefore, brain integration is the dynamic synchronisation of the timing of neural and mental events. Any loss of synchronisation represents a loss of integration. Loss of integration in turn, results in loss of some specific mental capacity, such as the ability to do maths.

THE STRESS FACTOR

When I tell people we are going to integrate their brain functions they tend to assume the change will be permanent, like pouring concrete. It is not. Brain integration may come and go depending on two factors: the stress in your life at that time, and the stress associated with whatever task you are doing *both* at present and in your past.

The difference between a well-integrated person (who learns easily), and a poorly integrated person experiencing learning difficulties is stress tolerance—the level of stress that triggers a loss of integrated brain function.

Following, or during times of peak stress in our lives, loss of brain integration may be global. There are times in your life when you totally lose it. You lose your ability to think straight and just can't seem to function. In this case you have lost synchronisation of most of your brain functions. The trains are off schedule, the roads are blocked and the drivers are on strike.

What is more normal however, is the loss of local integration: loss of synchronisation between functions that perform specific tasks. In these cases, only that task is compromised; the train system is running well, but some of the stations have closed.

The other factor to recognise is that there is no such thing as a universal *stressor* that causes loss of brain integration, rather there are stresses in people's lives and, depending on the context, they may or may not cause loss of integration. The same stressors that cause one person to lose integration may only represent a challenge to another person, a challenge to accomplish something. For example, some people who find maths easy might become dysfunctional when asked to write an English or history essay. Yet if you ask a person who easily writes English essays to pen something about literature, they'll be happily challenged. But if they are asked to work out a mathematical equation, they may fall apart. Whether an experience constitutes a stressor or a challenge is thus different for different people. Stressors are contextual within each person's life and life's experience.

This brings us to the real cause of learning difficulties: *the loss of integrated brain function, produced by a particular stressor in a particular circumstance. For some it may only be a momentary loss of integration when performing a specific task, while for others, it may be an on-going loss of integration in whole areas of function.*

We emphasise that this is an entirely new concept, not current in modern psychological or educational literature. Previously there has been no way to measure whether someone has integrated brain function or not. Hence, when people became dysfunctional it was assumed that they had become anxious and that their anxiety had inhibited their ability to think.

Kinesiology provides us with the opportunity to understand why a person becomes dysfunctional when trying to learn. Any stressor affecting mental functioning can also cause a change in muscle response. By matching the muscle response that indicates stress, against different types of stressors, the specific stressor causing loss of integration can be identified. I can tell, for example, whether the loss of integrated brain function is due to emotional anxiety or to the loss of synchronised brain function itself. I have found that the most common cause of learning difficulties *is* the loss of synchronised brain function.

Once you lose integrated brain function, you become dysfunctional—unable to perform a desired task and this then often generates an emotional state of anxiety. If you can't understand something, you often become anxious, and this generates further stress which causes further loss of integration, and further anxiety; a continuous feedback loop. I claim that it is the initial loss of integration that causes anxiety, not the anxiety that causes disintegration. In my clinical practice based on several thousand cases, in greater than 90 percent of these cases, loss of brain integration precedes the emotional state of anxiety. Loss of brain integration does indeed immediately generate anxiety, because once you have become dysfunctional there is plenty to be anxious about!

Anxiety can become a factor, but only after you have already lost integration, tried and failed. The more you fail, the more anxious you are likely to become because you are afraid of failing again. This anxiety created by the fear of failure may then cause more rapid and even greater loss of integrated function, guaranteeing that you will indeed fail again. Failure initiates a negative spiral of diminished self esteem and loss of confidence. This is the negative stress loop.

Emotional stress can, however, also be an antecedant factor to loss of brain integration. Traumatic emotional experiences, usually early in childhood, can effectively 'shut down' important integrative pathways or access to subconscious processing centres which underlies the loss of integrated brain function. The following sections expand upon this concept.

THE CORPUS CALLOSUM

The Routes of Integration
The most common site for loss of integration is the cortical areas connected by fibres passing through the corpus callosum, the lineal structure running from the front to the back of the brain. It contains between four hundred million and six hundred million interhemispheric neurons, which connect the functional areas of the right and left hemispheres.

We can regard the corpus callosum as the trunk cable connecting many telephone switchboards by which functions in one hemisphere are co-ordinated and integrated with functions in the other hemisphere. If the operators on all switchboards controlling individual cortical processing are all on duty, then the flow between the functional centres in the two hemispheres through these switchboards can be easily co-ordinated; all the messages can be transferred to the correct areas at the right time and processing can proceed unimpeded.

If 70 percent of the operators on any one of these switchboards suddenly walked off the job, few problems will be experienced as long as there is only minimal flow through the switchboard. But as soon as the functions dependent upon that switchboard are activated, the number of messages will rapidly exceed the number of available operators, lines start getting crossed, messages are cut off or mislaid and eventually the whole switchboard jams up. Functionally, this represents a loss of synchronisation of flow across the corpus callosum and hence a loss of integrated brain function.

If only one of these cortical switchboards is compromised then only those messages that are usually processed through this switchboard will be affected. Because of this block to straightforward communication, the brain will seek an alternate way to process the information, the next best route. If it cannot integrate the Gestalt and Logic functions that are required to most easily perform this task, the brain will then process the information in the Logic or Gestalt area that is the next most accessible.

If you are already Gestalt dominant in your mental processing, then the Logic functions with which you would otherwise integrate are unavailable. Your brain takes the line of least resistance and processes this information in the Gestalt processing centres that are available. It may not be the optimum method but in your brain it constitutes the most efficient mode possible. If the processing is not possible at all, or only with great difficulty, the brain may just opt out and stop processing this type of information altogether as it is just too stressful.

When you set out to solve a problem in algebra, you look at the problem, and the symbols and spatial arrangement of those symbols are interpreted and decoded by your Gestalt processing. This should stimulate flow across the corpus callosum to activate the areas of Logic function that can appreciate abstract proportionalites. If the integrating areas (switchboards) of the right and left hemispheres connected through the corpus callosum are blocked, suddenly you will not be able to bring on line the Logic functions needed for abstract problem solving. Your conscious response may be, 'My God, this is difficult. I don't see how I can do this. It's too hard.' This will either result in you feeling very stressed, perhaps to the point of perspiring, or, you might just give up altogether.

Emotional stress or other stressors can cause the cortical areas linked via the corpus callosum to go 'off-line', shutting down effective information transfer between the hemispheres, or the stressor may alter the timing of transmission disrupting synchronised activity. Whether it is 'blocked' transmission or 'desynchronised' transmission of information through the corpus callosum, the result is the same, a loss of brain integration. From here on, I will call this loss of brain integration due to transmission problems across the corpus callosum—corpus callosum shutdown

Shutdown in one or more of the cortical areas linked via the corpus callosum may occur when a child is as young as two or three, in fact this is one of the most common ages associated with corpus callosum shutdown. The most common result of this is poor access to Logic functions. If it happened before the child reached the age of reason (about four to five), then there is little stimulation of the Logic areas and these areas never develop fully. After age five, most children have developed their Logic functions at least to some degree. In other words, they become more logical and can be reasoned with, and they can now use rationalisation and reason to effectively reduce the stresses in their lives.

Once access to Logic has been blocked such children can be literally locked into their Gestalt functions. They will then attempt to handle the vast majority of their mental processing by Gestalt means. These are the people who are run by their emotions, with little understanding of cause and effect in their lives. Yet these people are also often highly creative even though they may have difficulty expressing this creativity in their lives.

THE TERRIBLE TWOS:

A Crucial Age in Loss of Integration

Why is the age of two so critical in human development? When you consider it, this is probably the most emotionally stressful period you will ever face in your life. Very little in the years that follow can ever match the level of emotional intensity and trauma experienced by two-year-olds. How many times as an adult have you thrown yourself on the floor in a rage?

Children do not only tantrum for attention, they do it because they are emotionally distraught. Adults can rarely appreciate the level of distress a young child feels: all we see is irrational, obnoxious behaviour. Adult minds can rationalise stress, but children two to three years of age do not have the Logic abilities to do so. They respond in the only way they know.

Several factors are working against the young child: By the age of two, most become egocentric. They know 'I' and what 'I want'. Because they live totally in the moment, if they want something, they want it Now! And they want it with every fibre of their beings. It becomes their sole focus. Two-year-olds are not only egocentric they are also totally unable to understand rational explanations. If they ask for something they simply cannot understand a refusal, no matter how reasonable the refusal may be. The frustration of not understanding why they are being denied the one thing in the world they want often reaches high levels of intense frustration, which is then expressed as a tantrum.

A real life example: I had a young patient who couldn't learn to spell because when he was two and a half years old his mother wouldn't give him a cookie. That sounds ridiculous to a rational adult. Yet if you consider it from a toddler's viewpoint, it is logical. It was the only choice the child could make in responding to the stress he was experiencing at that time.

It was about Christmas time and the boy's mother always made special cookies for the occasion. She had only just pulled a batch out of the oven when Johnny came into the room. He smelled the cookies, he saw them and wanted one. 'Cookies!' He knew they were special cookies. 'I want cookies.'

His mother said, 'No. You can't have these, they're for Christmas.' That was only a few days away but to a two-year-old, there are only two times: Now and Not Now. A few days from now is not a real time, not now equates to never! What Johnny heard his mother say was, 'You're never ever going to get one of these cookies!'

Now, the Gestalt mind also has a keen appreciation of non-verbal clues and Johnny had observed in the past that when he was a good boy his mother often gave him a cookie. Cookies equated to mother's approval. So from his distressed non-rational perspective, Johnny was not only hearing that he was never going to have that biscuit, he was also hearing, 'I'm not going to give you my special approval. Not now or ever.'

The child interpreted this response as rejection, now and forever. Rejection by the most important person in your life is tantamount to annihilation, bringing fear fully on-line. This rejection and fear activate punishment programs in the amygdala which then become encoded in subconscious emotional memory. Not able to handle his fear of being rejected put him into a tantrum that his mother could not believe. Inside his brain he was experiencing a tremendous emotional stress. Adults expiate stress by rationalising it but Johnny could not rationalise and he had to do something to cope.

There is no physiological proof for this, but it was as if his brain said to itself, 'What am I going to do with all this stress? How am I going to cope?' It looked about for a place to put the stress and located the otherwise unused integration pathways in the corpus callosum. At this age they weren't doing much integrating because there was, as yet, little Logic to work with.

In a sense, the brain located an empty room, threw the stress in, slammed the door, locked it and threw away the key. Johnny felt better and the tantrum ceased. But what he had done to cope with the stress was to shut down part of the information flow through this important integrative pathway. He popped the circuit breakers in the cortical switchboards transmitting through this part of the corpus callosum—in effect creating subconscious loss of brain integration.

Later, when he was trying to learn to spell, he could not access these areas of corpus callosum shutdown by this traumatic childhood experience because it was blocked by an emotion that was too fearful to look at again.

If you look at such a fear as an adult, it's ridiculous. But because the memory has been emotionally encoded at an early age it still feels too frightening to be let out. And while it is locked away, the function is also blocked. The child therefore had no access to the Logic functions involved in spelling and compensated in the best way he could using the Gestalt functions he still had available. Hence he was a phonetic speller.

Once the corpus callosum shutdown occurs, all the evidence I have from my clinical work is that people whose functions have been blocked at the ages of two, three or four can still have those functions blocked in their teens, middle-age and perhaps for their whole lives. Blocks do not go away as we grow up because the stress remains unresolved at a subconscious level.

If you recall that the amygdala encodes punishment programs and stores them in the subconscious, they are then outside of cortical control. No matter how hard you might try to change it consciously, the function is off limits and that part of the mind cannot be unlocked consciously. The end result is that the person has blocks to certain types of learning.

By far the most common stressor for shutting down flow across the corpus callosum is the birth of a sibling when a child is aged between two and three. In many cases of integrative dysfunction that I have treated, the birth of a younger child turns out to have been the causative stress factor. Why would this be so?

From a child's point of view, one of the most stressful things that could happen is to be replaced in your parent's attention by a rival, particularly if you were the first child. Until the birth of your sibling, you had probably been the centre of your parent's universe, and because you are intensely egocentric and thrive on all the attention, you actually perceive yourself as being at the centre of the universe. Suddenly, this strange pink blob arrives in your life from out of nowhere and a lot of the attention of the household shifts away from you and on to it.

This is the basis of sibling rivalry and often the reason some siblings may hate each other for years, even a lifetime. Because there is no ability to understand rationally why the new child is commanding so much attention, children who are presented with a new brother or sister will often regress behaviourally, even to the point of losing their toilet training. Sometimes they will try to physically harm the unwanted rival.

We were told by the wife of a 40-year-old male client that her husband was still experiencing sibling rivalry with his 38-year-old brother. When this was mentioned to James he said: 'I don't have any issues with my brother. When he enters a room, I leave.'

When I use age recession techniques to deal with learning blocks and find they have arisen at these early ages, the emotions I commonly find are rejection, disapproval or feelings of being unneeded, unwanted, or unloved. Children of two and three cannot rationalise displacement, they usually interpret the birth of another child as an indication that they are no longer good enough or no longer wanted, and these feelings can be intense enough to shut down cortical functions and integrative flow across the corpus callosum resulting in long-standing loss of brain integration.

There is, of course an interplay of other factors at work here: Genetic disposition is one of them. I tend to find that when a child comes to me with a particular type of integrative problem, one or both of the parents will often say, 'I was just like that as a child.'

Part of what you inherit from your parents is a personality structure based on a constellation of hundreds of thousands of different genes. That personality structure, when stressed, will make certain choices about how to cope with that stress. Introverts will internalise and withdraw. Extroverts will act out. Your genetic structure will determine the ways in which you will be predisposed to dealing with major stressors in your life. So for people with a particular personality structure, intense emotional stresses will tend to cause a loss of integrated brain function as a mechanism of coping.

The birth of a sibling is definitely not the only factor blocking integrative flow across the corpus callosum. Any intense emotionally-charged circumstance that occurs during this critical period may block functional flow through the corpus callosum. Hospitalisation when the child is very young is another common stress associated with corpus callosum shutdown. Sometimes young children have to go to the hospital. Suddenly, they are separated from their mother and home, which generates a feeling of being abandoned and often intense fear. Not only are they separated from their protectors, and in an unknown place, but unknown people are doing unknown things to them, some of which may even be painful. This is a tremendous emotional trauma for most children, which in susceptible people may trigger corpus callosum shutdown.

Just because you or your child has undergone one or more of these stresses does not mean that their brain integration is compromised, as these factors do not necessarily cause loss of brain integration. Many people can undergo such traumas and manage to maintain fully integrated brain function.

OTHER INTEGRATIVE PATHWAYS

There are several other important pathways involved in integrating brain functions. We will look at them briefly:

While the corpus callosum links most of the cortex of the right and left hemispheres, the anterior temporal lobes of both hemispheres have their own special commissure (set of cables) providing for their integration. These cables are known as the anterior commissure.

The anterior temporal lobes are richly and reciprocally wired to the two hippocampi, amygdalae and surrounding medial temporal lobes and function together to integrate information from various areas of the cortex. Hence, this anterior temporal lobe-hippocampal complex, can be considered a major processing centre for each hemisphere.

The integration of these two important processing centres is therefore essential for normal brain function. Anything that compromises the information flow between them may inhibit efficient function. But like the corpus callosum, stressors may block either permanently or intermittently, transmission of vital integrative flow through these essential pathways.

When these pathways are blocked, people often experience problems integrating aspects of their Logic and Gestalt functions, making all mental processing more stressful.

One of the other most important integrative pathways is the hippocampal commissure, connecting the right and left hippocampus, the sites of short-term visual and auditory processing, respectively. When this connection is lost we may suddenly be cut off from everything we know. Our mind goes blank.

This is because much of our long-term memory is stored in visual images in the Gestalt areas of the cortex. These images are laid down from information which is often first created by the digital/symbolic verbal processing in the left hippocampus, then transferred to the right hippocampus via the hippocampal commissure. The image of the information held in the short-term memory circuits of the right hippocampus, if relevant enough or rehearsed often enough, becomes interleaved into long-term eidetic (picture) memory.

Recall of that information reverses this path, with activation of the right hippocampal retrieving the images from long-term visual memory making them available to visual working memory. Or the remembered image may be directly imported to visual working memory from long-term memory. The image of the information held in visual working memory, may then elicit the verbal (word) representations of the image in the verbal working memory in concert with left hippocampal activity. Once the image has been represented as words, you can then say them. But before this image-to-word transition has occurred, you can 'see' and know the information, you just can not talk about it. The famous it's on the tip of your tongue syndrome.

You know the situation: You are introduced to the new bank manager from whom you are about to request a loan. 'This is Frank Parsons.' You take note of Frank's face, which has a particularly large nose. This information travels via the pathways outlined above and is stored in the Gestalt areas of the cortex involved in facial memory.

At the same time, you are telling yourself, 'This is Frank Parsons, the bank manager. I need to remember his name'. The relevance of this information to your life causes you to rehearse his name in your auditory short-term memory in the left hippocampus for long-term storage in the auditory association areas of the left hemisphere. When you meet your business partner the next day, you remark about Frank Parsons' extremely large nose.

But would you believe it, the next time you come into the bank to confirm the loan, you recognise the nose and know you know the face, but for the life of you, you cannot recall the name! What has just happened is a breakdown in the information transfer across the hippocampal commissure.

Blanking out in exams is another life circumstance in which loss of integration via the hippocampal commissure can have disastrous consequences. You have studied for your exam, you know you know the information; in fact, immediately before entering the room you were explaining to your friend the details of the subjects you were going to be examined on.

You walk into the room, pick up your exam paper, sit down, and the teacher says, 'You now have one hour in which to complete this examination. No additional time will be permitted. You must put your pens down and hand in your paper in exactly 60 minutes. Start now.'

You look down at the paper, read the first question and suddenly you go blank. But you know you know the answer. It just won't emerge in writing because the verbal thoughts won't form.

What occurred was, the stress of the exam itself and of the time limit caused a loss of communication across the hippocampal commissure, and perhaps the corpus callosum as well. All that wonderful information stored in your visual long-term memory is suddenly out of reach of your ability to express. When this occurs in the creative act of writing it is called 'writer's block.'

In my clinical practice I often treat children for exam anxiety. They are generally well integrated, and can learn the material, but they just cannot express it during an exam. In virtually every one of these cases, the function that is lost is indeed communication across the hippocampal commissure. As soon as this connection has been functionally restored, the student no longer experiences exam anxiety and can now express the knowledge he or she has learned.

THE ROLE OF SUBCONSCIOUS PROCESSING CENTRES IN BRAIN INTEGRATION

While access to integrative pathways is important in the maintenance of brain integration, of equal importance is access to, and the full function of, the subconscious centres involved in mental processing.

As we have stated earlier in the book, the vast majority of brain activity takes place in the subconscious. The desire to perform a mental task is a conscious decision but the ability to perform the mental task relies on an integrated set of subconscious functions involving visual and auditory processing. Even though the auditory processing may not be overtly verbal, we talk to ourselves in our head all the time. And whether you are externally verbalising a thought or only thinking it, you would find many of the same neural pathways are activated.[6]

Thus we rely upon the subconscious visual and auditory functions to do most of our mental processing, particularly when it comes to academic pursuits. Most of the words we see in our inner speech, before speaking or writing, exist as auditory or visual images in our consciousness. If they did not become images, however fleetingly, they would not be anything we could know. The same is true of symbols, which if they were not imaginable, we could not know them to manipulate them consciously such as in doing mental arithmetic. Again, in the words of Damasio, 'thought is made largely of images'.[7]

The simple act of reading one word involves a complex cascade of neural processing. It begins with the control of pupil dilation and contraction to provide exactly the right intensity of illumination on the retina. This initiates a vast flow of visual impulses through optic radiations to the back of the brain where they are assembled into a rough image. Then, through a series of steps the rough image is developed into a full-blown conscious perception of the word via references to images in our memory. All neural events, up until the moment of conscious perception of the word, took place outside of consciousness.

If any of the subconscious processes preceding conscious perception were not easily accessed and well synchronised, then we may have difficulty forming an accurate conscious image. For example, you may have difficulty reading a word on a sign if you have suddenly come from deep shade into bright sunlight because your pupils have not yet constricted properly. They are letting in too much light, and that decreases the sharpness of your vision.

On the other hand, even when there is proper illumination of the retina, the streams of neural impulses flowing back to the visual centres follow different pathways and move at different speeds. If these should arrive at the visual processing centres out of sync, you may still have difficulty knowing what the word is. Or, the image may be properly formed in the visual cortex, but problems with accessing referents (images in memory) within the other areas of the brain, may cause you to misinterpret the word on the page. You might read the word 'through' as 'thought'.

This has been a specific—if simplified—example, demonstrating just how many layers of processing are involved and how many potential points of dysfunction there are in the perception of a single word. This is equally true of all other sensory perception. At this point we must acknowledge how truly amazing it is that we are able to perceive the world with such clarity.

Although mental processing is consciously initiated (I look at a book with the intention of reading) most of the actual process of reading is subconscious, right to the last level of visual perception, where it once again becomes conscious. If something should interfere with any of these subconscious processes, I will only be aware that I cannot read, not why I cannot read. This is equally true of difficulty in any other academic area.

If access to these subconscious functions is blocked, then clearly our ability to perform conscious mental activity is compromised. As it is in the case of the corpus callosum, one of the primary factors found to block the subconscious functions is emotional stress. And again, emotional stress is contextual for each person and unique to their personal history.

THE LOSS OF BRAIN INTEGRATION

From a functional point of view, the primary factor controlling our ability to learn is the maintenance of integrated brain function. Since the components of both our learning and memory systems are widely distributed throughout the brain, involving both subconscious cortical and subcortical functions, it is the synchronisation and timing of neural events that permits the brain to operate as an integrated unit. Loss of timing or synchronisation between two or more parts results in loss of brain integration, and the ability to 'think' in certain ways. It is like an orchestra that has lost its conductor. The symphony musicians are still playing, even playing well, but just not together, and the symphony disintegrates into meaningless noise.

But what can be done about this loss of brain integration that can have such devastating effects on our learning, our sense of self-esteem, and our lives? The next two chapters introduce techniques that you can do for yourself (Chapter 8) or have done for you (Chapter 9) to re-integrate a disintegrated brain. These techniques were developed in the field of kinesiology or borrowed from other fields, and are largely based upon the re-synchronisation of neural activity either via movement exercises or acupressure stimulation, hence the description of the acupuncture meridian system in Chapter 2.

Chapter Eight

LOSS OF BRAIN INTEGRATION: WHAT YOU CAN DO ABOUT IT

FACTORS CAUSING A LOSS OF BRAIN INTEGRATION

Now that we've discussed how a person under stress can lose brain integration (and it tends to happen at the most inopportune times) the next obvious question is, what can you do about it? That depends largely on the factor or factors causing this loss of integration. They may range from the simple loss of integration in specific circumstances, to things that occurred in early life which have resulted in on-going disintegrated brain function.

While there are as many causes that underlie what creates stress for each person, and all are uniquely personal, there are several common factors that can cause loss of brain integration. Four major classes of factors that cause loss of brain integration are:

Instantaneous circumstantial stress: This can occur in a particular situation and often only persists for the duration of that situation. Everyone has in their life another human being in whose presence they tend to disintegrate. It can be your boss, your mother, or some significant other. Even as a powerful and successful adult we can go to see our mother or father, and suddenly, in their presence, find ourselves acting like a five-year-old.

Or, there might be a particular circumstance, such as being called upon to speak in public, that may generate great stress. As soon as you walk onto the stage you might find yourself falling apart. But as you leave the stage later, you can talk to a friend and feel totally normal.

Disintegration of a specific brain function: This can result from exposure to a particular type of stressor. For example, academically you only lose brain integration in maths and only when you are attempting to do maths more difficult than algebra. You can do arithmetic, fractions and percentages with ease but somehow, when you attempt to do algebra, you disintegrate. You just can't seem to understand the first thing about it. This describes an area of function rather than a situation.

Corpus callosum shutdown: Brain disintegration resulting from corpus callosum shutdown often originates as a coping mechanism for stresses occurring in early childhood, and is usually an on-going state. In this case you also tend to poorly access functions of one hemisphere or the other to varying degrees. Since, in early childhood the dominant mode of processing is Gestalt, the usual result is poor development of Logic functions, causing difficulties with reading comprehension, spelling and problems with abstraction such as mathematics.

Deep level switching: This is a deep level of confusion in mental processing. Metaphorically it is as though there is a cable that carries the Gestalt information to the Gestalt processing centres, and a similar cable that conveys Logic information into the Logic processing centres. And, in deep level switching these cables somehow become crossed. Logic information is then sent to the Gestalt processing centres, which can only process such information with difficulty, if at all. Deep level switching is the least common factor related to poor brain integration, but it has the most profound effects. Children who demonstrate it are often delayed in their language development.

Acupressure techniques and movement exercises often provide a stunningly simple means of dealing with these problems. These corrective techniques can be applied in two different ways depending on which of the factors is being dealt with. For loss of brain integration caused by instantaneous or circumstantial factors, self-help techniques may be enough. Even for the third type of factor, corpus callosum shutdown, self-help techniques can be useful if done repeatedly and on a routine basis. When addressing the last factor, deep level switching, self help techniques may have little on-going success, because the level of confusion in brain processing is so great that it may undermine their efficacy.

Deep level switching and corpus callosum shutdown can be more permanently addressed using treatment protocols administered by a professional kinesiologist or Applied Physiologist. Application of a multi-faceted protocol can often eliminate or defuse the factors causing corpus callosum shutdown or deep level switching. Because similar acupressure techniques and movement exercises are used in both self help programs and by professionals, we will first introduce how these techniques work. Then we will elaborate on the self-help techniques and, in the next chapter, on professional treatments.

ACUPRESSURE TECHNIQUES THAT AFFECT THE BRAIN

All acupressure techniques are based on stimulation of specific acupoints for the effects they have on physiological function. It is important to note here the distinction between *acupuncture*, which is the use of needles penetrating the skin to stimulate acupoints, and *acupressure*, the use of gentle physical pressure to stimulate acupoints.

When there is physiological disturbance within the body, specific acupoints in the acupressure energy system become spontaneously active. In many cases, this activity will be registered as pain when that point is pressed firmly. In fact, many of the acupoints were initially discovered because they were what the Chinese call, 'Ah Shi points', literally translated 'Ouch!' or sensitive points. The term Ah Shi points is now generally reserved in acupuncture for acupoints not located on meridians.[1] A specific acupoint on the skin will often be painful while a point immediately adjacent to it will demonstrate no such sensitivity. This shows the specificity of the acupressure system.

Sensitivity, as indicated by pain, is clearly a physiological response. The acupoints can therefore indicate disturbance in physiological function. Indeed, one class of important acupoints are even called the 'alarm points' and there is one alarm point for each major meridian energy flow. They are called alarm points because when that meridian has an over-abundance of energy (known as over-energy) representing stress or disease in the associated organ, these points commonly become painful, even to the lightest touch.[2]

A friend told me he believed kinesiology and acupressure must really work because many times when I would go to a correction point, it would be very painful to touch. Yet, until it was touched he was unaware of its existence. He said: 'It's incredible, you can find every painful spot in my body, even when I'm not aware of them.'

Using muscle response in kinesiology, it is possible to locate active acupoints before they have become painful. If the point is in balance, merely touching it will produce no muscle response. If it is out of balance, there will be an immediate response, alerting the kinesiologist that there is an imbalance and that this point is now 'active', that is, causing a muscle response when touched.

Stressors of any type can activate acupoints. For example, if you tend to be confused about left or right you will often find that the 27th point on the Kidney meridian (K-27), will be tender to rub. The K-27s are located just beneath the end of each collarbone where it meets the sternum. If you move your finger across the bottom of the collarbone until it runs into the edge of the sternum, there you will find a soft dent, the centre of which is the K-27.

Stimulation of K-27s by gentle massage, while holding your navel, which is another important acupoint (Central Vessel 8) is said to reintegrate brain function. How can this be true?

Recent research has demonstrated that in animals when a specific acupoint is electrically stimulated it will cause a change in the firing rate of individual neurons within specific parts of the amygdala, a deep subconscious brain centre. Stimulation of other acupoints causes different patterns of firing. Further, stimulation of other areas of the skin (sham points) does not cause any change in the firing rate of the neurons of the amygdala. Again this demonstrates the extreme specificity of this remarkable system.[3]

Other research has demonstrated that acupuncture stimulation of the acupoint 'Heart 7' produced long-lasting increases in the P300 wave, a late evoked EEG potential that has been associated with cognitive activities. Stimulation of another acupoint 'Large Intestine 4', did not change the P300 wave, suggesting the cortical response to acupoint stimulation is highly specific. As in other studies, stimulation of non acupuncture 'sham' points had no effect.[4]

Early kinesiological research showed that the K-27 points were indeed related to mental function, particularly to the integration of right and left processing.[5] An imbalance in this processing results in the confusion of right and left and the reversal of letters, as commonly observed in dyslexics. It was noted that immediately after stimulation of these points, people who were

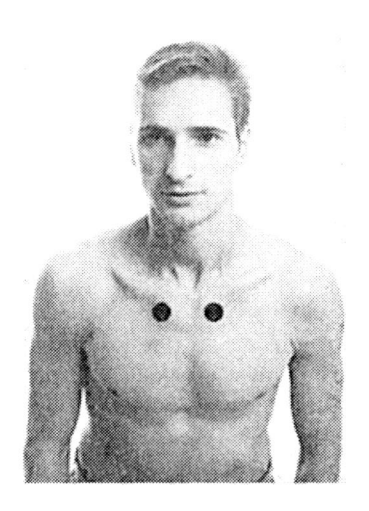

Figure 8.1. Location of K27s. The K27s are the last point on the Kidney meridian and lie in a soft dent just beneath the end of the clavicle (collarbone) where it meets the sternum.

confused in this way would suddenly no longer mix right with left and would stop letter reversal, at least in the short term.

To illustrate this in an even more physical way, I was once sharing a house and one morning one of my housemates came out of her room and said: 'Charles, this is really strange. I've just woken up. I can see from the welts that I have been sleeping on my left arm, but it feels normal. It's my right arm that is asleep. How the hell could that happen?' I told her to massage her K-27s, (which she said were indeed tender), until the sensitivity disappeared. This only took 30 to 40 seconds. She then said: 'This is even more amazing. As the tenderness of the points disappeared, suddenly, my right arm felt normal and my left arm now has needles and pins.'

What this showed is the true nature of brain function, which is to project back to the source of stimulation the nature of the experience the brain is having. In this case the sensory receptors in her left arm were sending a stream of impulses to areas in her right brain which then interpreted this as a feeling of needles and pins. In the normal course of events, it would have correctly projected this sensation back to her left arm. But due to confusion on the part of the brain, the signals of the feeling were switched and projected to the wrong side of the body—so the wrong arm was experiencing the sensation.

This illustrates how the brain has reference to itself and may become confused with respect to itself. Right becomes left, top bottom, and front back. A sensation coming from here is perceived as coming from the wrong place. In fact the brain creates its own reality from the sensory information it receives. Its creation may be true to the world of the sensory input or, it can just as easily be an illusion based on its confusion.

A well known phenomenon that exemplifies this propensity for illusion is the case of the 'phantom limb'. People who have lost an arm or leg will often still feel sensory events in that missing limb. One of my clients, who had lost his left leg above the knee, was still feeling pain in his left foot. The nerves that had gone to the foot were clearly still firing sensory information into his brain after the amputation, perhaps due to the physical trauma and the scar tissue formed. His brain was then creating an illusionary pain that it was projecting to the missing foot. When I used kinesiology to locate the active acupoints on his stump, and rebalanced them, his phantom limb 'disappeared'.

MOVEMENT AND THE BRAIN

One might question what movement has to do with learning and higher mental functions? In fact, when the initial evidence was presented that movement was controlled from the cerebral cortex, scientists of the day considered it controversial because to them it was well known that the cerebral cortex was exclusively the domain of thought.[6] But as direct neurological experience demonstrated, stimulation of specific areas of the cerebral cortex did indeed relate directly to activation of specific parts of the body. This region of the cortex has been called the primary motor cortex and is laid out topographically similar to the way in which related parts of the body lie next to each other (see Fig 3.9). Stimulate a certain area and the thumb might move; stimulate an adjacent area and the index finger moves, and so on.

Whether to move is a conscious decision; how to move is another matter. Consciousness is involved in planning of the intended movement and initiating its activation, but does not play a direct role in its execution.

You consciously decide to walk to the refrigerator to get another slice of that chocolate cake. You consciously initiate the action of standing up and walking. But from that point on you are only thinking of how good that cake is going to taste and whether anyone would miss it if you took just another teensy piece. Clearly the motor activity involved in walking to the refrigerator is of no concern to your consciousness. Instead, an extremely complex and integrated set of subconscious functions is taking care of the business of walking.

To summarise what is really going on in your brain: the conscious intent was sent probably by the frontal lobes of the cortex, via projection fibres to the subconscious centres controlling movement, namely the basal ganglia and cerebellum. Because you have already learned to walk, the basal ganglia has a how-to-walk program stored in the putamen, which is activated by your conscious thought. This sends a co-ordinated stream of messages encoding the walking program to the globus pallidus, another part of the basal ganglia, which in turn relays this information to the substantia nigra and subthalamic nuclei (feedback centres in the brainstem).

The circuits running between the basal ganglia and the substantia nigra/subthalamic nuclei modify the walking program on the basis of this feedback, largely by inhibiting extraneous movement. (What happens in Parkinson's Disease is that the neurons secreting the inhibitory signals in the substantia nigra are lost, resulting in the characteristic tremors of this debilitating disease.)

At the same time these messages are sent to the ventroanterior and ventrolateral nucleii of the thalamus, which relay them back to the premotor areas of the frontal lobes. From there they are relayed to the primary motor cortex. The primary motor cortex then sends out the actual movement message to the muscles of your legs via the corticospinal fibres, down the spine. Then you walk.

But that's not all. When the initial message went to the basal ganglia, the intended movement was simultaneously sent to the cerebellum, where the balance programs for maintaining equilibrium are stored. On the basis of the feedback from the vestibular nuclei received from the organs of balance in the inner ear, the cerebellum activates compensatory muscle activity to balance the body while walking. These balance programs were then activated at the same moment that the muscles began to move for walking. It must be recognised that as a toddler it took you a while to integrate the balance programs of the cerebellum with the walking programs of the basal ganglia. Witness any toddler taking its first steps.

But there's more. The proprioceptors, the subconscious sensors in the muscles, tendons and joints, send a volley of information back into the cerebellum and basal ganglia about what movements are actually taking place. The cerebellum then compares the intended action—received from the cortex, with the proprioceptor feedback about what is actually happening in the body and adjusts muscle activity by feedback to the ventroanterior and ventrolateral thalamic nuclei.

One of the major functions of the cerebellum is to act as a misalignment detector, smoothing out motor movement by turning off muscles at the appropriate time so the limb goes where you intended it to go and stops where you intended it to stop. Loss of this feedback due to cerebellar or spinal damage results in a loss of synchronisation of the actual and intended action.

I had personal experience of this breakdown between the intended and the actual movement. When I was recovering from my spinal injury, I first regained gross motor control of my arms and could move them to my face. But I had lost the cerebellar control of the action. So while I intended to scratch my nose, I actually thumped myself in the forehead because once my arm started moving towards my face I could no longer dampen down the action.

Another example of this loss of control of the actual movement by intent, is called intention tremor and results from cerebellar damage. Intention tremor is the shaking of, say, the hand and arm when you intend to reach and pick something up. Because the cerebellum can no longer inhibit the muscles in a co-ordinated way, often quite violent shaking occurs. However, when the same person is making a similar movement without intention they may not demonstrate the tremor.[7]

In a simplified graphic form, the neurological wiring and the sequence of impulse flow would look much like Figure 8.2.

This whole sequence could be likened to a highly trained fighter pilot flying a sophisticated computer-controlled jet. He is the conscious mind and intends the plane to fly a particular course and so he pushes the controls to the right. The electrical signals generated by his action race to the onboard computer (the subconscious) which sends signals out to the ailerons and rudder (the muscles), sending the jet into a steep turn: the intended action. The ailerons and rudder have sensors relaying messages back to the onboard computer (proprioceptor feedback), and on the basis of this feedback it constantly makes

214   A Revolutionary Way of Thinking

adjustments so that the pilot's intended action becomes the trajectory of the plane.

I MOVE, THEREFORE I THINK

From what we have just discussed it is clear that even simple actions require a great deal of mental activity both at the conscious, and particularly at the

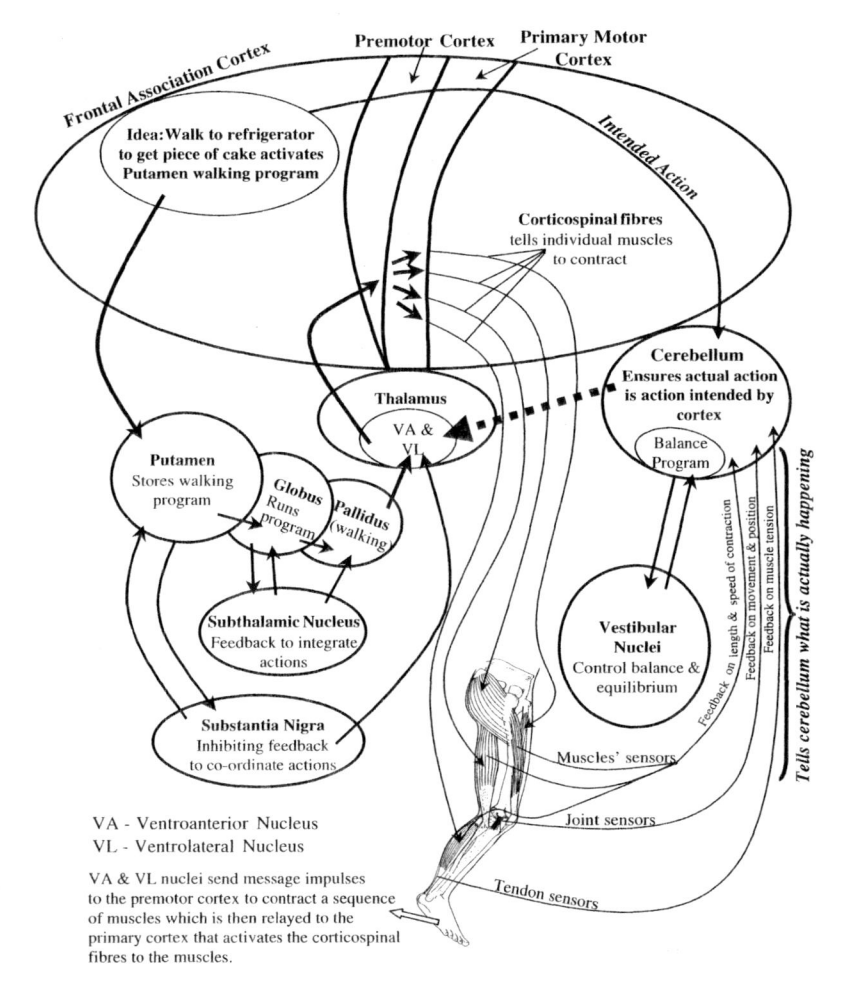

Figure 8.2. Simplified wiring of walking.

subconscious levels. The more specific the intent, the more the frontal lobes of the brain are involved. In the example above, we have been talking about a largely automatic process: walking. But activities that require novel motor activity, such as learning to juggle; or very precise motor activity, like trying to thread a needle, are controlled by conscious action to a much larger degree, supported by the subconscious movement centres.

Every movement is a sensory-motor event. Approximately 70 percent of all proprioception is from movement and provides much of the raw sensory data about our environment. In fact the brain is said to be 'proprioceptively driven'.[8] This constant input maintains activation of the reticular activating system, the system within the brain that allows you to be alert and pay attention. Learning can only occur if we can pay attention.

Movement, in fact, is one of the major reinforcements to learning. To really 'get something down' mentally, some type of movement activity is usually involved; either speaking, writing or physical action. Thoughts that are not spoken out loud, hence not involving muscle movement, are much less likely to be remembered than those you have voiced. For most people, a major reinforcement to memory is to write down what they have thought about.

Have you ever woken up in the morning after an amazing dream, one full of fantastic thoughts? Because you didn't share the details of it with someone else verbally, nor write them down, within a few hours all you could bring to consciousness was the essence of the dream. On the other hand, if on waking, you had related it to your partner ('You wouldn't believe the weird dream I just had') you would certainly be able to remember the details perhaps days later.

Why is movement so essential to learning? Part of the answer lies in the fact that the constant sensory input and processing maintains active development of neural networks within the brain. These networks are constantly being sculpted by dendrite formation and pruning. New mental or motor activity generates an outburst of dendritic formation, creating new connections within the brain. If these new connections are not reinforced, they will be pruned, literally reabsorbed by the cell body, because maintaining neuron function is an energetically expensive business. The brain only puts energy into maintaining those connections it is actively using.

Another important benefit to the nervous system of movement is that muscular activities, particularly consciously controlled co-ordinated movements, appear to stimulate the production of neutrophins, natural substances that stimulate nerve growth and increase the number of nerve connections in the brain.[9] The more precise the movement the more developed the neural networks become.

As previously discussed, there are strong links between the motor cortex and the reasoning/thinking parts of the frontal lobes. Initially, most planning/thinking is object and movement related. This is particularly true for children.

'I want the ball over there'. The brain is now occupied with neural activity to plan a movement strategy to fulfill this conscious desire. Even in later life, most people find the need to turn conscious thoughts into motor activity by discussing, writing, or drawing pictures of ideas to further refine them. When people tell stories, notice how often they gesticulate to reinforce the words with actions. Movement stimulates increasing diversity of the connections, allowing thought to spread beyond its original focus.

MOVEMENT AND SENSORY EXPERIENCE

Movement is critically important for vision. The eyes are never still because the retinal receptors only fire by changes in contrast. Every time the eye is moved horizontally across a vertical edge, the vertical field cells fire, informing the brain that there is a vertical edge. This rapid, constant oscillation of the eyes is not seen when you look at another person's eyes because it is below the flicker-fusion threshold so your vision melds the eyes you are looking at into a static image. Nevertheless without this continuous tremour or microsaccades, vision ceases.[10]

If you find yourself staring, how much information are you taking in? For active learning to occur, the external eye muscles are constantly moving the eyes to take in new information.

One of the marvels of human experience is our ability to take in visual information while our bodies are moving. This is due to the vestibulo-ocular reflex (VOR) that coordinates body and head movement with eye movement to provide a stable platform for vision.[11] Attempt to read this book while you hold the book still and move your head back and forth about three times a second. Did you have any trouble reading?

Now hold your head still and moving the book back and forth at three times a second. You are certainly going to find it much more difficult to read because while your VOR was compensating for your head movement and keeping your eyes fixed on the words on the page in the first instance, in the second, the words were blurred because they are moving back and forth through your visual field.

Likewise when you are walking or running, your head is constantly moving and yet, you perceive a stable visual environment. This is due to the VOR linking your eye muscle movement to the vestibular system controlling body movement. In fact, 80 percent of the nerve endings in the muscles of the body are directly linked, via proprioception and the vestibular system, with motor nerves running to and from the eyes.[12]

Since approximately 70 percent of sensory input for humans is visual, vision plays a large role in learning. Movement initially leads and shapes vision as a baby develops awareness of itself and its environment, largely by movement. Then it begins to watch the movement of its limbs, creating neural networks linking movement and vision. But later, vision plays a major role in the elaboration of neural networks involved in the conscious activation of movement. This is the basis of hand-eye coordination, which develops as babies reach for objects. Hand-eye coordination allows them to bring the objects closer for observation and learning. In these early learning experiences the hand tends to lead the eye.[13]

It is interesting to note that people blind from birth represent perspective when drawing in the same way that sighted people do. For instance, edges and angles are similarly represented and a table drawn by such a blind person is readily recognised by a seeing person. Clearly the blind person's knowledge of shape and form must be almost entirely proprioceptively derived.

As the child develops more elaborate neural networks, by myelination (insulation) of tracts in the brain and spine, through practice and maturation, hand-eye coordination develops to the point that the eye leads the hand movement. We learn to connect movement to our sight. This connection can then be internalised, allowing mere visualisation to actually provide a template for movement.

Visualisation techniques are currently used in modern sports training to improve motor performance. There have been studies done in which athletes, who only visualised in detail the motor functions involved in their sport, were compared with other athletes who physically practised their sport. As long as the visualisation was specific and complete (each individual movement was fully visualised) it proved to be as effective as actual physical practice.[14]

Other research has shown that precise internal visualisation of an action causes microstimulation of the muscles involved in performing that action.[15] If we look at this feedback loop from the other direction, physical movement can also stimulate the thinking areas of the brain. This is the basis of the exercises we use to help co-ordinate mental activity.

Hearing is also very dependent on movement. The ability to orient to a sound in our environment is critical for our survival. In fact, hearing is one of the first of the complex senses to fully develop in the womb. It has been found that a foetus can orient itself to sounds in the near vicinity. After birth, between six and nine months of age, the vestibular control of the neck muscles and the auditory system become linked in a neck-righting reflex designed to co-ordinate head movement with sound.[16]

The development of these neural networks allows us to turn our head towards the sound source, so the eyes can 'see' what made the noise and evaluate it for potential meaning. For example, you are stepping on to a roadway and you hear a car horn. You turn your head to locate the sound source and decide what to do next.

Sometimes, after a child is hit by a car, the driver will swear: 'He just stepped off the curb in front of me. I was beeping the horn like crazy! I can't believe he didn't hear it.' The child may have had such confused neural processing in his sound-orienting mechanism that he mistook the direction of the sound. The child had heard the sound as coming from the right and so was looking that way. Seeing no danger he proceeded to step off the curb.

To give a remarkable illustration of this phenomenon, a 13-year-old girl I saw in my practice was having a correction using sound. She wore a pair of headphones connected to an audiometer, an instrument that generates pure tones of different frequencies and volumes. A tone of 3000 Hz (in the middle of the speech range) at 80 decibels (bordering on the pain threshold) was played into her right ear. She reported only hearing the sound in her left ear. She was so convinced that the sound was only in her left ear that I put the headphones on myself to check. The right earphone said Right, and had a red cable going into it. The left earphone said Left and featured a blue cable. When I turned on the audiometer, I heard a loud sound in my right ear. I put the headphones back on the girl, turned on the audiometer, and she said 'It's still in my left ear.'

The audiometer was being used for auditory stimulation as a corrective technique for the auditory confusion the girl displayed. After 90 seconds of stimulation at this frequency and volume, suddenly she stated, 'It's in my right ear.' And thereafter she correctly oriented to sounds. That exact frequency at that volume for that period of time apparently caused her auditory system to entrain and reorient to the correct side.

Because of the extreme auditory confusion she displayed, I asked her mother if her daughter had ever suffered a head injury. Her mother replied that she had a 360 degree skull fracture as the result of going through the windscreen of a car. The mother also said the auditory confusions I had demonstrated might explain why the girl had not been able to stay in the same room if more than two people had been talking at the same time. 'She just gets distressed and goes to her room where she turns on her stereo very loudly.' Imagine having several people talking to you, and hearing the speech coming from the opposite direction each time. The stress would soon overload your ability to coherently process incoming auditory information. A prudent option would be to check out.

MOVEMENT AND THE VESTIBULAR SYSTEM:

Paying Attention.
Any movement also activates the vestibular system, which co-ordinates our equilibrium, balance and posture. The vestibular system is made up of three

parts: The vestibular apparatus of the inner ear, which provides information on head position and movement; the VOR linking eye and head movement; and cerebellar feedback from proprioceptors of the neck, which give information about head movement relative to the body.[17]

Sensory input from all three of these systems is fed into the vestibular nuclei, which are four nuclei lying on each side of the medulla oblongata and pons of the brainstem (see Fig. 8.3). The vestibular nuclei integrate the sensory inputs and then adjust the muscular tone of the body, especially the core muscles controlling posture to maintain our balance and equilibrium. Whenever the vestibular nuclei are activated, they stimulate the reticular activating system (RAS) of the brainstem. The RAS is a reticulum (mesh) of nerve pathways carrying impulses from the sensory systems; medulla, and pons to the midbrain and cerebral cortex.[18] RAS stimulation is like a 'wake-up call' to the brain, alerting it to the receipt of relevant sensory information.

As long as the sound in our environment is constant, it constitutes a background noise to which we pay no attention. An unusual noise, however, activates the RAS, sending alerting signals to the cortex to pay attention. 'What was that bang?' Once you've identified that it was just a car back-firing, the traffic noise will once again merge into the background. Turning on the RAS is like a nudge in the ribs, notifying the brain that some sensory or motor event of note has just happened. The call to attention from the RAS is essential to allow us to take in information and to respond to our environment which is, by definition, the basis of all learning.

The integration of the cerebral cortex, eyes, hearing, the vestibular system and feedback from the core muscles, is central to the learning process as all are important in maintaining attention to the world around us. Therefore movement, particularly of the core muscles, provides an external means of stimulating the RAS, alerting the brain to pay heed and prepare to take in and consider the information received. When the RAS 'turns off' or is not stimulated, our attention wanders and we tend to fall asleep or have difficulty concentrating. If the cerebellar, auditory and visual inputs are suppressed or confused, the vestibular system, through movement of the body, is the wake-up call of last resort.

Children who can only activate their RAS by movement can't sit still and concentrate. This may be one of the factors behind hyperactivity. As soon as they sit still, the RAS tends to turn off, which means their attention wanders and in order to wake up their brain, they move. Then they are told to sit still and pay attention. To them, this is an oxymoron or a contradiction in terms. Research has shown that 94 to 97 percent of children with dyslexia and specific learning difficulties displayed electronystagmograms (ENG) indicating cerebellar/vestibular dysfunction of some kind.[19] ENG measures co-ordinated movement of the eye muscles. This difficulty in co-ordinated movement of the eyes often leads to reading problems as the eyes tend to both overshoot and/or undershoot words on the page. The eyes tend to jump rather than track smoothly. Often so much effort goes into the control of eye movement that reading comprehension is poor.

As you can see from Figure 8.4, which depicts the actual tracking pattern of a person with ENG dysfunction, people with disturbed eye muscle co-ordination, tend to jump back and forth along a line, and often jump between lines as they attempt to control the tracking of their eyes across the page. A normal reader would move their eyes in a co-ordinated sequential pattern across the page. Just notice how long it took each reader to complete the same line. You can also compare the order in which the information is presented to their brain as each numbered vertical stroke indicates a fixation, or a place where the eye stopped to take in information.

Clearly movement both defines and activates the brain, establishing the state of alertness necessary to pay attention to relevant information. At the same time, movement is important for the establishment of co-ordinated visual and auditory reflexes essential in the learning process. Hence, movement is

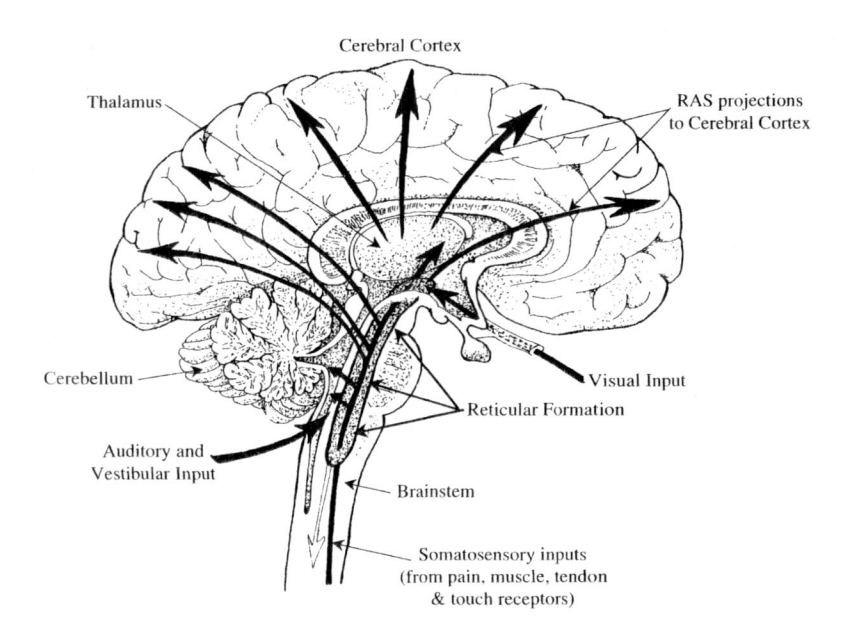

Figure 8.3. The Reticular Activating System. This system is a diffuse network of brainstem and midbrain nuclei involved in maintaining conscious arousal necessary to pay attention.

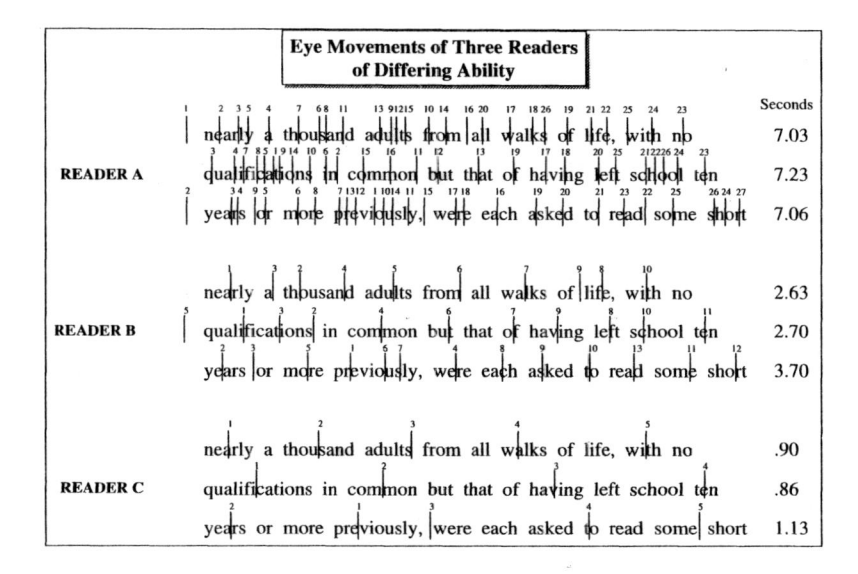

	Eye Movements of Three Readers of Differing Ability	Seconds
READER A	nearly a thousand adults from all walks of life, with no qualifications in common but that of having left school ten years or more previously, were each asked to read some short	7.03 7.23 7.06
READER B	nearly a thousand adults from all walks of life, with no qualifications in common but that of having left school ten years or more previously, were each asked to read some short	2.63 2.70 3.70
READER C	nearly a thousand adults from all walks of life, with no qualifications in common but that of having left school ten years or more previously, were each asked to read some short	.90 .86 1.13

Figure 8.4. Electronystigmograms giving the number and order of fixations for three different readers. Reader A, a poor reader, demonstrated ENG dysfunction, while Reader B is an average reader and Reader C a fast reader. Note how long it took each reader to read the same line.

critical to the development and maintenance of the neural networks by which we learn. All the processes described here explain why people with severe physical disabilities often have difficulties fully developing their learning potential. They can often observe the world with sight and sound, but cannot engage their world through movement.

SELF HELP FOR A DISINTEGRATED BRAIN

A number of techniques are available to an individual who has lost brain integration. They are based on three forms: acupressure techniques, physical movement and emotional stress defusion.

Acupressure techniques, as we have explained, basically involve either the rubbing or holding of specific acupoints to stimulate electromagnetic reintegration of the brain. Physical movement techniques can activate neurological flow within the nervous system, which can then help to reintegrate neurological flow within the brain. Emotional stress defusion techniques can serve to dissolve blocks causing brain disintegration that have arisen from emotionally traumatic events in your life, many experienced in early childhood.

As we explained in Chapter 2, many of these techniques originated with, and have been developed most fully in Educational Kinesiology, or Edu-K, and in One Brain Kinesiology. Dr Paul Dennison, the founder of Edu-K, was a person who had great difficulty learning, but, as is often the case with such people, he also recognised that he was quite clever. As a young adult, he became exposed to Touch for Health and Applied Kinesiology techniques and these had a profound impact on his ability to learn. He saw that by doing these techniques he could improve his function beyond anything he had previously been able to achieve.

He spent the next years of his life investigating and working out new techniques by borrowing from various practices like yoga and acupressure. By integrating these findings, he developed Educational Kinesiology and, with his partner Gail Hargraves (now Dennison), further developed a practical self-help program known as Brain Gym.[20] Brain Gym concentrates on acupressure stimulation and more particularly on physical movement to improve brain function. Because he wanted the young children he worked with to use these techniques, he prudently avoided calling it 'homework', instead calling it 'homeplay'.

Gordon Stokes, one of the founders of Three-In-One Concept's One Brain Kinesiology program, was also very dyslexic as a child. In fact he considered himself one of the dumbest kids in his class. He completed a stint in the navy and later came across kinesiology, which profoundly improved his learning skills. Stokes got deeply involved in kinesiology and, with his partners, evolved a program similar to Dennison's. They applied it to correcting dyslexic dysfunction, focusing their program on the emotional basis of dyslexia. Using kinesiology, acupressure techniques and especially emotional stress defusion and age recession techniques, they showed that the emotional causes of much dyslexic dysfunction may be overcome.[21]

FURTHER ACUPRESSURE TECHNIQUES

Simple acupressure techniques can be used to stimulate reintegration of brain functions. Physical massage or even just holding specific acupoints stimulates the flow of Ch'i along the related meridian pathways. Flow of Ch'i, as demonstrated earlier, stimulates underlying neurological flow and causes physiological response within the body.

Acupressure for Switching
One of the first set of acupoints that was shown to affect brain function was the K-27s. Applied kinesiologists observed that whenever K-27s were active

there was also usually right/left confusion and very commonly letter reversal. Merely massaging these points would often eliminate the right/left confusion. Clearly, brain function had been changed in a positive way via this incredibly accessible technique. It was later found that by holding Central Vessel 8 (the navel) at the same time, a more complete circuit was established and better effects resulted.

This type of brain confusion was termed 'switching' by the early Applied Kinesiologists. Switching indicated by active K-27s was found to be only one of three types of brain confusion. Other types of switching were soon discovered, which could also be corrected by acupoint stimulation. Although switching represented physiological and mental confusion, it was also believed to represent electro-magnetic polarity reversal within the brain.

The body and the brain have polarity, which is a predominance of positive or negative charge within one body region. For example, the right front quadrant of the body, the right side of the face, trunk, arm and leg, are all slightly more positive in charge than negative. Likewise the left side is slightly more negative than positive. In the brain itself, the right side of the brain tends to be more negative than positive and the left more positive than negative. In Chinese terms these represent the qualities of Yin (negative) and Yang (positive).

Right/left switching: Everybody has experienced giving directions when they pointed right but said, 'Turn left here'. This is not deception but mental confusion. They genuinely became confused about the location of right and left. Often this is only a momentary circumstance, but for others it may be a constant state of confusion. I have a friend who told me, 'Don't tell me to turn right or left. Point which way you want me to go because I always get them mixed up and will invariably turn the wrong way.' Stimulating acupoints, it didn't take long to straighten him out, and he's been able to follow directions accurately ever since.

Acupressure for right/left switching: Hold Central Vessel 8 (the navel); then take your thumb and index and middle fingers and locate the twin depressions on the chest below the end of the collar bones at the sternum (K-27s). Press gently and note any tenderness. Then, massage them gently in a circular fashion. Sometimes when you start rubbing, one or the other of these points, or both, may become tender, indicating an energy block of some kind. Even when there is no tenderness present, continue to rub these points for 15 to 30 seconds. At the end of this time or when the tenderness has disappeared, the reversal of polarity will have been corrected, at least temporarily (see Fig. 8.5).

Neurologically right/left switching appears to represent blocked flow in the commissural pathways; the corpus callosum and the anterior commissure, or deeper subconscious brain areas. The simple acupressure stimulation appears to reinstate the neurological flow through these important connections as the previous confusion is instantly eliminated.

An alternate procedure for correcting right/left switching is taken from the ancient science of yoga. It has also been observed that when we breathe air in through our nostrils, the air becomes ionised, or charged. Air flowing in through the left nostril becomes slightly more negatively charged than positively charged. In contrast, air flowing in through the right nostril becomes slightly more positively charged than negatively charged.[22] In the eastern traditions it is believed that breathing predominantly through the left nostril (negative ionization) will activate right hemisphere functions. Likewise breathing predominantly through the right nostril (positive ionization) will activate the left hemisphere functions. Research has shown that a simple breathing exercise enables the alteration of brain dominance in the short term.[23]

It is interesting to note that the flow of air naturally alternates from one nostril to the other in approximately 90 minute cycles.[24] First more air flows in through the left nostril than the right, activating predominantly the right hemisphere. Then it changes to more air flowing in through the right nostril, activating the left hemisphere. Yoga has taken advantage of this natural cycle. By alternately blocking one nostril and breathing in, and then blocking the nostril you just breathed in through and breathing out the other nostril, you cause activation of only one hemisphere.

Reversing the procedure causes activation of the other hemisphere. This very powerful yoga technique is called 'Nadi Shodan', or alternate nostril breathing, and is practised precisely to balance right/left brain function.[25]

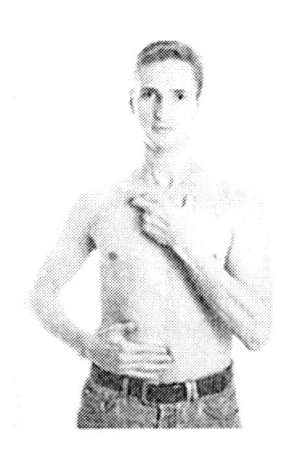

Figure 8.5. K27s for Right/Left Switching. The right and left K27's are rubbed with the thumb and index and middle fingers of one hand while the other hand holds CV8, the navel. This process is done for approximately 15-30 seconds and then the hands are reversed and the process repeated.

Doing five to 10 rounds of this exercise is often enough to reintegrate right/left brain functions, thereby eliminating mental confusion (see Fig. 8.6).

I know an older woman who had experienced two fits a year apart, both at Christmas, when a lot of family tension surfaced. She was then placed on an anti-epileptic drug, which caused problems with her physical co-ordination and appeared to increase her mental confusion. Prior to the treatment for the seizures she had been a sprightly, alert person who enjoyed creative writing. After some time on the drugs she became so shaky that she could not even lift a cup of tea to her lips without spilling it. She could no longer write and was told she should never drive again.

After she was advised to practice Nadi Shodan by a swami, which she did

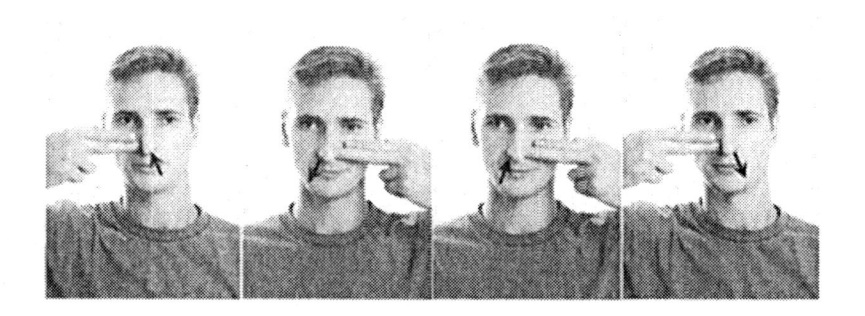

Figure 8.6. Nadi Shodan. Alternate nostril breathing balances ionisation and right/left brain function. First the right nostril is blocked and you breathe in through the left nostril, then blocking the left nostril you breathe out through the right nostril. You then breathe in through the right nostril and then blocking the right nostril you breathe out through the left to complete one round of nadi shodan.

several times each day for six months, she slowly withdrew her medication. She then found she could go back to creative writing, could once again work happily in her garden and drink a cup of tea. She was driving again within a year and has not had another fit.

Top/Bottom Switching: While top/bottom switching does affect mental processing its results are not as apparent as right/left switching. It is perhaps best appreciated for its physical effects. If you sedate an upper body muscle, such as the biceps, it should immediately relax or unlock. But if top/bottom switching is present, instead of the biceps unlocking, a lower body muscle, the hamstrings, will relax or unlock. This is because there has been confusion in the brain about the location of the upper and the lower body.

226 *A Revolutionary Way of Thinking*

Mentally, this is usually represented by people demonstrating a lack of integration between the top of their brain (the thinking cortex) and the deeper lower brain (the limbic feeling centres). When this switching is active and ongoing people may demonstrate one of two behavioural patterns. They will tend to be 'all in their head' and only able to think about things. They will have little ability to 'get in touch with their feelings'. When you ask them how they feel about something they will either answer with, 'I don't know', or 'I think . . .'.

The other pattern is someone who cannot get out of their emotions. They will tend to be so in touch with their feelings that most of their life is lived as a reaction to their feeling states. When you ask what they think they will tell you, 'I feel . . .'

Acupressure for top/bottom switching: Hold the index finger of one hand to the dent just below the centre of the nose on the upper lip, which is the 26th acupoint at the end of the Governing Vessel. With the thumb of the same hand touch the dent below the centre of your lower lip (the 24th acupoint on the Central Vessel). At the same time, hold the other hand on Central Vessel 8 (the navel). Hold these points for 15 to 30 seconds and usually a gentle pulse will arise under the fingertips, indicating a reintegration of top/bottom brain functions. Then the hands are reversed and the process repeated.

Neurologically, top/bottom switching appears to represent blocked flow in the projection fibres that carry information from the cortex to the sub-cortical

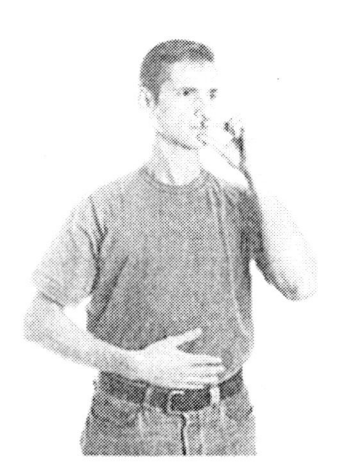

Figure 8.7. Top/bottom Switching. The thumb and index finger of one hand are held to the dents just underneath the lower lip and just above the upper lip (CV24 & GV26) while the other hand holds CV8, the navel. These points are held for 15-30 seconds and then the hands are reversed and the process repeated.

areas of the brain, including the limbic system, and from these sub-cortical centres back to the cortex.

Front/back switching: As in the case of top/bottom switching there is no overt indication of this type of switching. However, again it is represented physically. If the biceps is again sedated, instead of it unlocking or turning off, the triceps muscle on the back of the arm will turn off instead. This indicates confusion in the brain between the front and back of the body.

At the mental level this refers to processing within the frontal lobes of the brain versus the lobes at the back of the brain. The frontal areas are where

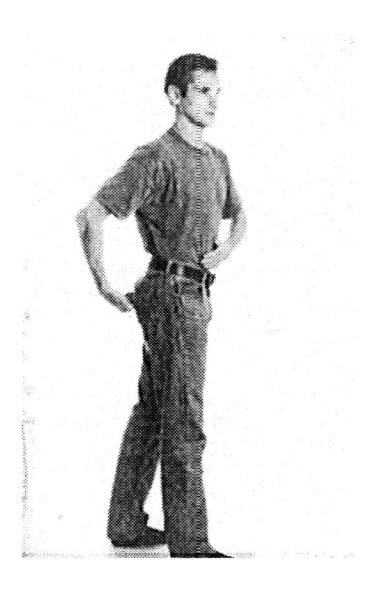

Figure 8.8. Front/back Switching. One hand is placed on CV8, the navel while the index and middle of the other hand massage the tip of your tail bone (GV1) for approximately 15-30 seconds. The hands are reversed and the process repeated.

we do our associational thinking, planning and synthesizing of new experiences. The lobes at the back of the brain are more involved with storage of memories of what has happened and the processing of on-going sensory events involving sight, sound and touch.

For mental processing to proceed normally we need to be able to effectively link our thinking with our memory and our on-line sensory processing. When there are any blocks to information flow between the front and back of the brain, what is usually lost is our 'now-time' thinking and we get trapped in our memories, which means we are largely left reacting to life out of what has happened in the past. People who demonstrate this on a continual basis can never seem to learn from life's experience; they just seem to repeat the same behaviour over and over because they are largely living from the past.

Being able to access the processing area of the frontal lobes, in a sense, allows you to be present in now-time. When this integration is lost, people tend to relate everything that happens to them in the moment to something that happened in their past. Thus life becomes a pageant of 're-actions' that prevents them from having truly dynamic 'inter-actions' with their life. While right/left switching strongly affects academic learning, because of the need to integrate right/left hemisphere functions, front/back switching has less observable impact on academic learning. It does however, have significant impact on learning life's lessons.

Acupressure for front/back switching: Hold Central Vessel 8 (the navel) with one hand and rub the first point on Governing Vessel, (the tip of the coccyx) with the other hand. Continue this rubbing for 15 to 30 seconds. Then the hands are reversed and the process repeated. This will reintegrate front/back brain function. Note that the tip of the coccyx is located below the shallow depression where the two buttocks meet at the end of the tailbone.

Neurologically, front/back switching appears to represent blocked flow in the association fibres that connect the front and back parts of the brain. Some of these fibres only flow for short distances while others run all the way from the back to the front of the brain.

When the brain is in a state of full integration, it can identify right, left, top, bottom, front and back, and they are all communicating with each other. Switching of any type results in loss of integration between some of these brain areas. Fortunately, this can be quickly rectified by the application of these acupressure techniques.

But the obvious question is, how long will this integration last? Quite simply, it depends on the nature of the factors causing the switching. If it is an instantaneous stressor, related to a particular circumstance, the correction may be long lasting. If, on the other hand, the switching resulted from an on-going stressor, it is likely to be a short-term correction with switching reappearing in a short time. Even though it may need to be repeated, at least you can put yourself into a more integrated state when you need to be fully functioning.

The next time you find yourself confusing right and left or feeling mentally jumbled, just rub these points as we have outlined above, and notice any difference in how you feel.

Acupressure for vision

Much of our learning is dependent on our visual processing. Reading is one of the most important life skills and is totally dependent on our ability to take in information through the medium of our vision. People may say we take in information with our eyes but vision involves much more than our eyes. The eyes are merely the portal through which visual information enters the brain, as we have already discussed, there are many layers of visual processing that must occur before we have a conscious visual perception.

Many people recognise that they have some difficulty with reading. This may be with the actual act of reading: stumbling over words, misreading words, or not comprehending what they read. When a person says I am having difficulty with reading, it means at one level that they are having difficulties integrating their visual processing.

Often difficulty in taking in visual information originates with poor teaming of the eyes. When we look at a word, both eyes should focus exactly on the same spot, as we move from word to word across the page, the eyes should operate together as a 'team', a process termed conjugate gaze. If however, the muscles that move the eyes are not synchronised with each other, the eyes may not focus accurately on each word and may jump as they track across the page. This can profoundly affect the inflow of visual information to the brain, compromising our ability to comprehend what we read.

Acupressure for integrating visual processing: The acupoints to help reintegrate eye muscle function are located on the front edge of the deltoid muscle, which is the muscle running from the crest of the shoulder down to the middle of the upper arm. The points can be located by moving your fingers down the front edge of this muscle until you feel a slight indentation. To make sure you are on the point, gently massage the muscle. If you are on the point it will usually be tender to almost painful. If the point you are touching is not at all tender you are probably not on the correct point. Keep moving your fingers until you locate a slightly sore spot.

Having located it, now rub up and down vigorously, while simultaneously moving your eyes from side to side for 10 to 15 seconds and then up and down for 10 to 15 seconds. Then alternately focus on your nose and then on a point in the distance for a further 10 to 15 seconds. When you subsequently return to any reading task, you should find it easier. Often people find their comprehension of what was read has also improved, often significantly. Again, this reintegrated state will remain only as long as there are no on-going factors causing a further loss of integrated function.

One of my earliest introductions to kinesiology was during a demonstration of Edu-K in which a young man was asked to read for the group. He read falteringly, pausing often and displaying very poor fluency. When asked what he had read he also revealed poor comprehension. These simple acupressure and visual integration techniques were applied and a little cross crawl (which we will describe later). He was asked to read again. I couldn't believe I was listening to the same person. He now read fluently, with no hesitation and with good intonation. He could also give a verbatim account of the text.

Acupressure for hearing

The other major channels for information flow into the brain are, of course, the ears. Hearing is the process of turning sound waves into information. When we are capable of hearing and understanding we say we are 'listening'. Many times children and adults have difficulty with listening. They can often hear what is said but have difficulty comprehending it.

Fortunately, there is an easy way to reintegrate your brain so that you may 'listen' rather than just hear. There are between 300 and 400 acupoints on and in the ear and when these points are stimulated the result is often improved auditory comprehension.[26]

Acupressure for auditory integration: Place your index finger behind the top of your ear, then take your thumb and gently unroll the curl of your ear, while simultaneously pulling the ear out and back. Continue to do this right along the curl of the ear from the top to the lobe. Doing this three times will activate reflexes that allow you to suddenly hear and listen more effectively. In fact, the ear will warm up which indicates that you have activated blood flow to the area.

Acupuncturists have identified more than 140 points along the back of the

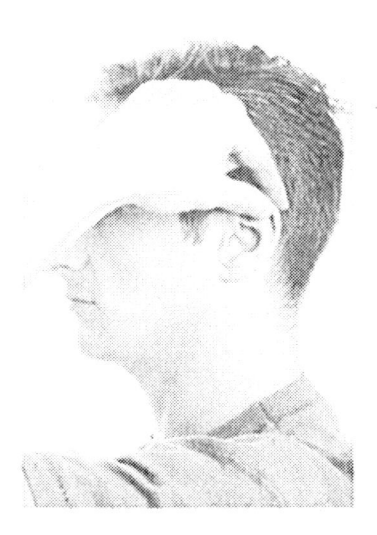

Figure 8.9. Thinking Caps. The thumb is applied to the top of the curl of the ear while the index finger is slipped behind the ear. The thumb is then rolled up and out pulling on the ear against the index finger behind the ear. This process is repeated pulling out on the curl of the ear from the top all the way to the lobe and is usually done three times.

ear that relate to motor functions of the body, starting with the feet near the top of the ear with the point representing the head lying at the lobe.[27] Stimulation of these points is said to activate and improve function in the associated muscles. Thus massaging all of these points is tantamount to giving yourself an acupressure body massage.

PHYSICAL MOVEMENT TECHNIQUES

As we have learned, much of the brain is involved in movement. Movement is essential for the development of the human brain. Witness a baby or a young child exploring their environment. They may use vision for distance information but they use touch and movement to understand their place in that environment.

Because the movement of the body is so complex there are a number of automatic reflexes that control much of our movement. Some of the most important of these control our posture and equilibrium, an integrated set of reflexes called the gait mechanism. If you should take a baby immediately after it is born and hold it vertically so that its feet touch a horizontal surface, it will automatically go through the motion of walking. Thus the reflexes that control walking are developed very early, long before the musculature and neurological fine control for this action are operational.

Other reflexes, the VOR, (vestibulo-ocular reflex), control head movement relative to the eyes in order to provide a stable platform for vision. Still others are involved with orienting the head with respect to sound. This arrangement clearly has survival value. Since we have right and left arms and legs, eyes and ears, it is obvious that the two sides need to work together. There are mechanisms to integrate the activity of the limbs and senses and indeed, the gait mechanism and the vestibulo-ocular reflex are two of the most important.

As we have explained, the right hemisphere receives sensory information from the left side of the body and controls the muscles of the left side, while the left hemisphere receives information from the right side of the body and controls the muscles of the right side. Clearly then, for the body to work in a co-ordinated way it requires that the brain can integrate the information coming from the right side with information coming from the left. Based on integrated sensory input, the brain then co-ordinates muscular activity. Hence, by initiating bilateral muscular activity, we are obviously stimulating integrated brain function.

Using this principal, cross-motor (opposite side) activities have been employed to integrate brain activity for more than a century. Several pioneers working with people who have severe learning or physical disabilities have developed successful programs designed to improve mental and physical function and these programs are based on a form of cross-lateral motor-patterning called 'cross-crawl'.[28]

There is a strong correlation between children who did not crawl as pre-toddlers and learning problems, in particular, reading difficulties. Often these children merely went from sitting to standing and then to walking. Others did not do normal cross-lateral crawling, but rather scooted on their bottoms or performed some variation of a crab scuttle. Due to the lack of development of certain types of integration within the brain they did not crawl normally. Because these same types of integration are also important in the co-ordinated eye movement involved in the process of reading, and apparently, in the mental coordination necessary to read and comprehend, lack of development of integrated motor function affects integrated brain function.

It is obvious why cross-crawl and muscular repatterning can so powerfully assist the re-establishment of integrated brain function. While for most people cross-crawl is a useful activity, there are individuals whose motor development is not sufficiently stimulated by cross-crawl for it to affect positive change.

Cross-crawl for brain integration

Cross-crawl is quite literally a matter of marching on the spot; moving your feet and knees up and down, in co-ordination, while moving your arms back and forth. The right arm must be coming forward when the left leg is coming up and the left arm has to be coming forward when the right leg is coming up. It is a simple, cross lateral muscular activity. Cross crawl is basically consciously walking on the spot.

Because it is a bilateral muscle activity involving a larger number of the muscles of the body, it creates considerable flow across the corpus callosum. When this is done routinely, the activity stimulates the development and myelination of neural-networks connecting the two hemispheres. Through this activity communication between the two hemispheres at both physical and mental levels is facilitated.[29]

These cross-crawl movements should be done consciously and slowly because it requires more mental involvement to run precise fine movements. Also when done slowly, the automatic compensations are much less likely to intrude. As the activity becomes easier the speed can be increased until it is a reflexive, fluid movement. It is best to do at least 20 strokes of cross-crawl per session, and two to three sets per day. For children, it is best done in the morning before school, after they return from school and again before doing their homework or going to bed. By a stroke we mean completing the whole right-left movement (i.e. right arm with left leg and left arm with right leg).

It is very important that the arms move freely from the shoulder and not from the elbow. The reason for this is that the gait mechanisms controlling arm and leg movement relate to specific muscles of the shoulder and hip, not the elbows and knees. Many people tend to move their arms from the elbows and fix their shoulders as a compensation to prevent the stress of trying to co-ordinate shoulder and hip movement.

While this sounds quite simple, for some people it can be very difficult not to move homolaterally (same side arm and leg). Such people sometimes require considerable practice for cross-crawl to become smooth and reflexive.

People who are very strongly homolaterally patterned often find it extremely difficult and, sometimes, almost impossible to perform cross-crawl, which is the normal marching action. It is unfortunate if such a person joins the army because they are often hounded mercilessly by the drill-majors and called 'square gaiters'. This is not to mention the havoc they cause to others in their squad.

While cross crawl practise may help these people to some degree, cross-crawl alone will not be enough to integrate their motor and mental function. In these extreme cases, they should seek the help of a qualified kinesiology practitioner or Applied Physiologist to provide repatterning procedures to help reorganise their gait mechanism imbalances.

Following acupressure stimulation for brain integration, cross-crawl acts as

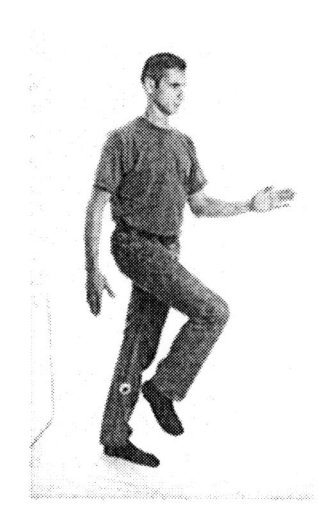

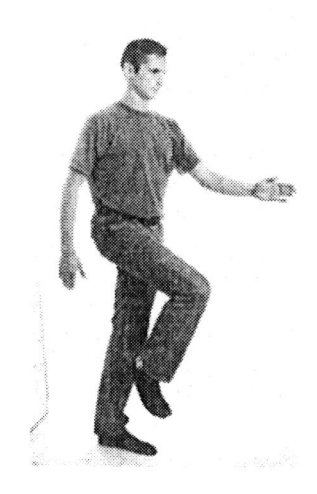

Figure 8.10a. Cross-crawl the wrong way. Arm moves predominantly from the elbow with shoulder held still.

Figure 8.10b Cross-crawl the correct way. Arm moves freely from the shoulder not the elbow.

a mechanism to reinforce this integrated state. Whenever you are feeling mentally disintegrated, stimulate the acupoints as above and follow it up with 20 strokes of cross-crawl. Notice how you feel now?

Lazy 8s for integrating visual function.
Drawing the Lazy 8, or infinity sign requires the person to cross the visual mid-line without interruption. In this way both right and left eyes are activated integrating the right and left visual fields. When the 8 is drawn on its side, it has a definite mid-point as well as distinct right and left areas joined by a continuous line.

Tracing or feeling movement along a small infinity sign, or Lazy 8, has been used for several decades in educational therapy to develop kinesthetic or tactile awareness in children with severe learning problems. Often this simple exercise has produced significant improvement. In 1974, Dr Paul Dennison adapted the Lazy 8s as part of his vision-training program and had students use the large muscles of their arms and upper body to draw the 8s on a chalk board or other graphic surface. Only when they had mastered these large muscle movements were they instructed to make smaller Lazy 8s using only the hands.[30]

Lazy 8s are good for people who have difficulty crossing the mid-line in vision, the most stressful area to visually integrate because it is the region of greatest overlap of the two visual fields. To take in information from the mid-line requires the two hemispheres to fully integrate their visual inputs.

People who have difficulty crossing the visual mid-line will have difficulty tracking, or smoothly moving the eyes from far right to far left and back again, which is precisely what you do when you read. For some, approaching the mid line becomes so stressful that their eyes will tend to jump to the other side of the page and then, when they are scanning back the other way, jump again. This of course can make reading very stressful and can affect reading comprehension.

I had a 12-year-old female client who demonstrated an extreme of mid-line jumping. When tracking a finger from right to left, her eyes would stop at the mid-line, and then loop over the mid-line and continue tracking on the other side. When moving from left to right her eyes would repeat this looping action at the mid-line and then move again smoothly to the right. After watching her do this for several passes I began to feel dizzy myself. When I asked her: 'Jane, do you ever lose your place when you're reading?' She replied, 'Oh, all the time. I'm always skipping lines.' I was astounded that she could even stay on the same page.

Another young lad, when asked to read, held the book in front of him, turned his head to the right and then moved his whole head back and forth while keeping his eyes stationary. When his head was held still he merely moved the book back and forth in his left visual field. Clearly he could not cross the mid-line.

To perform the Lazy 8s, the symbol is drawn on a piece of cardboard, chalkboard or whiteboard. It should be big enough and positioned at shoulder-level so that the full movement of shoulders, arms and upper body is required to track it. The accurate model gives the child something to trace accurately.

Beginning with the right side, you look down along your right arm to the point of the index finger and starting in the middle of the symbol, begin tracing the figure up to the left, down around and back across the mid-line, up to the right and down, around and back across the mid-line again and so on. This activity should also be done slowly and with full concentration at first. As the action becomes smoother and more fluid the speed may be increased but it should always remain a fully conscious activity.

Lazy 8s for vision should be done 20 times with the right hand, 20 times with the left hand and 20 times with both hands working together, with eyes looking directly down the point of the fingers.

For people who do have difficulty crossing the mid-line, it can take practice to make it accurate and it may initially require effort. But we have found this

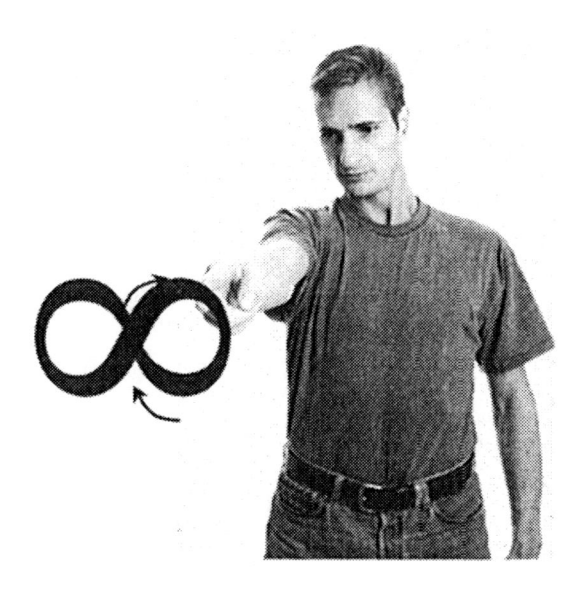

Figure 8.11. Lazy 8s for the Eyes. Sighting down the right index finger with the hand in the midline of the body, the hand is moved up to the left, down back through the centre point, up to the right, down around, back to the centre point and up to the left again in a continuous motion.

exercise helps children who have reading difficulties because the brain is being forced to move back and forth across the mid-line in a coordinated fashion. Apparently, having the finger to follow helps the eyes to resynchronise their co-ordinated function, while at the same time integrating eye and hand movement. It also appears to smooth out the neurological flow, improve co-ordinated eye movement and to enhance binocular and peripheral vision. This activity also strengthens the teaming of the eyes and their co-ordination with hand and body movement.[31]

It may also be done as a three dimensional exercise moving the finger close to and away from the eyes. Starting with the finger about 30 centimetres from the nose, the finger traces up and away from the face almost to the extent of the arm, down around toward the ground and then back up through the starting point toward the face, and then down in front of the nose toward the feet and then back up to the starting point.

Lazy 8s for eyes should be done before any visual activities such as reading, driving or watching films. Also, after you have been performing a visual function for some time—working on a computer, take a break and do some Lazy 8s for eyes. You will usually find that any eye strain will be greatly reduced.

Lazy 8s for integrating hand/eye activities

When we are writing we are using our hand, but the movement is controlled by the eyes. So once again you draw a Lazy 8 on a suitable surface as a model. It is often useful if an accurate model of the Lazy 8 is drawn in indelible marker on the white board with the child using an erasable marker. It should be traced as accurately as possible. If a white board is not available a chalk board or a large piece of paper or cardboard will suffice. The paper may be laminated so that the model remains intact and can be reused.

Start slowly with the right hand, moving up to the left as before. It is important to check the tendency to make one side bigger or squarer than the other. Once this has become a smooth activity, change to the other hand and repeat the process about 20 times, again until it is smooth and fluid. Finally, do it while holding the pen in both hands for a further 20 times.

Again it is important to consciously use large muscle movements initially in order to relax the muscles of the hands, arms and shoulders. Then reduce the size of the Lazy 8 as the action becomes more reflexive. Finally, they should be done on as small a scale as possible. Decreasing the size of the Lazy 8 shifts control of the action to smaller and smaller numbers of motor units of the hand and wrist—the same motor units which are used to write. Lazy 8s for writing should be done before performing any written work. These may be done as doodles. They are particularly good for children who have difficulty learning their alphabet, and also improve hand/eye co-ordination.

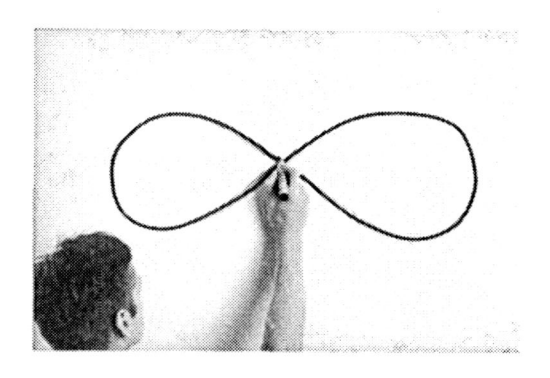

Figure 8.12. Lazy 8s for Writing. *The pen is held to the centre point of the lazy 8 on the board and moved up to the left, down in a circle and back through the centre point, up to the right, down around, back to the centre point and up to the left again in a continuous motion.*

They are helpful for writer's block and may be useful during exams.

For children, we sometimes call this 'doing racetracks', telling the child the pen is a car racing around the track. Of course, the driver at first must go slowly to make sure he stays on the track. Then he can go faster and faster but to win, he must stay on track.

Lazy 8s for integrating hearing: 'the elephant.'
In Edu-K, this is an exercise known as 'the elephant' because although it is similar to the tracing process of the last two exercises, this time you are putting your ear to your shoulder and extending your arm like an elephant's trunk. In this way your neck, shoulder and eye are engaged in one action.

Since the elephant predominantly relies on the core muscles involved with posture it strongly activates the vestibular system and as eye-body co-ordination is involved, it also stimulates the vestibulo-ocular reflex. Practicing this body-eye-hand movement involves establishing programs in the basal ganglia in conjunction with the cerebellum and the sensory and motor cortices of the parietal and frontal lobes.

You again trace the Lazy 8s about 20 times with the right ear/arm and then again with the left ear/arm. It is very good to get as much body movement into the exercise as you can comfortably manage because you are trying to integrate as much neurological flow as possible. This activity aids hearing because by putting your ear onto your shoulder you activate all the neck musculature related to orienting to the source of sound.

This exercise should be done before any language or auditory experience

238   A Revolutionary Way of Thinking

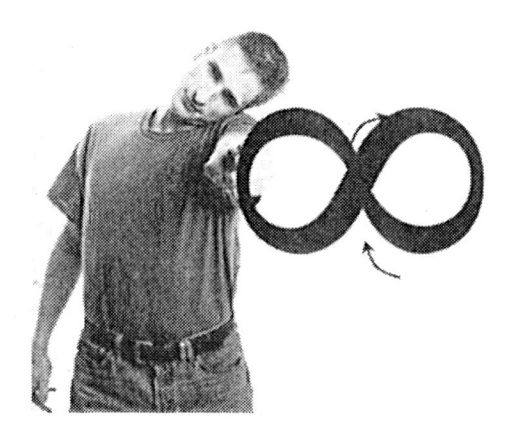

Figure 8.13. The Elephant for hearing. With the ear resting on the shoulder and sighting down the index finger with the arm extended in front of the body, the arm is moved up to the left, down back through the centre point, up to the right, down around, back to the centre point and up to the left again in a continuous motion.

and you can do it facing towards the sky or the horizon line with each side of the body. While you are performing the exercise, become aware of the changes in the energy flow in the neck which may be realised as a release of neck tension. The elephant is particularly useful for children who have been diagnosed has having Attention Deficit Disorder (ADD) because it strongly stimulates the RAS, helping the children to improve their attention.

A movement/energy exercise for the mind and body
The Cook's Hookups were invented by Wayne Cook, an expert in electromagnetic energy, to counterbalance the effects of electromagnetic stress, such as being in front of a computer, television or other appliances generating electromagnetic fields. He found that by using the following postures a calming, harmonising and integrating effect was produced on the mind and body. It is believed that it stimulates limbic and cortical integration as well as balancing the energy flows of the acupressure meridian system.

Originally Cook and Edu-K used a sitting position for the Hookups. The right ankle was placed on the left knee and the right hand grasped the ball of the right foot. Meanwhile the left hand grasped the right ankle. This pose was held for approximately one minute. Then both feet were placed flat on the floor and the fingertips of both hands brought together, with elbows comfortably at your sides. This pose was also held for about a minute.

Dr Paul Dennison recently modified the Cook's procedure which he calls 'Hookups' and this is now done standing or sitting. This is a two part procedure. In the first part, you sit comfortably, crossing the left ankle over the right. You then extend your arms, crossing the left wrist over the right and interlocking the fingers. Holding the fingers clasped together, the hands are moved up and through to rest comfortably on the chest with the elbows at your sides. You should now close your eyes, breathe deeply and relax for about one minute.[32] Optionally, you may press the tongue against the roof of the mouth on each inhalation and relax the tongue on each exhalation.

In part two, you open your eyes, uncross your feet, put them flat on the floor. Uncross your arms and touch your fingertips gently together and breathe deeply for about one minute.

Hookups have been shown to be very effective for hyperactive children or when children have outbursts, as it seems to allow them to bring themselves out of survival mode and into more conscious awareness of their situation. Carla Hannaford, a US neurologist and author of the wonderful book *Smart Moves*, worked with children aged 5–15 years old, labelled 'learning disabled

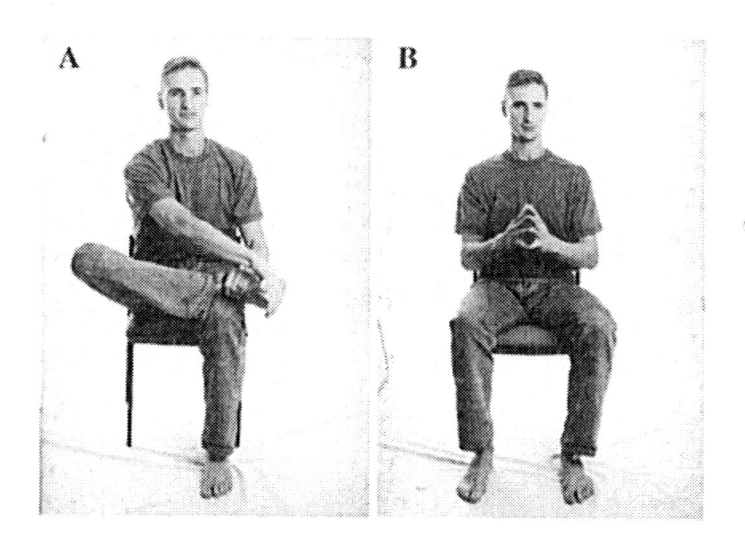

Figure 8.14. Hookups for Mind-Body Integration. Part A: Sitting comfortably in a chair the right ankle is placed on the left knee with the right hand grasping the right ball of the foot. The left hand grasps the right ankle and the person sits quietly for about one minute. Part B: The feet are then placed flat on the floor about shoulder width apart and the fingers tips of hands are held together with elbows comfortably at your sides for another minute.

and behaviourally disruptive'. She found Hookups an effective means of calming the children after fights or other emotional upsets. Whenever the children got into a skirmish she would have them do the Hookups for two minutes and by the end of that time often found them totally in control of their own behaviour.[33]

THE WHOLE IS WORTH MORE THAN THE SUM OF ITS PARTS

While we have presented these as individual exercises or techniques, of course they can be more effectively used together. When you become mentally confused, stressed or are having difficulty concentrating on your work, do a combination of these exercises. After a little experimentation, you will find a combination that works best for you.

As a suggestion, you may wish to sequentially rub your K-27s, hold the upper and lower lips, and rub the tip of your tail-bone while holding your navel. Then do 20 strokes of cross-crawl, followed by some Lazy 8s for vision. Then do the Hook-ups. You will be amazed at the difference in how you function and feel.

EMOTIONAL STRESS DEFUSION TECHNIQUES

There is another set of acupoints that can be used to reintegrate a brain that has become disintegrated as a result of emotional stress.

How many times in your life have you found yourself suddenly unable to think clearly when you are under a lot of emotional stress? You are having an argument with your spouse, or your child, and you find yourself just yelling at them. After the argument you may find yourself thinking: 'I should have said . . .'

The emotional stress of the argument had caused a momentary loss of your integrated brain function and in such a state you could not think, you could only react. At a later time when you had calmed down and the emotional stress had subsided, you were able to think straight again because your brain had reintegrated.

When we are able to access all of our brain functions and to integrate these functions, we look for creative solutions to problems in our life. We see life's issues as opportunities to be resolved and not as problems to be avoided. When we lose this integration, we tend instead to react on the basis of what has happened to us in our life. How can we overcome this tendency towards seemingly uncontrolled reaction?

In brief, whenever there is emotional stress, the blood flow is redistributed within the brain. The blood flow tends to be withdrawn from the frontal lobes where we plan and think creatively in a solution-oriented way, and is redirected to the deeper subconscious survival areas of the limbic system. These centres then activate memories of similar circumstance in our past and then merely replay what those past responses were to that circumstance. Hence we react rather than respond.

So how do we defuse these emotional stressors that cause brain disintegration? It would first require a change in the blood flow in the brain shifting us from survival mode into thinking mode. Fortunately, there are acupoints that allow us to perform this amazing feat.

Acupressure for emotional stress

By merely holding your thumb and fingertips to the centre of the broad bumps on the forehead, the 14th point on the Gall Bladder meridian (GB-14), with one hand, and holding the bony bumps at the base of your skull (GB 20) with your other hand, you will initiate this change in blood flow within the brain. If you are not sure where these points are, it may be easier to simply cover the forehead with your whole palm. Likewise cover the base of the skull with the other palm.

When you first hold the forehead points, you will generally be unable to detect any pulsations. After a period of time (the length depending on how stressed you are about what is on your mind), you will usually detect a subtle pulse at these points. It will be at the same intensity as a wrist pulse although it is not arterial. This is evidenced by the fact that the forehead pulses beat between 70 and 74 beats per minute, no matter how fast your heart is beating.[34] Once the pulses become synchronous and even, the defusion is complete.

It is interesting how people do this instinctively when they are under stress and having difficulty coping. You will see them bring their hands to their forehead and hold these points, even if it is only briefly. But in this time they have effectively reactivated the thinking and problem solving areas of their brain, giving them new options, allowing them to cope more effectively.

To test this technique, think about something that has happened to you within the last few days that has caused you either annoyance or irritation. Perhaps it was an argument you had with a friend. As you think about it, get a sense of what you really feel and where in your body you feel it. You will often find that you will have a tightness in the stomach, your jaw may clench and you may feel mental tension.

While continuing to think about this event, apply the acupressure techniques described above and be sure to breathe deeply. Once the pulses have appeared, or a minute or two has passed, then think again about the same event, and how you feel about it now. Most often you will find you just cannot

242 *A Revolutionary Way of Thinking*

contact those feelings again. The tightness in the stomach has disappeared and the mental tension has vanished.

If you wish to investigate this more thoroughly you can employ some basic kinesiology. When we are emotionally upset we feel it in our stomach—we get a 'gut feeling'. A pair of muscles that relate to stomach energy are called the clavicular division of the pectoralis major muscles (PMC). These are the chest (pectoralis) muscles attached to the collarbone (clavicle) that move the extended arm toward the midline.

To effectively monitor these muscles in kinesiology, the fibres of the muscle need to be straightened by holding your arm horizontally out to your side, with your palm open and rotated so that the thumb points towards the floor. With your other hand, feel just below the collarbone as you swing the straight arm to your front and then across the middle of your body. You will feel the muscle pop up.

If you then put both arms out, thumbs down and move the back of your hands together, both PMCs can be monitored at the same time by having someone try to pull your wrists apart. Since these are very strong muscles when they are locked they will strongly resist any attempt to part them. You

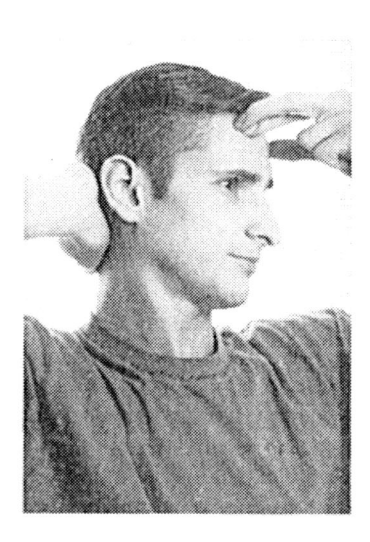

Figure 8.15. Emotional Stress Defusion—Frontal Occipital Holding. The palm of one hand is held across the base of the skull, while the thumb and index/middle fingers make contact with the broad bumps on either side of the forehead (the frontal eminences). These points are held until a gentle pulsing is felt beneath the thumb and fingers.

may wish to try this with a partner. Now, have the person whose PMCs were monitored locked and strong, think about a situation that has caused them annoyance or irritation and monitor the PMCs again. What happened? Most likely the arms just flew apart demonstrating the effects of stressful thoughts on your physical function.

Ask your partner to now perform Frontal Occipital Holding until they feel even pulses on your forehead, or until you feel the process is complete. Then once again, have them monitor both PMCs while you think of the issue. What happened this time?

Most likely the PMCs remained locked, indicating no further stress on this issue. Not only that, you will often be aware of a change in your feeling state, whereas before the defusion, whenever you thought of the issue you could feel it, usually in your gut. After the defusion, you can still think of it but there is just no feeling, no emotional charge in it.

You have not erased the memory of what happened, you have only integrated this experience into the greater context of your life, as one of life's little lessons. It doesn't matter what happens to us in our life, it is only how we feel about what happens that causes us distress.

A DAILY STRESS DEFUSION TECHNIQUE

The following simple emotional stress defusion procedure is offered as a means to reduce the stress in your life. All you have to do is use it—regularly.

Procedure one:
Every night when you come home from work or after a hectic day take a few minutes to do the following:

Step 1. Think of the day's events and if someone is available, have them monitor both of your PMC muscles at the same time (arms out, thumbs down, back of hands together). The person monitoring attempts to separate the backs of your hands by pulling gently on the inside of the wrists or forearms. If the PMC monitors unlocked (weak), you have carried stress from the day home with you. It would be best to resolve it now before it affects your interactions with your family and friends.

Step 2. If the muscles unlock, or you are aware that you feel stress, sit or lie down comfortably with your heels together and think over the day, particularly of any stressful situations. Really get into the feeling of the most stressful situation. Be aware of how you felt, any sounds, smells or sights that occurred and make it as real in your memory as possible because as you do so you will reactivate the neural circuits involved with these actual events.

Step 3. Move your heels apart about 45 centimetres. Now as you lie or sit quietly with your eyes closed, have the person perform Frontal Occipital Holding (one palm holding your forehead, the other holding the base of the back of the skull.) Wait until they, or you, feel gentle synchronous pulsations on the forehead. This may take anywhere from a few seconds to several minutes, depending on how stressful the situation was. Don't fret if you don't feel the pulsations, just remonitor the PMCs after a period of time. If the PMCs now lock, the stress has been resolved. Now, move your feet together and the defusion is complete.

Step 4. Then evaluate another stressful situation that has occurred in your day by repeating Step one above. Often the most apparently stressful situation will have been worked through during, or just after the time that it occurred. But there may be little things that remain unresolved, which will be stored away as emotional junk. Repeat Steps 2 and 3 for any event that still shows stress causing the PMCs to unlock. If there is no stress indicated on any situation, you have finished the defusion.

The whole process seldom takes more than five minutes so you will have the time to do it. All you need is the commitment. Just do it for several days and observe any difference in how you now respond to similar events in your life.

Procedure Two:
When issues arise at work that are stressful, take two to five minutes and do the following:

Step 1. Touch your heels together while thinking of the stressful situation (get the 'feel' of it). Then hold your own forehead and occiput and take your feet apart about 45 centimetres.

Step 2. Continue Frontal Occipital Holding until pulses appear equally on both sides of your forehead. Put your feet together.

Step 3. Reassess how you now feel about that previously stressful situation. You will often find a significant change in your feelings about what happened.

Step 4. Now take a deep breath, smile and get back to work.

Procedure Three:
This is a variation of Procedure One, which can be useful to resolve the stress of life's other tensions: problems in relationships, financial worries, or when you find it difficult to cope with challenges.

As in Procedure One, in step one evaluate the relevant situation for stress. If there is stress then continue with Steps 2 and 3.

Note. It is best *not* to do this with the person who is causing the tension in your life or who is involved in the on-going situation. In this case it is best if you do this procedure with a person external to the situation. From then on, you are better equipped to deal with the inevitable stresses of life.

While these self-help techniques may be a fantastic aid in dealing with many of life's issues and factors which may cause loss of brain integration, they are not the panacea to all of life's problems. For learning problems or issues generated by factors that have occurred early in childhood, and which may be causing persistent difficulty in coping with learning and life in general, the problems need to be addressed at a more proficient level by a qualified professional kinesiologist or Applied Physiologist.

The professional approach to resolving on-going brain disintegration on a more permanent basis will be discussed in the next chapter.

How to learn more
In this chapter we have only been able to give you a brief explanation and presentation of a few of the many types of self-help exercises and techniques you can do for your own brain integration and to relieve stress. There are several enjoyable workshops designed for lay people that enable them to learn more about these fascinating methods. For anyone interested in exploring more of these techniques, we highly recommend they attend an Edu-K Brain Gym workshop.

If you would also like to learn some basic kinesiology as well, we recommend that you attend a Basic One Brain, Touch for Health or Stress Release workshop. References for these workshops in your local area are given at the end of the book in Appendix C.

Chapter Nine

BRAIN INTEGRATION IN ACTION

DEEP INTERVENTIONS

In the last chapter we discussed a number of simple kinesiological and acupressure techniques that can help reintegrate brain function at the electromagnetic, neurological and emotional levels. For many of the simpler types of problems that are triggered by temporary stressors, these techniques may be just the trick to make the difference, at least in the short term.

For those people who have long-term on-going loss of brain integration resulting from experiences traumatic enough to permanently shut down part, or most of the communication across their corpus callosum, or who experience the massive brain confusion that we call deep level switching, more specific and direct interventions are required to resolve these more difficult causative issues.

This is where the role of the qualified kinesiologist or Applied Physiologist comes to the fore because at present we do not know of any other treatment modality that can so dynamically interact with on-line brain processing, or that allows the integrity of brain functions to be so directly assessed. Using only a few specific muscle tests, whole configurations of brain functions such as the integration of visual processes, can be accurately discerned.

THE EVOLUTION OF A NEW KINESIOLOGICAL PARADIGM

During the late 1980s, I was doing a lot of clinical work with children with severe learning problems, who were being referred by a child psychologist as a gesture of last resort. She described them as her 'basket cases' because no amount of remedial work seemed to make the slightest difference to their academic performance. Using the kinesiological tools I had available at the time, I was able to get fantastic, reproducible results in about 30 percent of these cases. Following treatment, three in 10 of the children improved their reading ability and comprehension, spelling and were better at maths. Moreover, these improvements were on-going.

In another 30 percent of cases, even though I did the same procedures, nothing seemed to work. And in the remaining 40 percent of clients, there would be significant changes while I was working with them but they did not last; as soon as they stopped the treatment and their self-help exercises, the children would resort to being just as dysfunctional as they had been before. As a scientist, I had to know why this was happening. Why were the results so variable? Why was it working for some and not for others?

To find out, I went back to first principles and began an exhaustive search of all the material I could find on the neurology of brain function related to learning, to establish exactly what processes were involved. The critical point turned out to be the subconscious, where so much of our actual mental processing takes place. So I looked carefully at the subconscious features of the brain that were not being addressed in the treatment models I was using. This meant the limbic system and its various nuclei and the paleocortex, the ancient part of the brain.

Kinesiology as it was then practiced, allowed me to access these structures only in a very general way. I could detect that there were stresses related to specific learning processes but did not understand how to go beyond this first step to tap into the hierarchical processing of the brain to determine which specific brain functions might have gone off-line. What had become clear to me is that the brain processed in a modular fashion, with single functions antecedent to many other functions. If one of these antecedent functions was compromised, all the processes dependent on this function would also show deficits. I had to find a way to get into these processing modules.

Just as these problems were arising for me, synchronicity stepped in with the solution. In 1989 I travelled to America to learn the new techniques of brain physiology formatting that Richard Utt had been developing at his International Institute of Applied Physiology. Utt had added to the existing model of kinesiology by focusing on the physiology of the brain itself and he showed that the readout of brain function seldom revealed itself in single active acupoints. The biofeedback from the brain would often show up as a patterns of acupoint activity.[1]

With Utt's brain physiology formatting at last I had the map of the primary neurological processing modules and a basic format to access them. Now I had a way in and from there on it was a matter of asking the right questions of the right structures. Now, for instance, I could ask the brain if there was any stress in the posterior hypothalamic nuclei? If a stress was present as indicated by muscle response, I could then proceed to determine if there was stress in the part of the posterior hypothalamic function that controlled dilation of the pupils in relation to the fight or flight response.

Once the stress had been identified then the factors causing that stress could be pinpointed. When I discovered what those stresses were, I could then apply kinesiological and acupressure techniques to resolve them. As we have outlined previously, in the case of dysfunction in communication across the corpus callosum, as soon as the stress, or stresses that have caused the block or shutdown of functions are resolved, these processes so vital to learning will come back on line.

I began to get much better results and consequently, many more patients. I was getting so busy that I needed a partner. Susan McCrossin, another Melbourne kinesiology student who had gone to America at the same time as me to do the Applied Physiology training, came to mind. I knew she was looking for a meaningful career change and was a highly motivated individual with a very rational mind, so I figured that we would probably work very well together. I asked her if she was interested in joining me as a clinical partner. She was.

As we began to work together we discovered that the more we refined application of the new formatting techniques, the more effective we were proving to be. But still we were running into children we couldn't help. We needed to do more research, more trialling of technique and application. We needed to head off together into the unknown with a fairly rudimentary set of tools. It was frustrating, exhilarating and amazing and every week we got new ideas and techniques that were working.

More children, by now between 80–90 percent of the referred cases, started showing positive changes yet perplexingly, there still remained a recalcitrant group that eluded our methods. What was it that we did not yet understand? To find out, we sent these children for assessment by a neurologist who specialised in epilepsy and learning problems. Using Magnetic Resonance Imaging and other assessment techniques, it was revealed that in all but one of the cases the underlying cause was organic brain damage.[2] Their problem was more than a glitch in the software. The hardware itself had been damaged.

DAMAGED HARDWARE

Organic Brain Damage
Some dysfunctions in the brain equate to brain damage, a term that generally conjures up the image of someone slobbering, unable to speak or who is quite obviously physically dysfunctional. A truer definition refers to a condition that we all have to some degree.

A few years ago, a neurologist friend was writing an atlas of the brain based on an improved method of Magnetic Resonance Imaging (MRI) to be used in the assessment of organic brain damage, particularly as it relates to epilepsy. Because there are so many different types of potential brain damage, he decided to try to find a 'normal' brain to scan slice by slice to which all damaged brains may be compared. The problem was finding a 'normal' brain. Every time he scanned what he thought was a 'normal' brain, there was some evidence of slight to major brain abnormality, even though the person possessing this abnormal brain behaved and functioned normally.

He scanned the radiologist who ran the MRI, a physicist by training, only to find a whole area of her brain was atrophied. The effected area is specifically involved in the spatial functions used to read maps. On seeing this, he happened to flippantly comment, 'You must get lost going to the toilet'. Her husband happened to be present, and he burst out laughing, 'You can say that again! If I took her two blocks from here and gave her a map to get back, and she was not allowed to ask anybody directions—we'd never see her again!'

Clearly she had organic brain damage, but because she was able to ask directions and all her other faculties were intact, she could compensate, and it was only people close to her like her husband that had any idea she had a brain dysfunction of any kind.

Another even more extreme case was a 32 year old accountant he met socially. Since he seemed a nice, normal sort, the neurologist asked if he would like to be scanned as part of his study, and he consented. But when they scanned his brain, much of the cerebral hemispheres proved to be just a large hydrocoele or fluid filled cavity. In spite of the absence of much of his brain, he functioned like a normal individual and was entirely unaware of having any brain damage.

On this evidence, all of us are probably brain damaged to some degree, but just not enough to make any significant difference to our outward function. Thus, it is a matter of degree not kind, that separates the 'normal' brain damaged from the overtly brain damaged.

Overt damage is therefore often only visible in someone who has a large degree of brain damage, which results in some pronounced physical or mental dysfunction. But there are many people with aberrations in brain structure that do not have any observable impact on function because the brain is such a brilliant compensator, with a large scope for redundancy.

When you think about the development of the human brain, from the stage of an egg and sperm getting together, to a structure the scale of 100 billion neurons, it is not surprising that some of the neurons become displaced. There is a point in the process of foetal brain development where billions of brain cells migrate from the inside to the outside, called neuronal migration.[3] The probability of this process being perfect in all cases is really quite low. It is remarkable that it happens as well as it does, as often as it does.

The brain can be damaged before, during or after birth. Birth is a dramatic passage into life and at any stage hypoxia, which robs the brain cells of oxygen, can become a hazard; the cord can wrap around the neck or the placenta can pull away too soon from the uterine wall, leaving the newborn critically starved of oxygen.

Brain damage can also result from a blow to the head that will either shear certain neurons from their axons, or cause microbleeding in small areas of the brain. We have all fallen on our heads, or hit our heads as children and if the right impact was just on the right spot, at the right angle, the result might have been permanent organic brain damage, as in the case of the radiologist. As long as the affected area was either small or in a non-critical centre of function, the brain was able to automatically compensate so the damage was not experienced as a conscious problem. Although not conscious it may have caused us to process in less efficient ways.

If, however, the damage occurred to a critical structure, such as the left hippocampus, it does become an overt problem because no other structure in the brain is as central to auditory short-term memory processing and nothing else can duplicate its function. As it happened, one of the processing functions that we were consistently finding that we couldn't change to any evident degree was the function of auditory short-term memory. We knew this because pre and post testing of digit span, a standard measure of auditory short-term memory, did not change.

SOFTWARE PROBLEMS:

Functional Shutdown

Clearly, something in our protocols did not address this function specifically enough to have any lasting results. We had to find out how to specifically format for the function of the hippocampus. Susan suggested a new application of Utt's hippocampal formatting that we might try. With the next child who was referred to us by the psychologist as displaying a very deficit digit span (having trouble retaining a sequence of information given verbally), Susan applied the new formatting with remarkable results. Post testing by the psychologist showed a return to the normal range of auditory short-term memory function and even more importantly, the child was from then on able to remember spelling words and retain multiplication tables.

One of the ways that deficit auditory short-term memory is displayed in children is the inability to remember their spelling words, even through they may have put enormous effort into the task of learning them. The other is that they can learn their multiplication tables by rote, but after a few days the information is lost because it was never effectively transferred to long-term memory. How frustrating to put such effort into learning the multiplication tables time and again, only to forget them.

Imagine our elation at having found the key to what had previously been an unfathomable question? What we had discovered is that the brain integration procedures we had developed to that time were effective but in some cases we needed to go beyond them to resolve these more difficult cases. We had established that we had to work with the brain's multi-tiered structure. Up to that time we had basically been laying an excellent foundation for higher-level brain functions but had not been able to address these higher-level functions directly.

In those cases where breakdown in basal brain functions (accessing visual processing), or integrating functions (corpus callosum shutdown), were the crux of the problem, our basic brain integration techniques produced brilliant results. Even after the basal functions were on-line, however, there were still many higher level mental processes that, although reliant on these basal functions, employ higher levels of integration that require access to still higher level brain functions.

Picture a twin towered office building. It has a right Gestalt Tower where the architects, artists and designers are busily creating new designs and ideas. In the left Logic Tower are the bean counters; the accountants, finance directors, operations managers and systems analysts, who are responsible for turning the brilliant designs of the creative team into a practical reality. The computer terminals in the Gestalt Tower used by the designers and the computer terminals in the Logic Tower used by the accountants are both connected to the central processing unit in the basement.

It is only by the effective integration of the information from the Gestalt and Logic Towers that anything gets done at all. If the designers and accountants cannot communicate with each other to integrate their complementary skills, the otherwise streamlined processes of creating a functional, marketable product, is disrupted. Functionally this communication between the two towers would flow through the corpus callosum in the brain.

On the other hand, if certain central processing units have functions that have gone off-line, it may compromise both Gestalt and Logic commands. However, even if the central processing unit is working perfectly and is able to integrate all incoming messages, there may still be problems with the connections to the individual terminals occurring at higher levels in the building. So the bean counter cannot save his budget sheets for future recall. He calculates the figures and gets everything to balance beautifully but when asked by the finance manager to produce the data a week later, he cannot recall them from the computer memory. The computer just keeps telling him it is suffering a serious disk error. The accountant, like a person with a learning

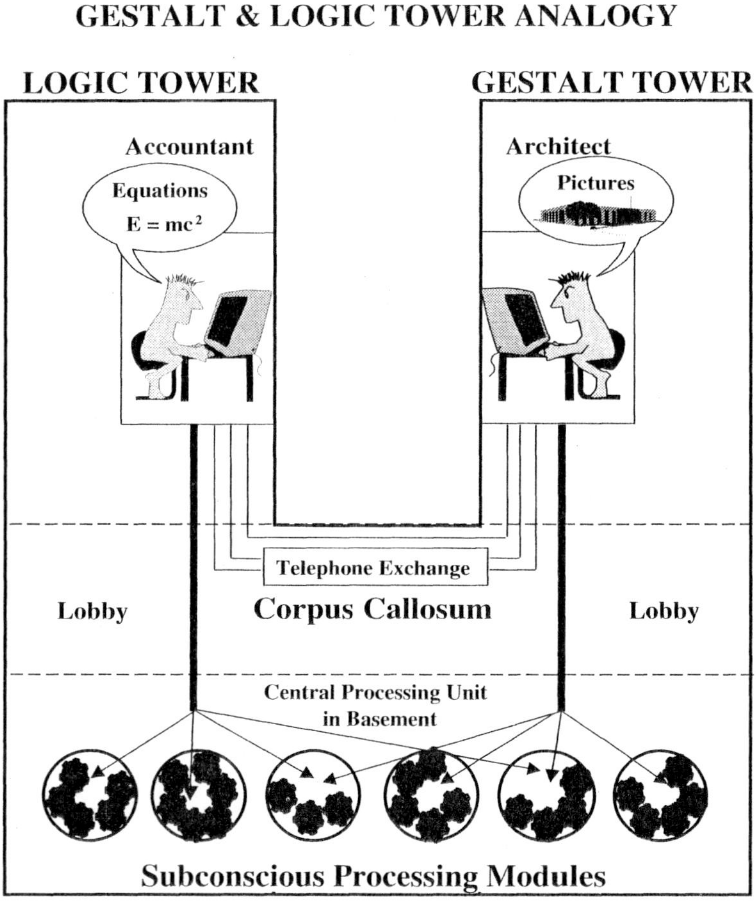

252   *A Revolutionary Way of Thinking*

GESTALT & LOGIC TOWER ANALOGY

Figure 9.1. Gestalt and Logic Towers Analogy. While the Logic and Gestalt lead functions allow you to perform conscious tasks, (like the accountant and architect), it is largely the subconscious modules that do the actual processing. For the Logic and Gestalt lead functions to work together, however, requires access to the interhemispheric fibres crossing the corpus callosum.

problem, only knows he cannot access the information he fed into the computer. He does not know why.

It may indeed have been Susan's background as a computer systems analyst that provided her with the critical insight. She had realised that there was nothing wrong with what we were doing, we just needed to go beyond the basic program. With this new understanding we developed new applications and witnessed another change in the pattern of response in our clients.

We had one child who came to us who was in the first percentile of same-age children for auditory short-term memory function, and was thus having extreme difficulty at school as she had basically no short-term memory. After applying the new hippocampal formatting techniques, she improved to the 50th percentile. She had gone from practically no useful function to average ability for her age, which meant she could now access enough short-term memory to learn adequately.

She began to remember her spelling words and for the first time in her life, could recall her multiplication tables even weeks after learning them. She literally went from the bottom of her class to the top of her class in six months. She had always been very clever, but with no functional short-term memory, she could never demonstrate the fine intelligence she actually possessed.

THE LEARNING ENHANCEMENT ADVANCED PROGRAM: LEAP

We were establishing a whole new paradigm and as the parents and some of our fellow practitioners saw what we were able to achieve, they began to ask us to teach our methods. We began teaching on a one-to-one basis and as we did so started to realise just how complex the system had become. We needed to write it down and to give it a name. It became 'LEAP', which stands for the Learning Enhancement Advanced Program. This program taught not only the brain formatting techniques, but where and how to apply them, and why they worked. An in-depth understanding of neurology was essential and, as you can imagine, the teaching began to consume hundreds of hours of our time.

We taught eight individuals how to apply the program and although it was certainly time-consuming we benefitted because those invested hours taught us how we needed to do the training. The demand from other kinesiologists increased and we had to create an integrated teaching program and manual. Several years on, with a 250-page manual in hand, we were asked to teach the program at the biggest kinesiological centre in the world, The Advanced Kinesiological Institute in Freiburg, Germany. This centre conducts 450 workshops a year in kinesiology training.

The complexity of the program we were teaching reflected the complexity of the human brain. Before any corrections could be made, the specific nature and types of learning problems had to be assessed and this protocol required 80 or so steps. Learning problems are unique mosaics of dysfunction, as distinct and individual as fingerprints. The techniques to unravel these patterns are just as varied.

Currently we have taught and teach LEAP in Europe and the United States as well as throughout Australia. Each year more kinesiologists are learning this powerful program and then helping to change people's lives. Together with our new students we find ourselves travelling into a frontier that is, in effect, rolling ahead of us. As the knowledge of neurology explodes with new information every week, we are constantly modifying our techniques and our teaching programs. Step-by-step we can go further and deeper, and be more effective. Fewer of our clients are falling outside the scope of our ability.

LEAP IN APPLICATION

A way of exemplifying the power and effectiveness of the LEAP program is to look at some of the cases to which we have applied it. Interestingly, Susan McCrossin, my partner and wife, is a case in point.

Susan's story
Generally, you can tell to a large extent how integrated a person is by knowing them for a while and by watching what and how they do things. Because Susan appeared to be such a functional human being, to the point of running her own computer software business successfully in both Australia and overseas, I assumed she was very well integrated. There was no evidence of any major learning dysfunctions.

As a first step in demonstrating the original program to her, I assessed access across her corpus callosum and to my surprise found that she had very little access across it. She had virtually only half a brain functioning and obviously, a major integration problem.

All through her schooling Susan had been a very diligent student who worked very hard. She could conceptually demonstrate to her teachers that she understood the information she was studying, yet each time she faced an exam, she would bomb out. She had a major problem in the fact that she could not adequately memorise dates, names and equations, all things that are crucial to passing written exams in many subjects.

But I knew she spelled very well. And how did she know her maths well enough to run her own computer business? Like most innately bright people she had managed to compensate by figuring out clever ways of by-passing, or compensating for her dysfunctions. Susan happens to have a very long forward digit-span capability. She can remember eight random digits where the average adult can only remember six. She also has an excellent ear for sound. What she had managed to do was remember the auditory pattern of words rather than word pictures, which is the usual mode of encoding words into memory. She could phonetically make patterns out of the words and hold these sound pictures in her mind. Susan understood that there were phonic representations in words that were not phonetic. For instance, when she saw 'tion', she recognised that phonically this sounds like 'shun', but it phonetically is 'tie-on'.

When it came to learning her times tables, she just couldn't make the images of the answers, and thus had nothing to store in long-term memory. Fortunately for her, her father was an actuary and would quiz her every day on the way to school about her times tables. She finally got so tired of not remembering the answers, she was motivated to work out a solution to her problem.

She managed to make up algorithms so that she could calculate her multiplication tables very quickly. Normally, people will simply recall the answer to the question, 'What is 8 × 8?' by looking up into their visual memory and seeing the symbol picture of the answer, 64. Susan would create an algorithm which built on 8, 16, 32, 64. She did it so quickly that her teachers never realised she had any problems remembering her multiplication tables.

To memorise poems, however, she would have to work for months on a piece that other students would have down in a week. She had no idea that her methods of compensation were not normal for others. It is the only way she could do it. Her willpower had served to overcome her learning problems and she was able to get by, but only with average grades.

It was not until her 10th year of school, when she took a standardised intelligence exam, on which she scored very highly, that her teachers realised how bright she really was. The teachers then began to pressure her to perform up to her abilities and stop being so lazy. They did not realise that she was already putting an extraordinary effort in to get the mediocre results she was achieving. When it came to her final year when she had to pass a set of matriculation exams to graduate, she failed the critical test in Ancient History that had required her to reproduce dates and names.

In spite of her failure, she came out of school with such good recommendations from her teachers that she entered the Royal Melbourne Institute of Technology to do a course in Industrial Design. After a year, she had failed again. Taking her mother's good advice she learned to type and secured a secretarial job. It soon became apparent to her boss that she had more potential than being a typist so she was moved into the data processing area of the company. There, having such logic dominance to her brain function, she excelled.

When we unravelled the stress that had primarily shut down flow across her corpus callosum, we discovered that it was based on an incident that had occurred when she was 18 months old. At that time her father had been transferred to the United States for a six-month posting. To a toddler, even the temporary loss of a parent is tantamount to desertion, an unbelievable emotional trauma to someone who cannot rationalise even the temporary departure of a significant being. To deal with the perceived pain of her loss, she made a conscious decision never to be vulnerable to such pain again. The subconscious consequence of this decision was corpus callosum shut down.

Susan was rather lucky because, unusual for a child so young, she already had good Logic development and this became extremely well developed, if at the expense of her feeling Gestalt functions. Computing was a stream that suited her functional style exactly, and operating in a male domain in her own business was no problem because she was cool-headed and unemotional. Having a learning problem is, as Susan's experience shows, not always a barrier to being successful in the world. (Australia's richest man, media baron Kerry Packer is a dyslexic, who was held back in his academic function but not in his worldly achievements.)

From then on Susan became the perfect guinea pig for our program because every time we developed something new, we could apply it to her and watch what improvements took place in her performance. Over a year her progress was rapid and very gratifying. In 1993 she went back to university to begin a dual degree in psychology and neuroscience, neither of which is a soft option. She was a distinction student and has gone on to complete her honours degree in neuroscience.

She reports that since being reintegrated via the LEAP protocols, she is more intuitive, which reveals that her Gestalt functions are now more open, and thus she is more in tune with her feelings. She often jokes that she had never consciously experienced a feeling until she was reintegrated. She also finds she can remember facts much more easily and this has given her the first real academic success of her life: a university degree at age 42.

Julie

When I first saw Julie she was 15 and presented as being very Gestalt dominant, which is by far the most common outcome of corpus callosum shutdown. In our assessment protocols, Julie demonstrated only a 3 percent access to Logic function. She was attractive, charming and very witty, which is the way many Gestalt dominant people compensate for their high level of Logic dysfunctions. Everyone likes a charmer and will usually help them because they are so delightful to have around. Julie was progressing through school with her classmates but was consistently failing in maths.

In year 10, she could not add up numbers greater than 10. She did not know how to carry a digit and couldn't add, subtract, or do fractions. At 15 she could not abstract arithmetical concepts that a primary school student could manage easily, yet was so personable and popular that she had been promoted through the grades with her peers.

Over a series of appointments that added up to about 10 hours, we did the whole LEAP protocol, reintegrating her visual and auditory functions, and bringing on-line various memory processes. Once the stress on numbers and letters that also caused disintegration had been cleared, we started addressing her presenting problem, which was her difficulty with maths.

I showed her the process of adding and carrying numbers, a technique she had probably been shown hundreds of times before. She suddenly said: 'Oh, that's how you do it!' With her new access to Logic available, she could instantly grasp the concepts. I gave her harder problems, and she easily generalised what I was teaching her, and could now deal with elementary arithmetic.

Our job is not to tutor students, so having opened up her functions, we sent her to a maths tutor for remedial work. In the five weeks of her summer holidays she was able to come up to the maths levels of her classmates. She went from basic numeracy all the way to algebra. Her tutor told us that in 25 years of tutoring students she had never before seen anyone make such rapid progress. Julie's reading and comprehension also improved, as did her spelling. Her self-esteem rose alongside her performance.

Jane

An eight year old girl, Jane was also Gestalt dominant to an extreme degree. Indeed, she was so vague that you felt that she was hardly there; her body was present but she seemed to be off in her own fantasy world. She was incredibly creative but could never produce any work because she could not access the Logic functions required to organise herself. Jane could do no schoolwork; all she could do was retreat into the realm of creative imaginings.

I took her through the brain integration procedures and after I had seen her a few times, she brought us a present. It was a beautiful tie-dyed wall hanging, which displayed an incredible appreciation of form and color. She had made it herself. Her mother told us how, for the first time in her life, Jane had completed a task: she had decided to do something and had actually managed to organise all the necessary materials, and actually complete the project.

Jane was so proud of herself that she was beaming. She had finally found a way to express who she was. Like a lot of the outcomes I see in my work, the internal changes to functioning expressed themselves in a positive change in self-perception.

Steven

Sometimes subtle factors can be a major block to a person's function. Often they will be so subtle that they almost don't seem real. Stress that is triggered by either reading or hearing numbers or the letters of the alphabet can sometimes resonate with so much emotional loading that they can cause a total loss of brain integration. Steven was nine when he came to us for spelling problems. To him the alphabet was little more comprehensible than alphabet soup.

I took him through the alphabet to see what letters caused him stress and found the letter K was enormously loaded for him. I did an emotional stress correction and took him through the age recession procedure to find out why, when he saw the letter K, he would get so stressed. A major emotional stress was revealed at age five. His mother confirmed our findings saying, 'Oh, I remember. When Steven was five, K was the first letter that he learned and he scratched it into the side of his grandmother's cedar wardrobe.'

You can bet that grandma didn't congratulate Steven on mastering one letter in the alphabet. She justifiably hit the roof, and the whole emotional context of the event had been locked into that letter for Steven ever since. And since there are Ks in many words and scattered through even elementary reading material, was it any wonder that this boy had been having all sorts of problems with reading and spelling tasks?

David

I had another young lad who at 12 exemplified what happens when a similar stress becomes attached to a number. David could read, comprehend and spell well, but his maths was erratic. His father said: 'I just don't understand it. Sometimes he can do it well, other times he just can't do it at all.'

I gave him a series of maths tests to establish just where it was that he was having problems. First I tried addition. He added and carried quite well at a simple level, so I gave him bigger numbers: 3211 plus 179. He added them easily. Then I tried him on subtraction. Take 64 from 94. He sat and stared at the numbers for almost a minute. Nothing happened. I then changed the problem to 94 minus 74. Instantly he said '20!'. I tried again: 94 minus 54. Instantly he gave us 40. I tried 94 minus 64 again. He sat and stared blankly.

It turned out that any time there was a six in the digits presented, he would lose his brain integration and become totally dysfunctional. I could well imagine why he was driving his maths teachers nuts.

David's story demonstrates how a particular stimulus can bring an emotion back on-line and cause complete loss of brain integration. In his case the stress wasn't so much maths as the number six. David had an unresolved emotional issue that related to the number six. On his sixth birthday he had been given a bicycle with a big number six attached to it. He could not master learning to ride it. It may have been his frustration that had become so firmly linked to the number. It was this memory of frustration that I defused. After defusion of the stress on the number six, David could then easily do all the maths procedures he already knew, whether they contained the number six or not.

David's story illustrates an important point about brain integration, which is that it is totally contextual. David had brain integration and the ability to perform in maths—provided the context did not contain the number six. Once six was present, integration would be instantly lost. However, as soon as the six was removed, his brain would reintegrate. This was because David was basically functional, with full brain integration, except in the context of the stressor six.

Adding and subtracting are functions of simple arithmetic. It is not until you start doing fractions that you enter the realm of mathematics. Fractions require the abstract application of arithmetic principles. The symbol 1/2 is an abstract representation of half of anything. When children are being introduced to the concept of fractions, they will often be shown a big circle with a line down the middle and told that this represents a whole which is composed of two halves. Two halves therefore make a whole. For students who can abstract, the statement is perfectly logical and self-evident. For those who are totally Gestalt and cannot abstract, all they will be able to see is a flat circle with a line down the middle. Concretely, that is all there is.

I often meet children with learning problems who demonstrate few difficulties with basic arithmetic but who have insurmountable problems understanding fractions.

By the time they have consistently failed in maths for five, eight or 10 years, the subject has become so stressful for them that all you have to say is 'think of mathematics' and they will instantly lose total brain integration. Thus, they have become dysfunctional before they even look at a maths problem and there is no possibility of them successfully solving these problems. All the tutoring in the world is going to be relatively ineffective because of their inability to maintain integration when they attempt maths. Once you lose integration in a specific context you will invariably be dysfunctional in that area.

Aden

A variation on this theme was embodied by a 13-year-old boy, Aden, who was extremely bright. He was about to sit an exam that might win him entry to one of the best high schools in the state, but was having great difficulties in maths. He too would wax and wane. He could often complete a very complex maths problem successfully and then, in the next instant, be unable to add or subtract. It was obvious that he would not be able to maintain brain integration through the exam.

As I went through the steps of assessment, I found that most of his functions were truly on-line. But one function was dropping out: access to the hippocampal commissure, the structure that links both visual and auditory short-term memories, through which we access long-term memory. This meant Aden would literally become disconnected from what he did know.

He knew how to perform a lot of higher maths functions but because of the drop out of the hippocampal commissure, he couldn't express it. As in the case of trying to recall the name for a face you have remembered, the harder you try to remember the name you know you know, but cannot verbalise, the more profound the breakdown in communication across the hippocampal commissure becomes and the more the vital information recedes into the distance. As soon as you relax or change topics, the information may suddenly pop into your mind, as integration across this vital structure is once again re-established.

When integration dropped out Aden became incapable of doing even simple arithmetic. He must have been a great source of frustration to his maths teachers, who probably wondered whether they were dealing with a clever but lazy student, or an occasionally brilliant dunce.

His treatment took me some time because I needed to re-establish access to his hippocampal commissure in many different contexts. I would clear the blocks to particular functions and he would go to school and test them in the context of the class environment. He would report back in what contexts he now experienced no difficulty, and which contexts were still proving to be problematic for him. I would then work on another specific learning context and when he sat the exam, six months later, he held brain integration and achieved one of the highest marks. Without integration, it was highly unlikely that he would have been able to perform at this level, if at all.

These outcomes are very gratifying. However, while we do have about a 95 percent success rate (excluding known cases of organic brain damage) we need to understand that learning is a voluntary activity. Even if you have good brain integration you may chose not to use it for a variety of personal and emotional reasons. There are some children who unfortunately live in extremely dysfunctional family situations. Emotional and physical survival is their paramount concern, and academic learning is a secondary consideration. Even when these children have been treated and have full brain integration, they may not improve in their academic performance.

Unfortunately, too, teenage boys can be some of our least satisfying clients because in many cases they are brought to us under protest. Also if you have not been able to learn to spell since you were six and you are now 16, you have 10 years of spelling and thousands of words to catch up on. And they have other interests such as girls and football that can distract them from wanting to learn to spell. Learning to spell therefore often comes at the bottom of 'must-do' items. Even if these teenagers currently choose not to take advantage of their new state of integrated brain function, reintegration does give them one big advantage: they now genuinely have the ability to develop a function if they want to use it in the future. Before integration they had little chance of ever spelling well.

For example, during a follow-up visit after completing the brain integration program with a 15-year-old named John, his mother told me: 'He doesn't spell any better than when he started.' I then asked John: 'How many spelling words did you learn last week?' His reply was, 'None.' How many had he learned the week before that? None. And the week before that? Again, none. I then checked John's ability to learn to spell words, which he easily demonstrated. I then asked him to spell some words he had learned as part of the program months before, again there was no problem.

I told his mother that John had demonstrated his ability to learn to spell any word quite easily and to remember it, but that he was just choosing not to do so at this time and for his own reasons. What John did recognise was that he had gained an enormous benefit from the program. The integration was showing up elsewhere: He was now making seven out of 10 baskets in basketball while before the treatment he had been making only two to three.

An encouraging counterpoint to John was the case of a 16-year-old boy who passionately loved reading and who was desperate to be able to spell well. He came to me for integration and in the two weeks following the correction of his spelling functions he mastered 150 words that had always given him problems. At his next appointment, he bought in a list of the 50 most difficult words and asked to be tested on them. He got all but one right. Six months on, he had no spelling problems of any note and continued to be highly motivated to succeed in an area where he had previously experienced only failure.

BRAIN INTEGRATION UNDER THE MICROSCOPE

As part of her neuroscience degree, Susan McCrossin undertook a study with five learning disabled adults using a very sophisticated form of an electroencephalogram (EEG) brain scanning device. These subjects ranged in age from 18 to 45 and each recognised that they had learning difficulties in certain contexts. Primarily they reported reading comprehension and short-term memory problems.

The EEG allows scientists to look at the patterns of electrical activity generated by the cortex when it is performing an activity. But the results of previous studies with traditional forms of EEG, using only three reference points, were notoriously variable, with little consistent correlation between the type of mental task and the areas of the cortex showing activity. Thus, patterns of EEG activity as a means of understanding cortical processing have been highly controversial because the brain is always involved in lots of simultaneous activities. How were the researchers to distinguish if activity was due to the stimulus they were initiating, or some other brain activity, such as random thoughts?

Susan's study concentrated on a new EEG method known as Steady-State

Visually Evoked Potential (SSVEP).[4] In this test, the subjects had a small red light flickering into the corner of their eyes, and because vision is a dominant sensory process, the flash rate entrained all brain patterns into a single brain wave. As long as the subject is not thinking of anything else but is just passively observing a visual stimulus, the brainwaves become a single pattern of 13 cycles per second.

In the SSVEP technique 64 electrodes are placed on the scalp, covering all processing areas of the cortex. In this way, specific areas of cortical activity can be identified, particularly against the constant stimulus of the flashing light. When the data from the electrodes is fed into a powerful computer, detailed maps of cortical activity can be constructed. While being SSVEP scanned, if you ask the person to consciously do a particular mental task, they will automatically activate specific brain areas related to the performance of that task. In the area that is active, the SSVEP signal is reduced and the degree of reduction is proportional to the degree of activation of that area.[5] This allowed us to draw an activation map of the brain.

The SSVEP machine had been used in a previous study comparing children with Attention Deficit Disorder (ADD) to normal subjects on two different mental tasks. One of these was an attentional task requiring the subject to pay attention and anticipate events. The other was a decision-making task. The SSVEP patterns of these two groups showed significant differences.

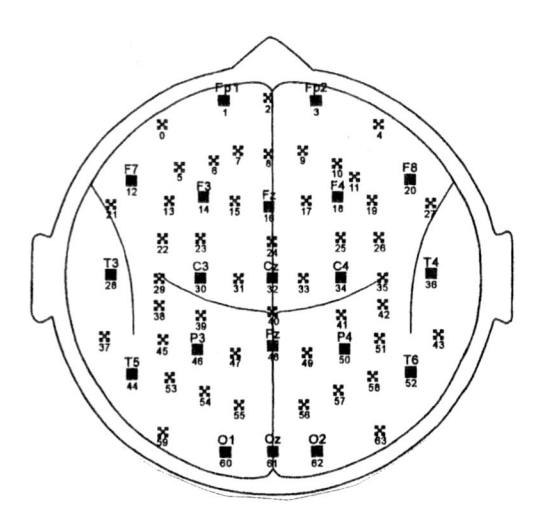

Figure 9.2. The 64 Electrode Pattern. Location of recording sites with International 10–20 positions indicated

When normal subjects were doing a purely visual task: observing a computer monitor displaying numbers, their brain showed activity predominantly in the occipital lobes in the back of the brain, where visual image formation takes place. When they were then asked to anticipate, or pay attention to a particular signal, their cortical activity switched to the frontal lobes, the area of the brain involved in attentional tasks. In ADD children, the brain activity did not change. Activity remaining predominantly in the occipital lobes.[6]

When Susan scanned her adult volunteers before they underwent brain integration, it was found that, like ADD children performing an attentional task, all of the activity was registered in the occipital region. Following application of the LEAP protocol, the activity patterns of all five adult subjects changed to the pattern observed in normal subjects. Now, when they were asked to pay attention, or make decisions, their cortical activity immediately switched to the frontal lobes, indicating a shift from passive looking to active mental participation in the task.[7]

Thus, it appears that children with ADD or adults with learning problems often just watch their world and react to whatever happens with little anticipation of what might occur because they cannot activate the brain areas involved in 'paying attention' which is required for anticipating outcomes. Likewise, since prefrontal activity is also required for 'planned' decision-making, and there is little prefrontal activity when people with ADD and learning problems make decisions, it would appear that these decisions must depend more on 'reaction' to stimuli than on planned actions based on considered decisions.

Along with these changes in cortical activity, there was concomitant improvement in the adult subjects' digit span and reading comprehension. Before integration, the reading comprehension of the group had varied from 33 percent to zero. One of the subjects could remember nothing of what she read because the stress she experienced in knowing she would be tested caused total loss of brain integration.

After the treatment, all had 100 percent reading comprehension. On the digit span test, all subjects changed from being marginal or borderline in their function to being above-average. Changes in both these mental functions is supported by the significant changes in cortical activity observed in the SSVEP results.[8]

In a year long study for her honors thesis in neuroscience, Susan performed a control study of children with learning difficulties, predominantly in reading, reading comprehension, spelling problems and demonstrable short-term memory deficits. She randomly selected 10 children for treatment and 10 other children to act as controls. All children were to be pre and post tested on a range of standard psychometric tests for intellectual performance.

Measures of intelligence are highly controversial because intelligence is a hypothetical construct and therefore, impossible to define in terms of 'an essence of intelligence'.[9] Never-the-less, a number of different standardised intelligence tests, such as the Wechsler Intelligence Scale for Children (WISC) and Stanford Binet Intelligence Test, have been developed to measure various aspects of cognitive function. Regardless of whether these psychometric tests measure 'intelligence' or not, they do provide reliable assessment of performance on certain types of tasks. The use of intelligence tests in Susan's study was not to measure intelligence but rather, to provide a standard assessment of performance in a variety of cognitively demanding tasks.

Intelligence has been defined as being composed of two distinct aspects: 'fluid' and 'crystalline' intelligence.[10] Fluid intelligence is the capacity to perform abstract reasoning which involves 'native' intelligence and is thought to be unaffected by formal education. This includes the ability to solve puzzles, memorise a series of arbitrary items such as words or numbers, as well as the ability to change problem solving strategies easily and flexibly. Crystalline intelligence, on the other hand, comprises the abilities that depend upon knowledge and experience or the amount of stored factual knowledge such as vocabulary and general information.

Susan chose three standardised tests of fluid intelligence; the WISC Block Design subtest, the Kaufmann Matrices and Inspection Time. She also tested them on short-term memory and reading comprehension. The WISC digit-span subtest was used as a measure of short-term memory, retrieval and

Before LEAP Treatment

After LEAP Treatment

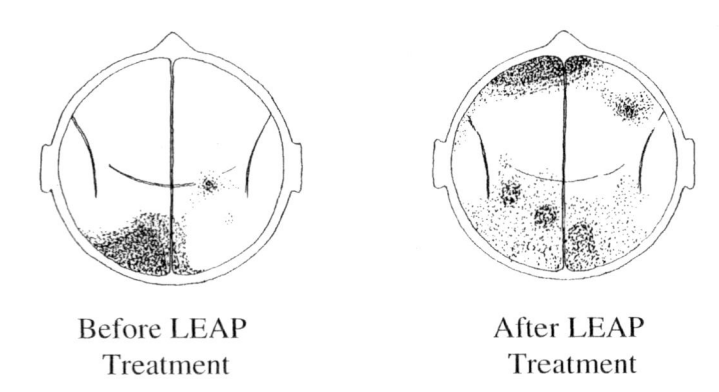

Figure 9.3. SSVEP Maps of typical subjects Before and After LEAP treatment. Degree of stippling indicates degree of activity. Before treatment subjects with learning difficulties showed the most activity in the occipital lobes when performing attentional and decision-making tasks. After treatment the cortical activity now switched to the frontal lobes on the same attentional and decision making tasks, the same areas active when normal subjects perform these tasks.

distractibility. The Neale Analysis of Reading, a standardised test to assess reading comprehension, was also applied. Tests measuring crystalline intelligence were not used as knowledge of facts is accumulated over a number of years and would not be expected to change substantially over the short time frame of the study.

All children were initially assessed on the five psychometric tests and then were retested six to eight weeks later. In the intervening period the treatment group had the complete LEAP protocol performed on them. The control group received no treatment but were retested at the end of the study.

The results were remarkable. Empirical observation and scientific validation of these tests show that fluid intelligence generally does not improve over time.[11] From this data it has been assumed that the person will in the future perform as they have in the past (or, allowing for growth, will hold their relative position amongst their peers), and therefore changes in performance in these subtests is considered unlikely. This appears to hold true for children with learning disorders even when they have received extensive remediation.

Rewardingly for Susan's thesis, there were statistically significant improvements in all of the tests of fluid intelligence between the pre and post tests for the treatment group. No changes occurred in the performance of the control group. Thus the LEAP protocol was shown to be capable of changing the innate reasoning capacity of these children. It was capable of affecting profound changes including the demonstrable ability to apply flexible strategies to solve problems in their lives. Surely, a valuable life skill.

Equally as important, the complex task of digit-span (short-term memory

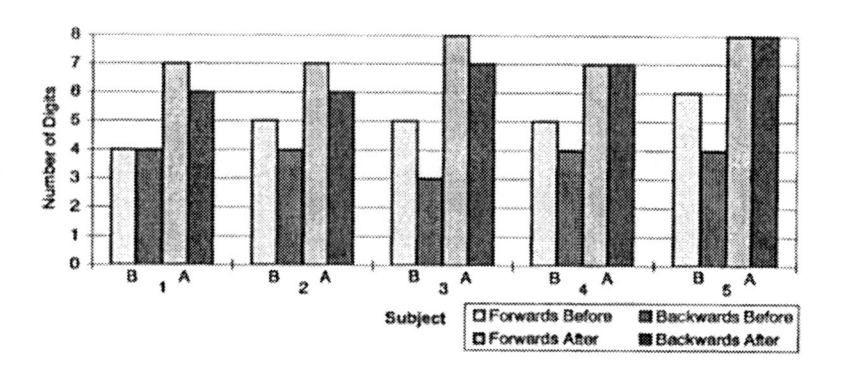

Figure 9.4. Digit Span scores for five subjects before and after LEAP treatment. In all cases the forwards and backwards Digit Span increased significantly following the LEAP treatment. B = Before, A = After.

and attention) also showed highly significant differences before and after treatment between the two groups. There was an increase in the forward digit span from 4.8 (before treatment) to 6.2 (after treatment) and an increase in the backwards digit span from an average of 3.1 (before) to 5.5 (after). Since the average adult digit span is six forwards and five backwards these children had clearly improved from deficit in this vital function to above normal.[12]

When it came to reading the results were even more striking. The treatment group contained two individuals who could not read prior to treatment. One, a 16 year old boy who had received weekly private tutoring for several years, still had not been able to read. Following the LEAP protocol, with the same weekly tutoring he was now able to read at an elementary level and is continuing to show steady improvement. Another 11 year old boy could only recognise a few small words prior to treatment. Following treatment he was able to read fluently at an elementary level and demonstrated the same improvement, even without special remediation.

In counterpoint, one of the individuals in the control group also could not read at the beginning of the study. At the end, he still could not read.

Reading comprehension showed equally remarkable improvements. The treatment group improved from an average of 27.5 percent reading comprehension to 94 percent following treatment, a massive change. The control group showed no change in reading comprehension.[13]

These tests graphically illustrate that LEAP does have significant and observable effects on the actual cortical processing in the brain and that these effects result in widespread improvement in perceptual and cognitive abilities.

HYPERACTIVITY AND LEAP

Hyperactivity, or children who display extreme distractibility, reckless impulsiveness and inability to stay still, has probably always been present in the population, but in recent decades these behaviours have been increasingly recognised as a major social problem. Hyperactivity not only impacts upon social and family interactions, but also on learning abilities with hyperactive children commonly displaying difficulties with spelling, reading and mathematics.

While hyperactive behaviour was previously given many labels, by the 1970s and particularly the early 1980s it was generally termed Attention Deficit Disorder (ADD). More recently, it has been defined more specifically with two types of attention deficit disorder recognised, attention deficit disorder without hyperactivity and attention deficit disorder with hyperactivity.[14] Children displaying the latter form are said to be suffering from Attention Deficit Hyperactivity Disorder (ADHD).

Initially, ADHD was perceived as a childhood behavioural problem that children grew out of at puberty. It is now clear that ADHD continues into adolescence, and that ADHD children merely become ADHD adults. ADHD was also observed to run in families, and thus appeared to be inherited but the mechanism was unknown. Recent research suggests that ADHD is most probably a genetic disorder that affects brain chemistry and is passed from one generation to the next.[15]

My own clinical observations certainly support that it is inherited from one or both parents. In several thousand cases, during the initial assessment as I explain the nature of their child's learning problems and the behaviours likely to be expressed by the child, one or both parents would often say 'that's just like me as a child'. Or the mother, who often brings the child, would say 'that's just like his father'. Many times until the parents listened to my explanation, they did not realise that they had been hyperactive or attention deficit because these terms were not in use in their youth.

In 1937, a Rhode Island paediatrician, Charles Bradley, found that giving stimulants, benzadrine, and later amphetamine, to ADHD children had the paradoxical effect of calming them down.[16] Since the 1950s amphetamines have been replaced by methylphenidate (Ritalin) because it has fewer side effects. In fact, now Ritalin use is becoming epidemic as more and more children are diagnosed as hyperactive. Between 1971 and 1987 there has been a consistent doubling in the number of children on medication every 4 to 7 years in a number of US public and private schools. By 1987 the use of medication had risen to between 1 percent and 6 percent of all elementary school children, and by the early 1990s, there were increasing rates of stimulant drug treatment in secondary school children as well.[17]

It wasn't until the latter part of the 1980s and early 1990s that an understanding of how Ritalin and other stimulants achieved the paradoxical results on behaviour began to evolve. It now appears that Ritalin and the other drugs, work through their effects on the important brain neurotransmitter, dopamine. As discussed previously in Chapter 4 (see Fig. 4.2) dopamine release in the reward system of the brain leads to feelings of well-being. Dopamine docks on the D-family of receptors (D_1, D_2, D_3, D_4, D_5), but most strongly with D_2 type receptors. Docking of the dopamine on the D_2 receptor gives rise to feelings of well-being and is calming, while at the same time augments the ability to maintain attention.[18]

An increasing body of evidence suggests that ADHD is primarily biologically based with studies indicating that people with ADHD may have at least one defective gene coding for the D_2 receptor making it difficult for the neurons in the reward center to respond to dopamine.[19] The reduced response to dopamine means that these people do not experience the normal reward feelings of well-being and have increased difficulty regulating their attention.

Kenneth Blum has termed this the 'reward deficiency syndrome', which leaves ADHD children and adults with feelings of restlessness, anxiety, feeling incomplete, difficulty focusing, and hypersensitivity.[20] These uncomfortable feelings may then be expressed as anger, aggressiveness, shyness, hyperactivity or deviant behaviour.

Perhaps equally important, in their recent book *Overload, Attention Deficit Disorder and the Addictive Brain*, Miller and Blum make a strong case for the connection between ADHD and alcoholism and drug abuse.[21] In 1990 Blum and his colleagues identified a deficit in the D_2 receptor gene that they found to be associated with alcoholism. Since then this D_2 receptor defect has been associated with other compulsive and impulsive disorders, including ADHD.[22] As discussed in Chapter 4, drugs of addiction appear to work by elevating dopamine levels in the synapses of the reward system, particularly the nucleus accumbens. While opium and cocaine do this directly, alcohol does so indirectly.

When alcohol is metabolised it produces molecules with the impossible name, tetrahydroisoquinoline, TIQ for short. When TIQ molecules are formed from alcohol, they flood the D_2 receptors and produce temporary feelings of well-being—the alcohol high.[23] This sets the stage for the ADHD—alcoholic connection. When ADHD people drink alcohol, the TIQ produced floods their limited D_2 receptors leading to normal feelings of reward—something they lack. Thus, for people experiencing the daily discomfort and pain of ADHD, use of alcohol and other addictive drugs can give them reward: pleasure and easing of the perpetual feelings of discomfort both physically and emotionally.

While alcohol produces pleasure and reduces physical and emotional pain for everyone, the payoff for people with ADHD is more intense and more dramatic. So they drink alcohol to feel more 'normal' only to get trapped in its addictive cycle of temporary relief followed by craving.

While all of this is most interesting, what does it have to do with LEAP? Many of the children we see have been diagnosed as ADHD and many are on drugs to modify their behaviour, most commonly Ritalin. As we proceed through the brain integration program, it is not uncommon to see these children calm right down, and often maintain this new state of more normal behaviour even after the withdrawal of the drug. While not observed in all cases, parents commonly report a long-term resolution of their child's hyperactive behaviour following the LEAP treatment.

Considering that the scientific evidence would suggest that ADHD is strongly linked to potential alcoholism as well as learning problems and deviant and delinquent behaviours based on a defective gene for D_2 receptors, the cessation of the hyperactivity and increased ability to learn following the LEAP treatment is remarkable. It suggests that the LEAP protocol somehow alters this reward deficiency syndrome. I postulate that the acupressure treatments and emotional defusions employed in the LEAP treatment either activate greater expression of the D_2 receptor genes, or increase dopamine levels by mechanisms that remain unknown at present. This then establishes more normal patterns of reward and attention in the brain.

Recent studies have found a significant correlation between abnormal P300 EEG brainwave activity and the A1 allele of the dopamine D_2 receptor gene.[24] This is the same gene defect associated with ADHD, alcoholism, drug addiction and compulsive and impulsive disorders.[25] When these findings are coupled with the recent observation that acupuncture stimulation can alter the P300 brainwave activity,[26] this may provide a possible mechanism by which the LEAP acupressure treatment may reverse or eliminate the reward deficiency syndrome.

Whatever the mechanisms, we see child after child go from ADHD behaviour, often regulated with Ritalin, to relatively normal behaviour without drugs. Susan's controlled studies confirm these changes in brain function both electrophysiologically with abnormal EEG patterns returning to normal patterns and in psychometric testing. Follow up observations even several years later show these changes in behaviour are on-going.

Since ADHD is associated with a greater likelihood of delinquency as adolescence[27] and alcoholism,[28] cocaine addiction[29] and stress disorders[30] as an adult, each ADHD child receiving the LEAP treatment may well reduce the human cost of these destructive behaviours both on the individual and society.

LEAP INTO THE FUTURE

We estimate that in the eight years we have been working with LEAP, we have probably seen more than 5000 people. Given that we have already taught 100 kinesiologists these methods in Australia, Germany, Belgium, the Netherlands and the US, probably double that number have by now been put through the program worldwide. Each year we travel around Australia and abroad teaching another 100 or so students. This means the LEAP program is spreading exponentially. The reason it has attracted such interest is because it gives such consistent results. It is not something only Susan and I can do; anyone adequately trained can also achieve the same results.

We could have made a very comfortable living doing LEAP exclusively in our own clinic. But what has been driving us to teach LEAP to others is that we perceive it to have profound effects on people's consciousness. They are suddenly able to realise more of their true potential.

If you are learning disabled, in a sense you are cut off from that which you could be in terms of your human potential. As you become more learning enabled you also become more able to fulfill the potential in your life. As well, if you understand why you have been dysfunctional, you can have more compassion for yourself and for other people with similar problems. When you have compassion for the difficulties someone else might be confronting, it invites that person to also have compassion for themselves.

One of the only common denominators that criminologists have been able to find between people who have committed violent crimes is that they are commonly functionally illiterate. By that we mean that even if they can read and write it is only at a rudimentary level. Many people sitting in prisons today are highly intelligent, clever individuals who are learning disabled. They have never been allowed to express their intelligence in an acceptable way. How many times have you heard the expression, 'If that so and so had only used his intelligence in a legal way he would probably be a very wealthy person today.'

He was never allowed to express his potential because he could not read or spell well, or pass the written interview test for the job. After making at least five spelling mistakes on his application, many employers just throw it straight into the bin. The applicant might have been the smartest person interviewed that day, but was rejected because he could not spell. He knows he is smart, but is frustrated when he is never allowed the opportunity to demonstrate his real abilities. This frustration often leads to anger and violence. If such people could enter society as equals and be taken seriously they would not have to vent their frustration about being locked out, a situation that often leads them to being locked up.

We truly feel that every time we turn someone around and help them access more of their function, they will utilise it in a way that is most harmonious for them and society. One 13-year-old boy I treated had been thrown out of five different schools in one year. He was being seen by a child psychiatrist for his violent behaviour and was considered a suicide risk. He was very bright but extremely dysfunctional in terms of his learning ability. He was very angry and very frustrated, and he expressed this by beating up other kids, setting fire to public buildings and physically threatening his teachers.

I was only half way through the LEAP protocols when I noticed he had calmed right down. His brain was coming together and he was beginning to realise that he could learn things that he had never been able to access before. By the end of the year that followed his treatment he was at the top of his class. Previously, he had been headed towards either suicide or delinquency and that would have been a loss for society either way. Society would have lost potentially a highly productive member. Instead, I was able to open up a highly productive future for this lad who is now in university and doing very well with his studies.

This has happened time and again.

To this point we have been talking about how limited academic functions can be improved. But brain reintegration can affect a person's life in many more (and perhaps more profound) ways. The most profound effect is undoubtedly a change in a person's level of self-confidence. Long before changes in academic performance have been perceived, parents often comment on changes in the child's level of self-esteem.

Indeed one mother told us that when she arrived to collect her son from school one afternoon, she saw a boy running towards her car. He looked vaguely familiar, but it was not until he reached the car she recognised this was her own son. 'He just moved so differently and with so much more confidence and co-ordination than he had before, I didn't recognise him until he was literally getting into the car.'

For a list of LEAP practitioners and LEAP training locations for kinesiologists see Appendix D.

THE SUCCESS LOOP

Dysfunction that results from brain disintegration can become a cycle. When you are starting a new, previously untried task, it is uncertain and uncertainty creates fear. If the fear is strong enough, or if it is linked to past failure, it can generate enough stress to cause a loss of brain integration. In a state of disintegration you are dysfunctional and will tend to fail again.

The next time you attempt that or a similar task, you are not only uncertain but obsessed by a fear of failure. This, ironically, can become a positive feedback loop of fear-dysfunction-failure, then fear of failure-dysfunction-failure. It leads unerringly to negative outcomes and the greatest loss is to self confidence and self-esteem.

On the other hand, if you are challenged with a new learning situation, and despite the uncertainty have managed to maintain your brain integration, you remain functional and figure it out. You are successful and with success comes reward, both externally and internally. Every time you figure it out and say 'Ah, ha! I've got it', endorphins are released in your brain, creating a sensation of pleasure. At the same time, praise generally comes from outside in the form of approval from a teacher, parent, peer or colleague, releasing more endorphins, further reward.

These positive rewards do two things: They make you feel good about yourself; and they make your brain integration more robust and resilient. After a series of successes you can even allow yourself to make an error and not lose integration. Instead, you can see where you went wrong, what you need to learn from the mistake, then try again and succeed.

You have met the challenge and you have succeeded. When we have a

Success Cycle
(created by Maintaining Brain Integration)

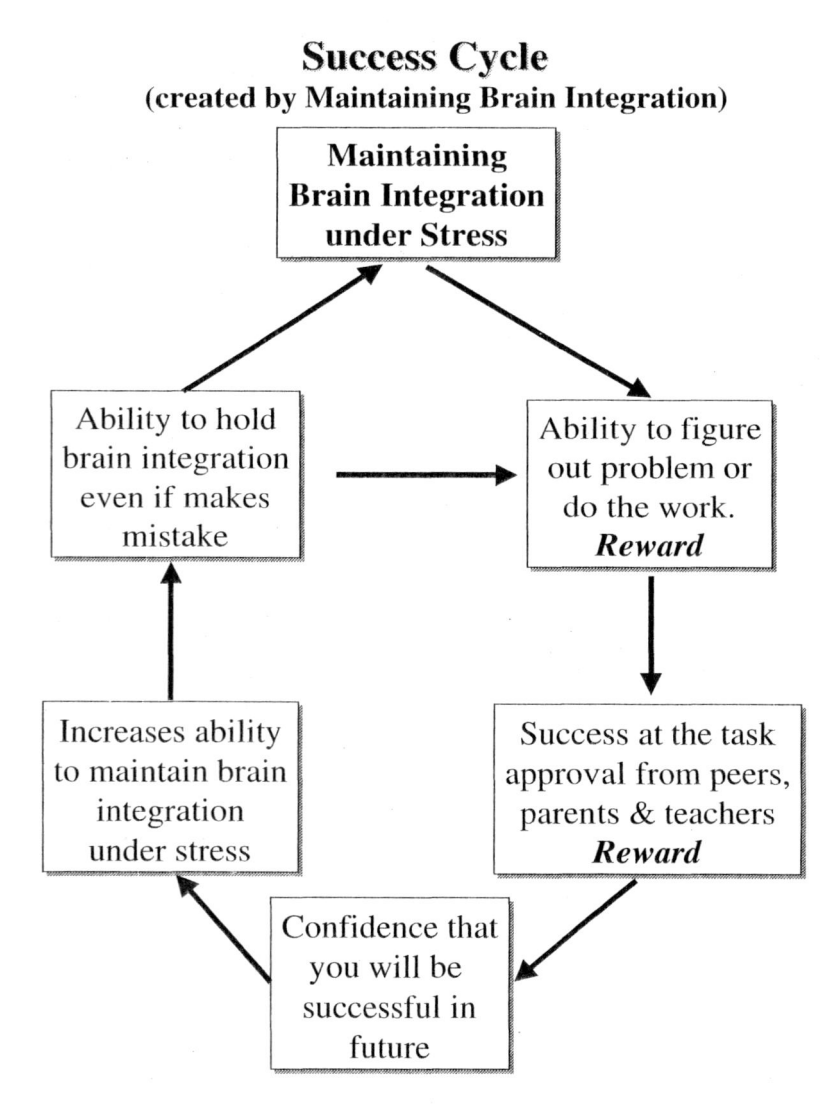

```
                    Maintaining
                  Brain Integration
                    under Stress
                   ↗            ↘
        Ability to hold      Ability to figure
        brain integration →  out problem or
        even if makes        do the work.
        mistake              Reward
           ↑                      ↓
        Increases ability    Success at the task
        to maintain brain    approval from peers,
        integration          parents & teachers
        under stress         Reward
             ↖                  ↙
               Confidence that
                you will be
               successful in
                  future
```

Figure 9.5. The Success Loop created by maintaining Brain Integration under Stress. When you can maintain your brain integration under stress you will be able to figure it out and receive the reward of being successful, which increases your ability to maintain your integration under even higher levels of stress and be successful again the next time. This leads to increased self confidence so essential for success in life.

history of success, challenges are no longer seen as problems but rather as opportunities to learn. People who are successful tend to continue being successful, whereas people who experience failure tend to repeat that failure. Success makes you confident.

In contrast, people who have tasted repeated failures tend to lack confidence in their abilities and in themselves. This is powerfully reflected in your states of motivation. If you believe you are incompetent and lack confidence, you tend not to give it a go—that way you can't fail again. If, however, you do have a sense of confidence, you will try anything because what do you have to lose except something new to learn? You're on a positive spiral (see Fig. 9.5).

If you can maintain integration, you can figure life out and get it right. Success is confidence. It's that simple.

In the next chapter I will discuss a number of environmental factors that may compromise effective brain integration, and hence learning.

Chapter Ten

ENVIRONMENTAL FACTORS THAT CAN AFFECT THE BRAIN

THE DELICATE BALANCE OF BRAIN INTEGRATION

Loss of brain integration is not only a consequence of emotional stressors within your life but can also be profoundly influenced by factors in the environment. Some of these, such as electromagnetic radiation, are external while others, like candidiasis, may be generated in the internal environment. In this chapter we consider some of the major environmental factors that need to be addressed to maintain brain integration. Some we can manage for ourselves; others may only be resolved through various therapeutic treatments.

INTERNAL ENVIRONMENTAL FACTORS

A proper diet is vital, not just to keep your body healthy, but to maintain a fully functioning brain. That means regular meals and, more importantly, keeping up your fluid intake. It is possible to go for days without eating and to overcome the distraction of hunger to some degree, but a day or two without water will have severe effects on your physical and mental function.

Maintaining Proper Hydration
Water, the universal solvent, is the most important and abundant inorganic substance in the human body. It comprises between 45 and 75 percent of our body weight and up to 90 percent of the brain weight.[1]

In the body, water plays a major role in all biochemical reactions, including nerve conduction. To function properly, nerve membranes require precise distribution of ions, which are dissolved in the watery medium of our bodily fluids. If we become dehydrated, it can affect nerve transmission, impacting very strongly on brain function.

Recent studies with elderly people reporting memory loss have shown that when they markedly increase their water uptake, their memory improved significantly because dehydration may specifically affect areas of the brain such as the hippocampus, which is involved in memory processing.[2]

A major system helping to distribute nutrients to the neurons of the brain and carrying toxins away is the cerebral-spinal fluid or CSF. Secreted from the blood, its composition and volume are controlled by the levels of water in the blood.[3] When there is insufficient water, CSF production is decreased, slowing the clearance of toxins and depriving the actively metabolising neurons of essential nutrients.

But what factors cause dehydration? The most common, ironically enough, is the drinking of fluids other than water. Many fluids commonly consumed in large quantities—coffee, tea, chocolate beverages and alcohol—are all diuretics, which inhibit the re-absorption of water in the kidneys and result in more water being lost in the urine. So while you are drinking cup after cup of coffee or tea you are actually losing more water than you are consuming. The tissues of your brain and body become increasingly dehydrated in the process.

Soft drink is little better, because sugar-loaded drinks bind water, making it less available for other functions.[4] Salt has a similar binding quality graphically illustrated by what happens when you eat salty chips. You can feel the thirst increasing with each bite as your body screams out for water to help balance the salts.

Consuming these masked diuretics has been implicated in headaches, and the most obvious is the headache of a hangover, which is partly just severe dehydration caused by the diuretic effect of alcohol. One of the most potent remedies for a hangover is to drink large quantities of water before bed, and again, first thing the morning after.

Physical exertion can also cause significant water loss, but another crucial factor that is often overlooked is psychological stress. Every time you become emotionally stressed, part of the survival response of fight or flight is the release of water through the skin.[5] We all know the sweaty palms and dripping armpits of nervous tension.

This subconscious release of water due to emotional stress enables lie detectors to work by monitoring changes in the electrical resistance of skin. When you are relaxed, the skin is dry and has a high electrical resistance. But as soon as you become emotionally stressed, the skin begins to sweat, imperceptibly. Thus, if you are holding the electrode of the lie detector, and are asked a question that creates any type of stress (and for most people lying is a stress) the sudden increase in skin moisture reduces electrical resistance causing the needle to deflect.

Dehydration stresses our system and many children and adults do not drink enough water. To survive and work properly, all cells need to be surrounded by sufficient water and that means pure H_2O because your body treats all other fluids in a different way. As soon as there are organic molecules present in the liquid, the body perceives it as food.

How much water is enough?

It is recommended that a person drink 20 millilitres of water for each kilogram of body weight daily. That means one litre per 50 kilograms or at least eight to 10 glasses. Double or triple these amounts if you are engaged in demanding physical activity or are suffering emotional stress. A good way to gauge the correct level of hydration is by your rate of urination. Ideally, you should urinate every two or three hours.

Diet

Diet and marginal nutritional deficiencies may play a significant role in our mental functions and physical behaviour. The following information provides only a brief discourse into what is an enormously interesting topic. What we are seeking to do is to highlight certain nutritional factors that have been correlated with hyperactivity, learning and attention problems, and which thus flag the possibility of the broader impact of nutritional activity on the brain.

The typical western diet, experts suggest, is too high in sugar, refined foods, salts and fats and too low in fibre.[6] A recent study showed that a single meal of fast food may provide up to 50 grams or 10 teaspoons of fat, accounting for 50 percent of the total calories in the meal. The same meal may also supply more than half the amount of salt, but less than 15 percent of the fibre recommended per day.[7] Other studies have shown that even people consuming a normal western diet do not consume the recommended amounts of fibre.[8]

This diet has several measurable problems:

Food processing destroys Vitamin B_6 and foliates which support the function of brain and the central nervous system.[9]

A junk food, carbohydrate-rich diet is deficient in thiamin and has been associated with increased levels of aggression.[10]

Iron is recognised as a major nutritional deficiency in the modern western diet[11], and iron is a co-factor for the synthesis of two important brain neurotransmitters, dopamine and serotonin, which affect our mood and behaviour.[12]

Sugar, although not proven to be a 'bad' food, provides only empty calories and yet may constitute much of the calorie content in a convenience-food diet.[13] This is not surprising when you look at the following list of the biggest selling items in Australian supermarkets and similar results were observed in basket surveys in the United States.[14]

1. Coca-Cola, 375 ml.
2. Coca-Cola, 1 litre
3. Coca-Cola, 2 litre
4. Diet Coke, 375 ml
5. Cherry Ripe
6. Nestle's condensed milk
7. Tally Ho cigarette papers
8. Mars Bar
9. Kit Kat
10. Crunchie Bar
11. Eta 5-star margarine—salt reduced
12. Heinz baked beans
13. Double-Circle tinned beetroot.
14. Diet Coke, 1 litre
15. Bushell's tea
16. Cadbury Dairy Milk chocolate
17. Pepsi Cola, 375 ml
18. Coca-Cola, 1.5 litre
19. Kellogg's Corn Flakes
20. Maggi two-minute chicken noodles
21. Generic brand lemon drink
22. Panadol tablets, 24 pack
23. Meadow Lea margarine
24. Generic brand lemonade.
25. Mrs MacGregor's margarine.

Although scientists have examined the link between diet and behaviour, and have shown a variety of often conflicting outcomes, there is no definite consensus. From our perspective however, there is considerable clinical and empirical experience to demonstrate that diet does have a profound impact on behaviour and learning potential.

Studies conducted in schools and correctional centres have provided us with a massive nutritional experiment that backs up our premise. Two different studies involving 12 correctional institutions and 803 public schools in the US reveal the pivotal influence of diet.[15] In both the institutions and the schools, the diet was changed from the 'normal' western diet (high in sugars, carbohydrates, salts and fats), to one comprising mostly fresh and whole foods.

The kitchens and canteens began serving unsweetened cereals instead of sugar-laden ones; fresh or canned fruits from which syrups have been removed; and unsweetened juices instead of cordials, colas and soft drinks. Honey was substituted for sugar and fresh fruits, nuts, cheeses and whole grain crackers were available instead of packaged snack foods and candy bars. Refined white breads and white rice were replaced by whole grain breads and brown rice. All other processed foods were replaced, where possible by fresh produce.

The results were stunning. In the correctional institutions, anti-social behaviour dropped 47 percent.[16] In the schools, students' national academic ranking rose 16 percentile points.[17] To confirm the findings, one of the correctional institutes reverted to serving the old diet and during the first six months found a massive 54 percent upsurge in anti-social behaviours.[18]

Before the study, 120,000 students in the 803 schools were reading two or more grades below their grade level. Three years after the diet change, 70,000 of those students—58 percent—had made up the two years and were reading at or above their grade level.[19] The implication is clear. A well balanced diet supports a well balanced mind. An unbalanced diet appears to lead to an unbalanced mind. But again, the people most prone to be affected by poor dietary habits are those who already have poor brain integration.

Sugar and Hyperactivity
Sugar has yet to be singled out as the ultimate culprit in hyperactivity, but it has been shown to be a factor in hypoglycaemia and to affect the endorphins or natural brain opiates that act as a virtual 'reward' system in the brain.[20] When we consume sugar we are giving ourselves a physiological lift which echoes the sense of well-being some people get from taking opium and its derivatives: morphine and heroin.[21]

Studies have highlighted these suggestions by showing that when a binge eater is given a shot of naloxone, which blocks the endorphins, they lose interest in consuming large quantities of sugar-rich foods.[22] They don't crave the sugar as such, what they appear to have been seeking was the effect the sugar has on their brain chemistry.

Sugar's empty promise appears to have a much greater impact on children than on adults. When 14 healthy children were given a dose of breakfast sugar equivalent to two sugar-frosted cup cakes, their blood adrenalin levels rose 10 times above the baseline.[23] This would make the children more prone to the adrenalin symptoms of anxiety, irritability and poor concentration. When adults consumed a similar dose of sugar for their body weight their adrenalin levels were not altered and no adrenalin-related behaviours were detected.

Sugar, in addition to high carbohydrate breakfast, increased deviant behaviour in hyperactive children, while the same amount of sugar consumed with a high protein breakfast, had no significant effect.[24] In another study, a moderate amount of sugar (28 grams for a 20-kilogram child), when eaten with a meal balanced in fat, carbohydrate and protein, improved classroom performance by decreasing reaction time, errors and activity levels.[25]

Children who eat sugar as part of a balanced meal are therefore less susceptible to these effects. Studies of boys with reported Attention Deficit Disorder, suggest that levels of aggressive-destructive or restless behaviour are exacerbated when they consume sugar in combination with meals that are unbalanced in carbohydrates, fats and proteins.[26]

The major point here is not that sugar causes the behaviour problems but rather, that sugar makes up much of these children's diet but does not nourish. The resulting marginal nutritional deficiencies may then affect brain function, which in turn affects behaviour.

Diet and Behaviour

Follow-on experiments conducted in some of the juvenile correctional centres correlated behaviour with the youths' intake of about 26 different nutrients. The worst-behaved consumed less of these nutrients than the best behaved. Further, those with average behaviour were consistently in the middle-range for consumption of these nutrients.[27]

When the staff supplemented the diet of all youths with these 26 nutrients, instances of anti-social behaviour by the worst-behaved group halved, and over the next six months misbehaviour overall decreased by 61 percent.

It thus appears that it is *simple nutrition*, or getting enough vitamins and minerals *and not less sugar alone* that accounts for most of the changes observed when hyperactive and aggressive people change to a low sugar diet. Why might this be so?

Figure 10.1 shows that cells use nutrients in complex biochemical pathways that produce energy from glucose. Forty nutrients are directly or indirectly involved in the production of energy including vitamin B_2 and B_3, and the minerals iron, sulphur and copper to mention only a few.[28] Included in this list are all 26 of the nutrients that were found deficient in the worst behaved youths.

The complex work of the brain is diet-dependent and malnourishment, which a high-sugar, highly refined diet fosters, may ultimately weaken energy production in the brain. Brain cells use these nutrients to provide the essential energy on which they function. This is crucial to understand when you consider that the thinking brain, the frontal cortex, requires two to three times as much energy as the limbic brain or the emotional centre.[29]

You can begin to understand that a lack of sufficient nourishment for the brain means that the cortex and higher mental functions suffer the most. The limbic brain, the reactive centre for sympathetic arousal associated with fear and anxiety, still manages to operate, a situation that clearly leaves the reactive or emotional brain in charge and which perhaps accounts for the hyperactivity and destructive or violent behaviour that can sometimes be observed in youth and children who routinely suffer from poor nutrition.

Dietary changes to support brain function

From such findings it is prudent for anyone, particularly a parent with a hyperactive or behaviourally-challenged child, to consider a dietary change that will provide the nutrients the brain needs to function well.

Such a diet should be:
- Low in sugar, less than 50 grams per day (less than half of current consumption). This amount appears to have no negative effects provided it is consumed in a diet balanced in fats, carbohydrates and proteins.
- Low in refined or processed foods, removing most fast or junk foods. Fresh fruit and vegetables should be encouraged.

280 A Revolutionary Way of Thinking

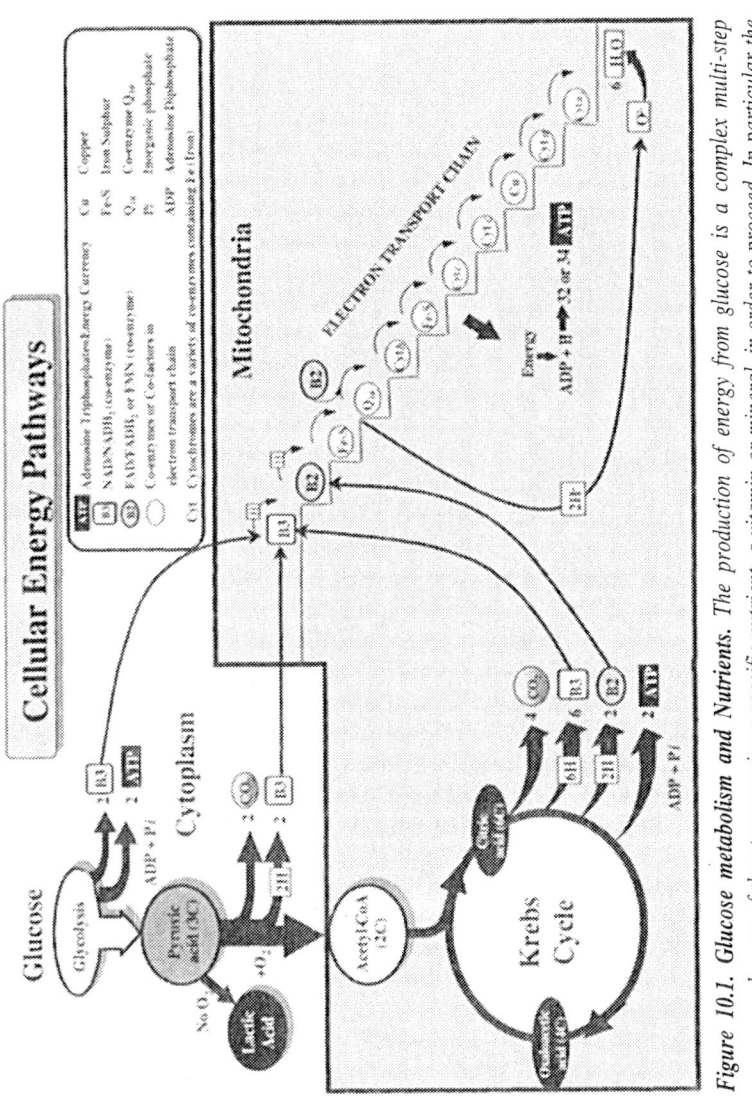

Figure 10.1. Glucose metabolism and Nutrients. The production of energy from glucose is a complex multi-step process, and many of the steps require a specific nutrient, a vitamin or mineral, in order to proceed. In particular the role of having adequate B-group vitamins and iron (Fe) is obvious from inspection of the figure above. Even marginal deficiencies of any of these factors will slow down energy production in the brain.

- High in proteins (meat, cheese, yoghurt, nuts and soya bean products), but balanced in fats. (Fats comprising less that 15 to 30 percent of the kilojoules consumed.) It may be important to check first for any dairy intolerances.
- High in fibre, at least 30 to 50 grams per day which is easily provided by the fresh fruit and vegetables.
- Low in food additives and preservatives, keeping highly processed, fast and junk food to a minimum.

We suggest that you, perhaps as a family, experiment. Change to the above diet for one to two weeks and observe any changes in behaviour or energy levels. If there are any doubts, switch back to the original diet for a same amount of time and watch what happens. Our experience suggests that the positive outcomes of the new dietary regime will be self-evident.

Supplementation for brain function
One means of eliminating or at least ameliorating nutrient-deficiency related behaviour and learning problems, may be the diet change we have suggested. However direct supplementation may both support and expedite these changes, and may be necessary is some cases due to inherited poor absorption of some essential nutrients by some individuals.

Vitamins. Vitamin B complex deficiencies have been implicated in hyperactive and aggressive behaviour. Vitamin B_6, which has a role in serotonin synthesis, is especially important because serotonin appears to calm the mind.[30] Hyperactive children often display low serotonin levels, but when their diet is supplemented with Vitamin B_6 their hyperactivity eases as their serotonin levels increase.[31] Some hyperactive children show a more marked improvement with Vitamin B_6 supplementation than those taking methylphenidate (Ritalin). In contrast to the Ritalin, the benefits of B_6 supplementation were on-going, even when supplementation ceased.[32] (A cautionary note here is that B_6 is only one factor involved in serotonin synthesis and simply adding this one vitamin may actually create other imbalances. Therefore, it is important to seek the advice of a well qualified nutritional therapist—a qualified naturopath or physician specialising in nutritional therapy, such as an orthomolecular doctor.)

Vitamins B_3 and B_6 have been found to be deficient in both disturbed children with behavioural problems and adult schizophrenics, and appear to result at least in part from malabsorption from a diet which may contain adequate amounts of these nutrients for people with normal absorption. One patient required B_6 supplementation of 1600 mg per day before measurable levels were detected in their blood.[33] This is more than 800 times the normal daily requirement of 2 mg per day for adult men and women.

Likewise, some people may require between 850 and 1800 mg of B_3 per day, far in excess of the normal daily requirement of 12 to 18 mg, and yet still have low B_3 levels in their blood. One schizophrenic taking over 3000 mg per day was borderline low for B_3 levels in his blood when assayed.[34] A similar situation was observed with children with behavioural problems dependent on B_3. As soon as a placebo was substituted for the nutrient, all children relapsed in their behaviour within 30 days, but recovered again when B_3 supplementation was restored.[35] It thus appears that for some people with poor absorption of B-group vitamins, which are often people displaying behavioural problems, supplementation is almost essential for optimum cognitive performance.

Niacin, pantothenic acid and thiamin supplementation have also been shown to help reduce hyperactive behaviour.[36] Since these B-group vitamins are essential for the effective metabolism of glucose in the brain (see Fig. 10.1), perhaps marginal deficiencies of these nutrients, or inherited absorption problems with these nutrients, reduces energy available to areas of the cortex involved in modulating behaviour.

Indeed, adults who were hyperactive as children showed both global and regional reductions in glucose metabolism compared with controls. Significantly, the largest reductions were in the premotor cortex and superior prefrontal cortex—areas known to be involved in the control of attention and motor activity.[37]

Perhaps, then, the primary effect of supplementation with B-group vitamins is to increase glucose metabolism in the brain, providing more energy to the cortex, the thinking brain, allowing it to once again reassert its modulating effects on the limbic system, the emotional brain.

The antioxidants, Vitamins A, C and E besides counteracting the toxins and pollutants that we inadvertently ingest, may play a significant role in facilitating the uptake of other important nutrients. A study done in a juvenile detention centre found that just making pitchers of freshly squeezed orange juice available at every meal resulted in a 47 percent improvement in behaviour.[38] Orange juice is a source of folic acid and thiamin as well as vitamin C, and all of these have been found to be low in delinquents.[39]

In addition, seventy-five mg of Vitamin C in a meal will cause approximately a six-fold increase in the absorption of heme iron[40], and iron is an important co-factor in the synthesis of serotonin and dopamine. The improved behaviour may thus have resulted from the increased iron uptake and additional nutrients in the orange juice, rather than the vitamin C alone.

Minerals. Calcium deficiency has ben reported in hyperactivity.[41] Magnesium deficiency can result in children showing excessive fidgeting, psychomotor instability and learning difficulties, even in the presence of normal IQ.[42] Magnesium is also an important co-factor in the activity of neurotransmitters linked to aggression, and magnesium deficiency is associated with a Type A behaviour pattern and aggression.[43]

Iron deficiency is associated with irritability and attention deficits in children, which may lead to cognitive dysfunctions including problems with visual recall, digit span, and performance on standardised IQ tests.[44] Studies in Thailand, Indonesia and India, of school children supplemented with iron, demonstrated significant improvement in IQ scores, cognitive function scores and learning achievement scores.[45]

In the brain, the most prominent feature of iron deficiency is the slowing down of neurotransmission or nerve signals in the dopamine neurons in various parts of the brain.[46] The consequences of this is a modification of dopamine-related behaviours and biochemical reactions, the most important of which is reduction of learning ability.

Zinc is a co-enzyme to many important neurotransmitters, such as serotonin and dopamine that are involved in the modulation of mood, and its highest concentrations are found in the pineal gland, where serotonin synthesis is stimulated. Zinc deficiency is also common in children with learning disabilities.[47] Foodstuffs high in zinc include shellfish, steak, eggs, sunflower seeds, sesame seeds, pumpkin seeds, pecans, legumes and beans, most of which are not high in the diets of children and adolescents today. While you should take in at least 15 mg of zinc a day, analyses of well-rounded diets served at cafeterias and hospitals show only 8 to 11mg per day is provided.[48]

Zinc is also useful for its quality of binding with lead, mercury and cadmium and can thereby aid heavy metal detoxification.[49] Elevated concentrations of lead, cadmium and aluminium have been associated with low academic achievement and low IQ scores.[50] Interestingly, when children with behaviour and learning problems were placed on a diet in which toxic metals, refined foods, sugar and fats were reduced and relevant vitamins and minerals supplemented, and whole grains, complex carbohydrates and unprocessed foods increased, significant improvements in intelligence, behaviour and learning were observed. In addition, cadmium levels fell 28 percent and lead by 49 percent over 22 weeks.[51]

In another study, children with learning problems were supplemented with vitamins and minerals and placed on a special diet which eliminated refined sugars and emphasized whole grains, unprocessed chemically free foods and fresh or frozen but not canned vegetables. Every child showed evidence of improved school behaviour and performance and parents noted relief from sinus problems, asthma, indigestion, 'nerves', and skin problems. While initial hair analyses showed 25 percent of the children to be in the medium to high range for lead by the end of the first year, none showed elevated lead levels. Likewise, 45 percent of the children initially were in the medium to high range for cadmium, but by the end of the first year, only 30 percent were in the middle range and 70 percent were now in the low range.[52]

Both of these studies highlight that it is children who may be deficient, often only marginally, in vitamins and minerals who are most affected by toxic metals such as lead and cadmium. Children who are deficient in magnesium, iron, vitamin D, calcium or zinc are affected more by elevated lead and cadmium levels than those whose nutritional status is good.[53]

Essential Fatty Acids and Amino Acids. Until recently there was no firm evidence of the behavioural effects of supplementation with essential fatty acids or EFA, such as Evening Primrose Oil and Max EPA (a fish oil derivative). A number of nutritionists however, suggested that supplementation may be beneficial.[54] The correct balance of essential fatty acids is crucial for childhood development. The active constituent of n-3 fatty acids, docosahexaenoic acid (DHA), is particularly important as development of the visual system is dependent upon adequate levels during pregnancy and infancy, and insufficiency of DHA has been found in Attention Deficit Hyperactivity Disorders and central nervous system disorders.[55]

In a recent study, children with dyspraxia (extreme clumsiness), became much better co-ordinated if they added fish oil to their diet. A nutritionist gave 15 dyspraxic children fish oil rich in essential fatty acids for three months and the result was a highly significant improvement in the children's balance and dexterity. To quote the author of the study, 'before the children couldn't catch a ball or learn to ride a bicycle. Now they can'.[56]

Supplementation is also recommended with essential amino acids as some amino acids, notably Tryptophan and Tyrosine, are important precursors to brain neurotransmitters, and are diet dependent.[57] Vitamin deficiencies may also be affected by amino acid deficiencies, as vitamin B_6 is necessary for the formation of vitamin B_3 (niacinamide) from the amino acid tryptophan.[58] A supplement with all 22 amino acids may be preferred, as conversions of some amino acids from the eight essential amino acids to these more complex forms, is not always efficient.

Supplementation for Hyperactivity & Learning Problems:

Based on the discussion above, it would seem prudent to consider supplementation for children demonstrating hyperactivity and/or learning problems. The following suggestions are only broad guidelines, and we suggest that you see a registered naturopath or orthomolecular doctor. We advise you to give the recommended dose for you or your child's age, or consult a registered nutritional therapist.

Vitamins:
Vitamin B Complex with reasonably high levels of niacin, pyroxidine (B_6), pantothenic acid, and thiamin. A good quality, non-allergenic, additive-free supplement is recommended.

Vitamin C, in electrolyte form (calcium, potassium, sodium, and magnesium ascorbates) also containing bioflavenoids that facilitate uptake of Vitamin C.

Vitamin A and Vitamin E, to provide for further anti-oxidant protection and membrane stability. A good quality, non-allergenic, additive-free supplement is recommended.

Minerals:
Multi-mineral complex with calcium, magnesium, manganese, iron, zinc, and trace elements. A good quality, non-allergenic, additive-free supplement is recommended.

Zinc supplementation may be considered in addition to the above, as many multi-minerals have relatively low zinc concentrations. Hair analysis or urine analysis may be needed to ascertain if your child is deficient in zinc, and you may wish to seek qualified advice regarding dosage. Vitamin B_6, magnesium, manganese, and vitamin A, all assist with the utilisation of zinc. Most good quality zinc supplements are available with this complex, although if your child is already taking the supplements as suggested above, this complex is not needed and a straight zinc supplement is all that would be required.

Essential Fatty Acids: Max EPA, Omega-3 Fatty Acids, Fish Oil (e.g. salmon oil), or Evening Primrose Oil.

Amino Acids: A good quality, non-allergenic, additive-free amino acid supplement containing all eight essential amino acids may be sufficient. A supplement with all 22 amino acids, however, is preferred, as the conversion of some amino acids from the eight essential precursors to more complex amino acids is sometimes less than efficient. Nature also provides nicely packaged, a complete protein source of all essential amino acids—an egg, and one a day would insure that this need is met.

Tissue Salts: Kali phos., Mag. phos., Nat. mur., Silica, Nat. Sulph., and Nat. phos. are the main tissue salts lacking in hyperactive children.[59] Kali phos. and Mag. phos. in particular appear useful with hyperactive children. If you are not familiar with Dr Schuessler's Tissue Salts, consult a registered nutritional therapist or homeopath.

What to Eliminate from the Diet:

Foods: All foods that you or your child have an allergy or intolerance to, for instance, dairy foods if there is a dairy intolerance. Reduce sugar, refined and processed foods (Junk and fast foods).

Food Additives, Artificial Colours & Preservatives: Try to keep these as low in the diet as possible.

Check for Heavy Metal Toxicity: Have yourself or your child checked for toxic levels of copper, manganese, lead, cadmium, mercury, and aluminium. Hair analysis, urine analysis, or blood analysis may be needed to ascertain if you or your child have high levels of these toxic metals. Eliminating the source of these metals is then important. Treatment with homeopathics can often be of considerable assistance in the elimination of toxic metals.

ALLERGIES OR SENSITIVITIES

Allergy is a term generally used to denote the observable physiological reaction to some food or environmental substance, but sensitivities also denote a physiological reaction, usually of a less specific kind. So although you would say someone has an 'allergy' to strawberries, because every time they eat them their face breaks out in a rash, you may say you have a 'sensitivity' to certain chemicals or foods, because you feel somehow different when you have been exposed to them.

The classic allergy response is the release of specific chemical compounds called immunoglobins into the blood. The most common allergic reactions result from large amounts of Immunoglobin E (Ige) in the blood or tissue reacting to the presence of the antigen or allergen. In many allergic responses there is a spillover of Ige into the blood, which is why many blood tests to detect allergies are actually detecting the presence of Ige or another immunoglobin in the blood.[60]

Food and chemical sensitivities, on the other hand, usually indicate that the adaptive enzyme systems responsible for handling these substances are not operating or functioning correctly.[61] Thus with many sensitivities, the exact biochemical mechanisms may remain unknown yet the responses are identifiable. If you have a sensitivity to wheat, after eating it you may feel a loss of energy that seems quite dramatic. In the context of this book, we are talking about allergies and sensitivities without distinguishing between them. Any factor that affects performance and function we will consider to be a stressor.

Allergies/sensitivities can arise in response to natural and unnatural factors. Some people have allergies/sensitivities to natural foods, like oranges and shellfish, while others react to unnatural factors such as food dyes and some food additives. Whatever the source, food allergies/sensitivities can cause a stress to the system and in some cases result in the loss of brain integration.

Food additives
Food additives are used to change the taste or texture of food, or to extend its shelf life. By far the most common additives that cause these reactions are preservatives such as Sodium Benzoate and Sodium Metabisulphite, antioxidants Butylated Hydroxytoluene (BHT) and Butylated Hydroxyanisole (BHA), and flavour enhancers such as Monosodium Glutamate (MSG).[62]

In sensitive people, these additives may cause overt physical responses such as itching or headaches. Others may demonstrate only behavioural responses such as hyperactivity or emotional outbursts. To quote a report in the journal Allergy, 'while true allergic reactions to food additives occur only seldom ... adverse effects due to various pharmacological (drug-like) mechanisms are much more common'.[63]

Sensitive people may even react quite overtly to the presence of these chemicals in natural foods, such as the salicylates in the skin of red apples.[64] I lived across the street from the grandmother of a child who was demonstrating extreme hyperactivity and uncontrolled behaviour to a degree that he would walk down a supermarket aisle willfully sweeping every item off the shelf with his arm.

What was remarkable was that his grandmother would receive the child early in the morning when his mother went to work and all day long the boy would be an amenable, agreeable three-year-old. She would put him down for a nap at 3 pm and when he awoke, would give him two red apples, which were his favorite food, for an afternoon snack.

By the time his mother arrived to pick him up at 4:30pm, he was already becoming hyperactive and this would continue until he went to sleep at night. This pattern continued for almost a year, with his mother blaming herself for failing to control his behaviour. His mother observed that the child seemed to be less hyperactive on weekends but attributed that to the presence of his father.

One day, his grandmother happened to read an article in the Reader's Digest which stated that salicylates in the skin of red apples had been associated with hyperactivity in some children. Suddenly she twigged: 'My God. I give him red apples every day before his mother picks him up.' Within days of removing the cause—red apples and other foods that contained salicylates—the child's behaviour changed profoundly and he remained the agreeable child his grandmother had always known.

Food dyes

To enhance the cosmetic appearance of foods, many manufacturers add colouring agents. The bright orange colour of most soft drinks and cordials is due to the presence of a food dye called Tartrazine. Some colourings are derived from natural sources. Others are synthetic chemicals. Tartrazine, for one, is derived from coal tar.

One of the groups of colourings that cause the strongest allergy/sensitivity reactions are Azo food dyes, synthetic organic colouring agents that make food brighter. Tartrazine is one of the best known members of this group but other Azo dyes, particularly the bright reds, greens and blues, can also have devastating effects on sensitive people. It is not uncommon for children with learning problems to demonstrate strong reactions to this particular group of food dyes.[65]

The mother of a child we were treating told us a story of being called to the school by her daughter's teacher. The teacher reported that after lunch that day, the girl had become so mentally confused and physically unco-ordinated that she couldn't manage to thread a big bead on a string.

Knowing her daughter to be sensitive to many food additives and dyes, the mother always sent her daughter to school with a lunch that was free of any of these substances. So she asked her daughter what she had eaten at lunchtime. The child reported that she had traded the apple from her lunchbox for a popular snack food that was loaded with Tartrazine. That single packet of snack food was enough to cause total loss of her physical and mental integration.

Another young client of 16 was so sensitive to food dyes and additives that if he had any foods containing Benzoates or Tartrazine he would be jumping out of his skin for a period of days. In his parent's terms, he would be 'floating around on the ceiling, he was so spaced out.'

After an exhaustive search, his parents had found that by giving their son a preparation of Tri-Salts, they could bring him back to earth within a few hours after exposure to the substance that so unbalanced him.

While there is considerable anecdotal evidence to support a connection between food additives and colourings and learning disabilities, hyperactivity in particular, much of the data generated in double-blind cross-over studies often fail to show effects of these substances on behaviour. In these types of studies, the child is usually put on a diet eliminating the suspected additive for one to several weeks, and then 'challenged' by having usually a single additive given to them in food or drink. In contrast, clinical and parental observations often *do* report major effects on behaviour.

In one scientific study, 24 children who had been confirmed sensitive to certain food additives were put on a diet that avoided these items. In all children there was a clear history that any lapse in the diet caused an obvious adverse behavioural reaction within two hours. Yet, when these children were challenged with the individual additives in a placebo-controlled double-blind experiment, in no case was there any change in behaviour noted by parents or nursing staff.[66]

In contrast, another double-blind study of 24 children diagnosed as hyperactive, showed many of the children also displayed allergies to a number of common allergens such as dust and pollens. Within one week of starting a food elimination diet, parents noted a moderate-to-marked improvement in 11 of the 17 children who stayed on the diet. This improved behaviour continued for at least 12 weeks. When later challenged with single food dyes (Tartrazine) and allergenic foods the children consistently displayed the previous symptoms of either hyperactivity or somatic (physical) complaints. Eighty-seven percent of the children who were on activity-modifying drugs

(Ritalin) were able to discontinue the drugs after 12 weeks on the elimination diet.[67]

Three other observations regarding the effects of food additives on behaviour are worth considering. In a carefully designed experiment, 82 percent of hyperactive children improved on a diet low in food additives and allergic foods, with almost one quarter achieving a normal range of behaviour within a number of weeks. Symptoms returned or worsened more often when suspicious foods containing additives were reintroduced. Of the 48 foods incriminated, artificial colours and preservatives were the most common substances provoking reaction.[68]

Tartrazine also appears to act as a chelating agent that binds to zinc in the blood causing an increase in urinary zinc excretion. In a double-blind study, a group of children classified as hyperactive and a group of matched control children drank a commercial orange drink containing tartrazine. The hyperactive children, but not the controls, showed a loss of zinc in their urine.[69]

This highlights two important aspects of the effects of food colourings on hyperactive children. First, hyperactive children appear to show abnormal metabolism, and thus may react differently to food additives relative to normal children. Secondly, food colourings like Tartrazine may not only have direct drug-like effects on these children, but may also cause marginal nutritional deficiencies of essential nutrients like zinc that have a major impact on brain function and behaviour.

Excessive phosphorus intake has also been associated with hyperactivity and aggressive behaviour.[70] If a phosphate-sensitive child is given a phosphate-free diet for several weeks, and then challenged with a dose of phosphate (75mg) mixed in food, the symptoms of attention problems and hyperactivity will return within one hour—usually within 15 minutes. Phosphate-containing foods include: processed and canned meats, processed cheeses, many baked products (phosphate baking powder), all cola and many other soft drinks, all instant soups, puddings, etc., and various toppings, seasonings.

Table 10.1 below summarises the food additives and preservatives that have been associated with various behavioural and physiological problems. It is not an exhaustive list, but it covers the additives or preservatives most commonly associated with these problems and hyperactivity.[71]

Table 10.1. Food Additives and Preservatives known or suspected of being associated with adverse behavioural or physiological reactions.

COLOURS	KNOWN/SUSPECTED OF BEING ASSOCIATED WITH ADVERSE REACTIONS
102 Tartrazine	*Hyperactivity*, migraine, asthma, rhinitis, blurred vision, insomnia, skin reactions
107 Yellow 2G	Asthma, *hyperactivity*, skin reactions
110 Sunset Yellow FCF	Asthma, *hyperactivity*, skin reactions, swelling, gastric upset, vomiting, possibly carcinogenic
120 Cochineal	*Hyperactivity*
122 Azorubine	Asthma, *hyperactivity*, skin reactions, swelling, water retention
123 Amaranth	Asthma, *hyperactivity*, skin reactions, possibly carcinogenic
124 Brilliant scarlet 4R	Asthma, *hyperactivity*, skin reactions
127 Erythrosine	Light sensitivity, *hyperactivity*, overactive thyroid, brain dysfunction, possibly carcinogenic
132 Indigo carmine	Nausea, vomiting, high blood pressure, skin reactions, breathing difficulty, *hyperactivity*
133 Brilliant blue FCF	*Hyperactivity*
142 Green S	Asthma, *hyperactivity*
150 Caramel	*Hyperactivity*, diarrhoea
151 Brilliant black BN	*Hyperactivity*
155 Brown HT	Asthma, *hyperactivity*, skin reactions

FLAVOUR ENHANCERS

620 L-Glutamic acid	Muscle tightening, numbing effects, thirst, nausea, palpitations, dizziness, fainting, headaches, cold sweat, asthma, *hyperactivity*
621 Monosodium glutamate	Muscle tightening, numbing effects, thirst, nausea, palpitations, dizziness, fainting, headaches, cold sweat, asthma, *hyperactivity*
622 Monopotassium glutamate	Nausea, vomiting, diarrhoea, abdominal cramps, headache, asthma, *hyperactivity*
623 Calcium di-L-glutamate	Asthma, *hyperactivity*
627 Disodium guanylate	Asthma, *hyperactivity*, gout

PRESERVATIVES	KNOWN/SUSPECTED OF BEING ASSOCIATED WITH ADVERSE REACTIONS
210 Benzoic acid	*Hyperactivity*, asthma, skin reactions, gastric irritations, brain dysfunction
211 Sodium benzoate	*Hyperactivity*, asthma, skin reactions
212 Potassium benzoate	*Hyperactivity*, asthma, skin reactions
213 Calcium benzoate	*Hyperactivity*, asthma, skin reactions
216 Propylparaben	*Hyperactivity*, asthma, contact dermatitis, numbing effect on the mouth
218 Methylparaben	*Hyperactivity*, asthma, skin reactions
220 Sulphur dioxide	*Hyperactivity*, asthma, gastric irritations
221 Sodium sulphite	*Hyperactivity*, asthma, gastric irritations, skin reactions
222 Sodium bisulphite	*Hyperactivity*, asthma, gastric irritations, skin reactions
223 Sodium metabisulphite	*Hyperactivity*, asthma, gastric irritations, skin reactions
224 Potassium metabisulphite	*Hyperactivity*, asthma, gastric irritations, skin reactions, collapse
250 Sodium nitrite	*Hyperactivity*, breathing difficulties, pallor, nausea, vomiting, dizziness, headaches, low blood pressure, collapse
251 Sodium nitrate	*Hyperactivity*, possibly carcinogenic

ANTI-OXIDANTS

320 Butylated hydroxyanisole	*Hyperactivity*, skin reactions, asthma, possibly carcinogenic
321 Butylated hydroxytoluene	*Hyperactivity*, skin reactions, asthma, possibly carcinogenic

Kinesiology balancing for allergies or sensitivities to food dyes and additives

Whenever substance to which someone is allergic/sensitive is introduced into their energy field, it will cause a distortion of this field. The distorted energy flow will in turn have a physiological effect. A momentary distortion of the energy field will only produce a subtle physiological disturbance; a prolonged, powerful distortion will produce an observable physiological effect.

For a person who is allergic to cat hair, as soon as cat hair is introduced into their energetic field it will immediately distort that field, which will be transduced to a physiological reaction, causing an observable kinesiological muscle stress response. The change or distortion in the field is unique to that person, as not everybody reacts to cat hair. In the western perspective, however, the allergen is usually considered the cause of the allergy rather than the person's reaction to it.

It is the electrical pattern induced by the energetic distortion that electrodermal acupuncture devices such as the Vega, Mora and Listen machines detect.[72] Once a person is balanced kinesiologically to the presence of that substance in their energy field, there is no longer any abnormal energetic reaction and the person no longer experiences an allergy/sensitivity, nor are imbalances registered on the Vega, Mora or Listen machines to that substance. It can be that simple.

I once went to visit a professorial friend, a cat lover, who had a student staying in his house. This boy was so allergic to cat hair that he was virtually reduced to staying in his room to avoid the house cats. As soon as he smelled a cat, his nose would block up and his eyes would run. If the cat scratched him, or if his skin came in contact with cat hair, it would often form pustules that would take weeks to disappear.

Because I was there, I offered to balance the boy for his allergy to cats. He was disbelieving. I asked him to lie down on the table, got some cat hair and placed it on his navel. The muscle immediately indicated severe stress. After going through a series of balancing techniques, the last of which was age recession, I found that the cause was an event that occurred at the age of two-and-a-half. Even though there was no conscious memory of this event, kinesiology identified an issue of anger with his father. There was also a cat involved and that was all we needed to know.

I then did Frontal Occipital Holding to defuse the emotional stress on this issue. As soon as I had finished, he no longer demonstrated any reaction to cat hair being placed on his navel. The boy got up and reported that he was feeling very strange.

He stated that for the first time in his life he actually wanted to pet the cats in the house rather than kick them across the room. He picked one of the cats up and smelled it. No response: no streaming eyes, no blocked nose. He put the cat on his shoulder and the cat began rubbing on his neck. Again, no physiological response. The cat slipped, digging a claw into his shoulder and again there was no response. His old reaction to cats had been eliminated.

He was so amazed that he rang his father to report what had happened. He asked his father why he might have been angry with him over the issue of cats at the age of two-and-a-half. His father said: 'I know what it was. When you were two-and-a-half I used to take you to a baby sitter's house and she had a cat that bit and scratched you. You would make such a scene about going that I had to stop taking you there.'

Somehow, this emotional state had been locked into the boy's system as a perpetual trigger causing his allergy to cats. Once it was balanced and defused, the boy no longer had a cat allergy.

As this example shows, it is possible to resolve some long-standing allergies fairly simply. But not all. Hayfever, a common seasonal allergy, is in a different category. Because there can be literally tens of thousands of pollens and mould spores in the air at any time and because these change seasonally, it is very difficult to find out exactly which particular pollen, or group of pollens, is causing the allergic reaction that results in that person's hayfever.

When specific pollens or moulds are identified as being involved in the hayfever response, these can be balanced and the hayfever resolved, yet there may be still other pollens or moulds that may trigger a reaction that remain unknown.

CANDIDIASIS

The presence of candidiasis, or Candida overgrowth, may profoundly affect brain function. Candida albicans is a yeast, that like the bacterium E. coli, is a natural component of the flora of the human intestinal system. This yeast is similar to baker's or brewer's yeast and normally maintains a growth pattern of budding asexually: one cell budding a smaller cell from its surface, and this cell budding a smaller cell from its surface and so on. Eventually the cells break off and the process begins all over again.[73]

This is a relatively slow process, slower than bacterial growth, and in the intestine there is constant competition for space. For organisms to remain in the intestines, they need a surface area on which to attach, otherwise they are carried out in the faeces. Since the yeast grow slowly and the bacteria grow rapidly, bacteria manage to usurp most of the surface space in the gut, thereby limiting the numbers of yeast.

These gut organisms are symbionts in our system. We give them space to live and they, in return, provide us with certain vitamins. Vitamin B_{12} is the product of Lactobacillus activity, and steroids, of yeast activity. Evidence suggests that the yeast produce steroids that may be absorbed and used as precursors to the formation of some human hormones.[74]

Sometimes, the balance between the yeast and bacteria can be upset and the usual catalyst is antibiotics.[75] Antibiotics not only kill bad bacteria, they also kill off the good bacteria in our gut. Because Candida is not a bacteria and is not affected by antibiotics, it suddenly finds itself in an environment in which there is a lot of space and lots of food, but nothing else to compete with. It grows more rapidly and the growth pattern changes.[76]

Instead of reproducing in the relatively innocuous budding form, these micro-organisms go into a mycelia overgrowth form, producing horizontal growth tubes which can penetrate the intestinal tissue. These rhizoids are similar to the fine white fibres that you can observe in mouldy bread when you tear it apart. These tubes can penetrate enough to enter the micro-circulation of blood vessels in the walls of the intestine, exposing the blood to the yeast and to other by-products of digestive activity.[77]

It is precisely because the proteins resulting from the partial digestion of foods can now enter the bloodstream that people often develop allergies or sensitivities to many of the foods they eat. When the partly digested proteins reach the bloodstream, the immune system sees them as antigens, and will respond by antibody formation. The body mounts a fight against this alien in the bloodstream and the next time the stimulant food is eaten there is an antigen/antibody reaction. Thus, the more often a person eats a particular food, the more likely they are to develop a sensitivity to it.

The most common food groups related to sensitivity are wheat, corn, soya and dairy products. When someone is suffering candidiasis a common pattern is observed: They will often eat toast for breakfast then feel a flagging of energy by mid-morning, as if someone has pulled the plug. They will then reach for something sweet to pick them up—a chocolate bar—and momentarily feel better. Then they eat a sandwich for lunch and the pattern repeats in the afternoon. Again they reach for a sweet stimulant. Since the yeast utilises simple sugars as its major food source, diets rich in refined carbohydrates and sugar foster yeast reproduction—maintaining the yeast over-growth situation. The two things interact and drive each other so a cyclical behaviour arises that effectively supports the yeast.

The yeast also produces a toxic chemical, acetaldehyde, that causes a loss of brain integration, and in that state the person will crave more of the foods that feed the yeast. The loss of energy due to the wheat sensitivity only reinforces the desire for the quick energy of sugar-laden foods. This initiates a vicious cycle of eating sugar rich foods and foods that you often have an allergy or sensitivity to that feed the yeast creating greater biochemical and immune system imbalance. The end result is a person that often appears neurotic or even psychotic and can not cope with life.

Progressively, these allergic reactions depress the immune system, making it less capable of dealing with other insults, such as infections.[78] Respiratory and ear infections can recur and these, in turn, have been shown to affect the vestibular system decreasing activation of the reticular activating system, part of the mechanism which allows you to pay attention.[79] In overgrowth, Candida also manufactures two very toxic chemicals, alcohol and acetaldehyde[80] which

Environmental Factors That Can Affect The Brain 295

can cross the blood-brain barrier, the unique structure of the walls of the brain capillaries, which is capable of resisting the passage of most other chemical substances.

While the effects of alcohol crossing the blood-brain barrier are well known—the state of inebriation, which predominantly affects the frontal lobes (our ability to think) and the vestibular system, (our ability to balance)—it can also compromise our ability to concentrate. In some individuals, the active metabolism of the Candida overgrowth can produce so much alcohol that even though they are teetotallers they are 'drunk' most of the time.

A 46 year-old man, Kozo Ohishi, kept becoming 'drunk' over a twenty five year period, in spite of the fact that he was a teetotaller. He was then found to have a massive colony of Candida albicans yeast in his digestive

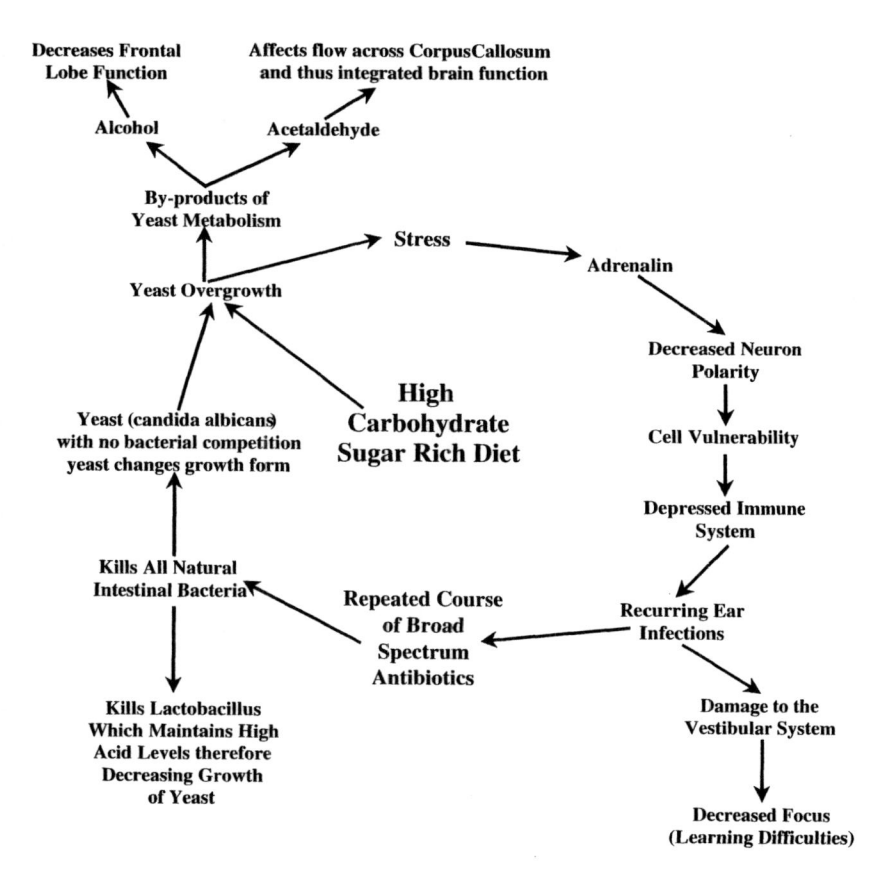

Figure 10.2. The Stress-Infection-Antibiotic-Yeast-Sugar-Toxins Cycle.

system. When he was placed on a low carbohydrate diet and treated with anti-Candida medication, he stayed sober. A number of other cases have been reported from Japan, with people ranging in age from three to 74 years, where the condition is called Meitei-sho, which literally translates as 'Drunk Disease'.[81]

A similar case reported in the Los Angeles Times 25 September 1983, was Duffy Mayo, a five year-old who had been diagnosed as autistic. He would stagger around, giggle and laugh very much like a drunk. Even his breath smelled of alcohol. After treatment with anti-yeast medication and special diets, little Duffy's behaviour improved significantly.

Alcohol has been shown to profoundly affect the neuro-development in the frontal lobes. In Foetal-Alcohol Syndrome, the alcohol crossing the placenta has far-reaching effects on brain development, producing symptoms that manifest in later life as decreased attention span, behaviour problems, sugar cravings, hyperactivity, depression and autistic behaviour.[82]

For children who develop Candida overgrowth, clearly the alcohol produced may significantly alter the development of important neural networks within their brain. While this may not be as permanent as Foetal-Alcohol Syndrome it certainly can affect their learning capabilities, especially if the on-going Candida overgrowth goes untreated.

When formaldehyde and acetaldehyde cross into the brain they affect the neurotransmitter function of the fibres crossing the corpus callosum, in effect producing chemically induced loss of brain integration. The subjective sensation of having Candida overgrowth is a feeling of being thick in the head or woolly headed. Why people feel so fuzzy-headed is because they are suffering a constant loss of brain integration. With many of the pathways of the corpus callosum shut down, it is no wonder they have difficulty thinking straight.

These two chemicals can sometimes cause quite dramatic mood swings, with people suddenly finding themselves bursting into tears for no known reason. In the past, it was common for women suffering Candida-induced mood swings to consult their doctor—and since candidiasis presents such a diffuse bag of symptoms—they could find themselves being treated as neurotics and being given anti-depressives or tranquillisers.

I once met a man socially who told me about his eight-year-old daughter who, he said, was becoming increasingly moody and irrational. I encouraged him to bring her along to my clinic and as soon as I saw her, I had to acknowledge that she did indeed look neurotic. Her eyes were bulging out of her head, showing what the Japanese term Sanpaku eye or 'three-sided white'.[83]

On-going emotional or mental stress may cause the eye muscles to vertically lift the pupil in the orbit so white shows beneath the iris when the person is looking straight ahead. If this occurs in one eye only, it indicates stress of short-term duration. In cases of long-term stress, both eyes will show white beneath the pupils.[84]

Based on my observations I thought I was looking at a case of long-term emotional stress, but the more information her father gave me with respect to her symptoms; sugar craving, bloating, flatulence and headaches, the more I heard the symptoms of candidiasis. Her father had also noticed that her mood swings were markedly affected after she ate certain foods, another classic Candida symptom.

I did the first few steps of brain integration on the child, balancing deep-level switching and opening up full access across her corpus callosum, and then spent a couple of hours balancing her energetic systems to eliminate Candida. She was also requested to restrict certain foods in her diet, especially simple carbohydrates, sugar, dried fruits and other mould containing foods, wheat and dairy products, except yoghurt, for about a month. Thereafter she could reintroduce most foods, but she would have to continue to restrict sugars and yeast or mould containing foods and wheat on an on-going basis.

Her father called a week later and reported: 'I don't know what you did but thank you. I now have a different daughter. She is the same happy child I used to know three years ago.'

Kinesiology balancing to eliminate the effect of Candidiasis on brain integration

People who have Candida overgrowth at relatively low levels, or people who have sound brain integration may not experience much of an effect of candidiasis on their brain function. For others, Candida overgrowth can have a significant impact on maintaining brain integration and mental function. It is important for these people that the effects of the Candida be eliminated before undergoing in-depth brain integration. Otherwise, we have the impossible situation where there are on-going chemical factors causing disintegration while the therapist is trying to promote reintegration.

Using muscle monitoring, a competent kinesiologist can tell if there is a resonance of Candida causing stress in the body. This stress is most commonly observed in the large intestine, the most common site of Candida overgrowth, and the liver and kidneys, the organs that detoxify and excrete Candida toxins, respectively. However, both the fibres crossing the corpus callosum and the frontal cortex may also show stress, because as we have explained, information transfer across the corpus callosum may be affected by the acetaldehyde, and cortical function, especially in the frontal lobes by the alcohol produced by Candida overgrowth.

Using vials of homeopathic preparations of Candida and placing them on the acupoint Central Vessel 8 (the navel) will cause a muscle response if there is a resonance of Candida present—a frequency match like tuning your radio. If this is observed, the alarm points can then be monitored to find which are active, indicating the organ systems affected by the Candida.

Once the priority organ system has been located, the imbalance can be entered on the biocomputer. Various acupressure corrections are then evaluated for a frequency match with the imbalance. Once the appropriate type of correction for the imbalance has been located it is simply a matter of applying that procedure.

Then the Candida vial is put back on Central Vessel 8 to challenge the body's response once more. If there are no further muscle stress responses to the presence of Candida, the body has re-established its balance with respect to this stressor. More commonly, another muscle stress response will indicate another type or level of balancing that is yet to be done. This procedure is repeated a number of times until there is no longer any muscle stress response from the challenge with Candida.

Kinesiology can be very successful in eliminating the effects of Candida on brain integration but it must be emphasised that once a body has had a chronic Candida problem, it can remain vulnerable whenever the mitigating circumstances recur. It is important, therefore, that in the period immediately following the Candida balance people restrict certain foods and stressors that either stimulate Candida overgrowth, suppress immune function, or stress liver function.

For this reason people may be asked to restrict certain foods in their diets. These include: sugar, alcohol, baker's and brewer's yeast, mushrooms, wheat and corn-based products, dairy products, dried fruits and some tropical fruits like papaya and rock melon, which may contain moulds. Fermented foods such as soya products and vinegars can also cause Candida to flare up and must also be avoided.

Foods that support the positive intestinal flora against being overwhelmed by Candida include: acidophilus (found in unsweetened yoghurts or yoghurt drinks) and caprillic acid: a naturally occurring anti-fungal that suppresses Candida growth and can be taken in capsule form. Garlic is another naturally occurring yeast suppressing food. Vitamin C, bioflavenoids and other antioxidants also support this process by scavenging free-radicals during the detoxification process and support the immune system. Zinc supplementation and a junk-food free diet which restricts the amounts of wheat, corn, yeast and mould containing foods and sugar is also recommended.[85]

EXTERNAL ENVIRONMENTAL FACTORS

Electromagnetic radiation

By electromagnetic radiation (EMR) we mean the radiation given off by various electrical devices. Every electrical current produces an electromagnetic field, so every wire in your house that has current running through it, has an electromagnetic field surrounding it. Every time you turn on an appliance or any electrical equipment, you are fluxed by EMR. Thus, even in our homes we are constantly moving through electromagnetic fields.

While the earth's geomagnetic field in the mid-latitudes is more than 1000 times greater than the EMR produced by typical electrical appliances in the home, there are two significant differences between the background EMR of the earth and the EMR of electrical appliances and commonplace equipment. Firstly, it has a primary magnetic component that is static and a much smaller secondary component represented by micropulsations in the 0.1 to 0.2 Hz (cycles per second) range.[86]

Secondly, human beings and their predecessors evolved for millions of years with this background EMR, and have adapted to its presence. In his important book reviewing the scientific literature on the effects of EMR on health, *Cross Currents. The Perils of Electropollution. The Promise of Electromedicine*, Robert Becker concluded that:

> 'the magnetic field of the Earth is an important physiological factor for living organisms. It appears that behavioural changes of an undesirable nature, either quite evident or subtle, may result from exposure to environments having lower or higher field strengths than 'normal' or *those having either no fluctuation or cyclic fluctuation at frequencies other than those to which we are adjusted.*'[87] (Italics added.)

Nikolas Tesla's invention of AC electricity forever changed the electromagnetic environment of man and other species. Telsa's AC electrical system, now the most commonly used electrical system around the world, operates at either 50 Hz or 60 Hz, frequencies that are *not* present in the earth's normal electromagnetic spectrum.[88] It is the phenomenal increase in the extent and range of electromagnetic frequencies generated by man-made electrical equipment from household electrical appliances to radio waves, TV transmissions, computer radiations and microwaves that now bombard man and his environment that Becker termed 'Electropollution'.

It is now generally accepted that these artificial EMRs can affect our body and brain processes because our body and brain also produce a low frequency electromagnetic field by the electro-chemical activity of our nervous and muscular systems and the membrane resting potential across every cell in our body. We can even measure these EMRs in the brain with the Electroencephalogram (EEG) and in the body with the Electrocardiogram (ECG).

As anyone who has tried to listen to their car radio while sitting next to a tram knows, one electromagnetic field definitely can interfere with another electromagnetic field. From a review of the scientific evidence, Becker concluded that 'the exposure of living organisms to abnormal electromagnetic fields results in significant abnormalities in physiology and function.'[89] What has been in question is the magnitude of the effects of these artificial EMRs on humans.

Presently, these fields are not acknowledged as posing any overt serious health threats, but there are questions arising as to the more subtle effects they may have on physiological function. Increasing evidence alludes to the idea that even low-level fields may produce stresses in our bodies and brains including:[90]

- Induction of chromosomal defects in mice spermatogenic cells (sperm- precursors) following microwave radiation in the gigahertz range.
- Changes in the calcium balance of living cat's brains exposed to microwaves modulated at extremely low frequencies.
- Alteration of nerve and bone cells exposed to extremely low frequency fields.
- Decreased activity of the immune cells of mice exposed to modulated microwaves.
- Apparent increases in deformed fetuses among miniature swine exposed to intense power-line frequency fields.

Since the 1970s there has been considerable scientific controversy about the effects of electromagnetic fields generated by overhead high-tension power lines. One of the first studies suggested that the EMR from overhead powerlines might cause childhood cancer.[91] Another study was done on cats, which have a small territory or home range. As anyone who has observed the fighting between male cats would be aware, cats stake out their own patch and spend most of their lives in this small area.

One researcher studied cats that lived within 500 metres of large power lines. He noted the incidence of feline leukemia in these cats was double that of cats which did not have territories near power lines. Because feline leukemia is considered an animal model of human leukemia, it was an alarming finding.

Other studies were undertaken to establish whether similar effects could be observed in human populations.[92] The earliest of these studies produced conflicting results, perhaps because humans, unlike cats, range over a large area and also move in and out of neighbourhoods. Also, the effects of low level

EMR appears to require long periods of constant exposure to produce observable results. Human mobility means it is difficult to ascribe the actual dose of EMR that people were subject to in these studies.

A more substantial Swedish study of about 500,000 people, controlled for the above variables, has established a clearer relationship between EMR and the rates of childhood leukemia. Children living within 300 metres of high-tension power lines showed double the rate of leukemia compared with control subjects residing more than a kilometre from power lines. Furthermore, a second study by the Swedish National Institute of Occupational Health found a link between high levels of occupational exposure to EMR and two forms of cancer—chronic lymphocytic leukemia and brain cancer.[93]

A report compiled over nine years by eleven leading American experts on EMR commissioned by the US National Council on Radiation Protection concluded that millions of people may face an increased risk of cancer and degenerative diseases because they are exposed to EMR from power lines and household appliances. The committee's chairman stated that there is now 'a powerful body of impressive evidence to suggest that very low exposures to EMRs has subtle, long-term effects on human health'. The report says that there is strong epidemiological and laboratory evidence to suggest that children exposed to EMRs from power lines are at greater risk of developing leukemia, and that adults exposed to EMRs at work run a higher risk of leukemia and brain cancer.[94]

Other studies have shown that the type and frequency of electrical current can have subtle effects on the structure and mutation rates of DNA. AC (alternating current) at 45 to 60 cycles per second showed the greatest effect on mutation rates, with cycles higher or lower having less effect.[95] It is interesting to note that all the electrical systems in the world operate on 50 to 60 cycles per second. This might sound frightening, but it is also worth remembering that most of us do not demonstrate any obvious effects from exposure to these electromagnetic fields, and most mutations observed in these studies were rapidly repaired by DNA repair enzymes.

Mobile telephones
Although highly controversial, there have been several law suits filed recently on behalf of people who developed brain tumors which they claim were the result of using mobile telephones. It was argued that the constant and close exposure of the soft tissue of the brain to the electromagnetic fields of the mobile phone led to tumor formation, and there is growing evidence to suggest that exposure to certain types of microwave radiation may indeed increase the incidence of brain tumours.[96]

The intensity of an electromagnetic field drops off with the inverse square of the distance from its source. That means if you double the distance, the intensity of the electromagnetic field is decreased by one fourth. Cellular phones, which are held in contact with the head, often for long periods, therefore may have greater physiological impact than other common appliances.

The effects of the electromagnetic fields of a mobile phone can be easily demonstrated using kinesiology. If you hold a mobile phone to your ear with the power off, and monitor a muscle, there will usually not be a stress response, the muscle will remain locked. If you turn the phone on, and particularly if it is engaged in a call, the muscle will immediately indicate a stress response by unlocking. This suggests that mobile phones may have a potentially distorting effect on our energy systems. As previously stated, when the energy structure is distorted by any stressor, it will have physiological effects, it is just the degree of these effects that may not be readily apparent.

Television and computer screens
The other electromagnetic devices that we all interact with these days are televisions or computer monitors. These use electron guns that fire electrons from the back of the tube at the screen. When the electrons hit the screen, they make the phosphorous in the screen fluoresce, resulting in both a picture and colour. While the electrons are captured by the screen and their charge neutralised by ions attracted from the air, the reason your TV screen attracts dust so strongly, the electromagnetic fields generated by this flux of electrons and ions is responsible for the EMR that may cause energetic and physiological stress.

If you have good brain integration and your body is energetically balanced, you will have a relatively strong resistance to these electromagnetic perturbations. But if you have poor brain integration, the constant flux of electromagnetic energy can cause a distortion of your energetic body, which can then cause mental confusion and other physiological effects such as fatigue. Even in people who have good brain integration, long exposures to these fields can cause a breakdown in mental function and fatigue.

I have noticed that while I have excellent brain integration and am generally a good speller, after a long period in front of a computer I will begin to make spelling mistakes. Also, I will get to the end of a line and find I have lost the thread of what I am saying. These are both symptoms of loss of brain integration. This is when I will often take time out to stand up and rub my acupoints for brain integration (K-27s, upper and lower lips and navel and coccyx) and do a few sets of cross-crawl.

The constant flux of electromagnetic radiation is one of the reasons people experience tiredness after working in front of a computer screen for long periods and why a lot of people fall asleep in front of the television set. If you are affected by these fields, prolonged exposure can disorient you enough that the brain will seek to escape the stress by putting you to sleep.

One of my clients told me of their neighbour who was so sensitive to the EMR from his television that when he sat in the same room with it he experienced physical discomfort that bordered on pain. He had to arrange a series of mirrors to reflect the picture into another room from which he could then watch TV comfortably.

People with poor brain integration and learning problems are the most susceptible to these environmental influences. Often such children will sit in front of the television before they go to school. At school they sit under fluorescent lights all day (another factor that may cause loss of integration) and when they return home, they once again sit in front of the television. These children are in a constant state of environmentally generated brain disintegration.

I heard an anecdotal report of a teacher in New Zealand who asked the seven-year-olds in his class to sign a contract saying they would not watch television for a week. At the end of the contract period, I was told that even the children reported they were able to work better.

Fluorescent lights

I had a client who was the most susceptible person to EMR of anyone I had ever encountered. This little girl was so sensitive that exposure to any electromagnetic stimulation would cause immediate loss of brain integration. She was particularly sensitive to fluorescent lights, which, even at several metres distance, caused measurable energetic stress. As part of the assessment, using kinesiology, I demonstrated to her mother just how sensitive her daughter was to this type of electromagnetic radiation.

It happened that the mother had an interview with her child's teacher the next day. She noticed the fluorescent lights in the classroom were switched off and asked the teacher about this. The teacher said she hated the fluorescent lights. 'As soon as the daylight gets long enough I turn then off early in the morning and leave them off all day.'

The teacher then reported how much better the girl had been doing in the spring term, improving particularly in the last several weeks compared to the winter term. The mother realised that the fluorescent lights had been on all day during the winter term and suddenly grasped that her daughter's improvements probably had a tangible cause.

Fluorescent tubes produce a lot of electromagnetic flux because of the way they work. There is an element in a fluorescent light called a ballast, which causes the tube to be highly ionised. Electric current is run through the tube, which contains an inert gas such as neon. The current flows between a positive and negative electrode, arranged at either end of the tube.

The positive ions race to the negative end and the negative ions race to the positive end. When they get there, the ballast reverses the field so that the ions immediately reverse direction, racing to the opposite ends. These polarity reversals are repeated 60 times each second and the charged ions rush past the inert neon gas molecules so quickly that the rubbing causes the inert gas to fluoresce, producing light.

This means that in the vicinity of a fluorescent light there is a very powerful oscillating electromagnetic field. The light itself also has a very unusual spectrum, being very strong in greens and blues but weak in other parts of the spectrum—particularly red wavelengths. This can be easily observed with a spectroscope that displays the visible light spectrum.

Both the electromagnetic activity in the tube and the quality of the light it emits can have a strong effect on sensitive people, causing a distortion in their energetic body. This distortion may cause a loss of brain integration and even noticeable physiological effects such as fatigue. Nevertheless, fluorescent tubes are found in most schools, most offices and most supermarkets because they are cheap to operate.

A recent study revealed the effects of fluorescent lighting on performance and productivity. In Reno, Nevada, there was a post office that had one of the worst sorting records in the United States. It also had older style fluorescent lighting that has a high green-end spectral bias that may cause a visual stress response.

To explain this further: Your interpretation of the brightness of light depends very much on the degree of greenness in the light. This may be because most of the natural environment is green and evolution has selected it as the best measure of brightness. Whatever the foundation, the brain interprets green-spectrum light as being extremely bright.

This is why supermarkets appear to be so brightly illuminated. But they're not. It is a trick of the eye. If you measure the actual lumens of light, a supermarket may be rather dim. For a comparison, natural daylight, even on an overcast day, is about a 1000 lumens per square foot, while supermarkets and the artificial lighting in the average office may only register between 60 and 100 lumens per square foot.[97]

Researchers at Cornell University exposed students to two independent light sources, one which was closely matched to simulate natural daylight (full spectrum light), while the other was an ordinary fluorescent tube of exactly the same 82 lumen illumination. After four hours exposure to each light source, significantly more students reported fatigue under the fluorescent tube.[98]

For many people, the spectrum bias and the electromagnetic flux of fluorescent lights will cause extreme disorientation or electromagnetic stress. Indeed, some people find that when they enter supermarkets they are unable to think straight. They lose their mental integration and can't remember why on earth they went there in the first place.

In the Reno post office, it was decided to upgrade the old lighting system with a new installation of $300,000 worth of high-efficiency, low-energy lighting. The post office administrators reasoned they would save money, but what happened was far more startling. Not only was money saved on the lighting bill but the sorting efficiency suddenly became one of the best in the country. The productivity soared and $500,000 a year was saved. Why were they now so efficient? Probably because for the first time the sorters could actually see what they were sorting, because the new lighting provided actual illumination, not apparent illumination. And secondly, more of the sorters, removed from the electromagnetic flux of the previous fluorescent lighting, may now have been working with integrated brains.

Because of the world in which we live, we are not going to be able to avoid fluorescent lighting, TV screens or computer monitors. How then, in face of this electromagnetic onslaught, are we to maintain our brain integration? There are two approaches: One is to have your energetic systems balanced with kinesiology to electromagnetic perturbations emitted from computers and common appliances. The second is to obtain devices that have been specifically designed to alter the type of electromagnetic radiation emitted by everyday appliances and electrical equipment.

Overall, it would appear that an individual's response to electromagnetic fields is similar to the variation in people's response to various allergens. In short, while one person may respond to a particular pollen, another may not. The culprit is not simply the stimuli, allergen or mobile phone, but rather, would appear to be the individual's energetic and physiological response to these environmental stimuli. I believe that it is only electromagnetically sensitive individuals who will suffer physiological harm from normal exposure to electromagnetic fields.

Since these electromagnetically sensitive individuals can be easily detected using kinesiology and this sensitivity greatly reduced by kinesiology balancing, this may have significant impact on their mental and physiological function, and perhaps even on their long-term health.

Devices for neutralising electromagnetic radiation

A number of devices have been developed in the last 20 years to neutralise the electromagnetic effects of appliances and electrical equipment. Most of these are based on electromagnetic and energetic principles that are not yet fully accepted by mainstream scientists. The principles on which these units operate were established by an Russian-American scientist, Nikolas Tesla, who in 1888 invented the electric motor in a form that is largely still in use today.

He was also the first to demonstrate that the earth itself is an electrical conductor and proposed that the electromagnetic fields of the earth, and of electrical devices, could have effects on human beings. He invented electromagnetic patterns that could be imprinted into plates and generated by various types of devices that he felt cancelled or counteracted the more negative aspects of EMR. While these fell into disrepute at the time, a new wave of energetic scientists has discovered his work and have created a number of devices which work according to his theories.[99]

The earth's electromagnetic background is basically long-wave, low-frequency electromagnetic radiation of approximately eight cycles per second. Electrical equipment and appliances on the other hand, emit a variety of frequencies of erratic EMR both above and below the frequency of the background radiation. Tesla believed that man-made EMRs could be harmful and current research is confirming his ideas.

Electromagnetic neutralisers are believed to work by either absorbing or converting the EMR from appliances and re-emitting them as low-frequency EMR, similar to that produced naturally by the earth.

However they work, kinesiology tends to verify their effectiveness. You can take a person sensitive to EMR, stand them in front of a TV and monitor their muscle for stress. When the TV is off, the muscle is locked, showing no stress. The instant the TV is turned on, and the person is fluxed by the EMR of the TV, stress is indicated by an unlocking muscle. If, however, one of these neutralising devises is placed on the TV or attached to the TV, the stress response disappears and the muscle locks once again.

From my personal experience, I can verify that people sensitive to these electromagnetic fields have gained considerable benefit from wearing neutralising devices or by attaching them to household appliances. I personally have an EMR neutraliser on my computer. It is somewhat like going outside when it's cold, that is into a thermally antagonistic environment. It is prudent to use thermal protection, for instance a heavy coat, when choosing to put yourself in that environment. Likewise, when I choose to sit in front of my computer and put myself in an antagonistic EMR environment, I choose to use a device to protect myself from the stressful effects of that EMR on my mind and body.

If you feel you might benefit from owning a neutralising device (and I suggest every computer owner needs one) I advise you to seek information about them (See Appendix E).

STRUCTURAL AND PHYSIOLOGICAL FACTORS AFFECTING BRAIN INTEGRATION

These are several other internal environmental factors that can also affect brain function:

Eye muscle balance
As you look to the left or to the right, the movement is controlled by external muscles attached to the eyeball. An integrated circuitry locks the two eyes

together so they work smoothly and both focus on the same point at the same time. This is called conjugate gaze and it maintains an integrated image on the retina.[100]

The six muscles on each eyeball are called the rectus and oblique muscles. The rectus muscles are located at the top, the bottom, on the outside and the inside of the eyeball. The superior rectus muscles roll the eyes up. The inferior rectus muscles roll the eyes down, and the lateral rectus muscles roll the eyes toward the ears. The medial rectus muscles pull the eyeballs towards the nose.

The oblique muscles attach to the top and bottom of each eyeball but pull at an oblique angle providing for rotation of the eyeballs. The contraction of the superior oblique muscles rotates the eyeballs up and inwards while contraction of the inferior oblique muscles rotate the eyeballs down and out.

When all the eye muscles are working together, the eyes are capable of movement in any direction, and proper alignment and movement of the eyes is essential for any visual task. In normal function, the lateral and medial rectus muscles work in pairs, allowing the eyes to move from side to side, which is the action involved in reading.

When you make yourself go cross-eyed, you are contracting both medial rectus muscles at the same time. If you have a squint or are cross-eyed permanently, it is because you have weakness in your lateral rectus muscles. The lateral rectus muscles are not too long, they are merely inhibited and therefore not pulling out against the pull of the medial rectus muscles pulling in. The result is a squint or turning in of one or both eyes. If these muscles are strengthened through exercise or kinesiological balancing, the squint may disappear.

On a number of occasions I have seen children who are cross-eyed, or who have a squint, and have been able to correct these problems completely by merely strengthening the lateral rectus muscles using kinesiology and acupressure techniques.

An academic friend, the chairman of a science faculty, had a daughter that demonstrated a squint. She was also observed to have a foot that turned in, which caused her to have difficulties running. She would often trip over. Her father had observed that when she woke up in the morning she walked well and had little or no squinting. But by late afternoon she would be stumbling and looking manifestly cross-eyed. She had a $600 brace made to straighten her foot and was scheduled for an operation to straighten her eye. I happened to visit her father at this time and discussed her problem.

After a one-hour kinesiology treatment for muscle reactivity, which results when one muscle inappropriately turns off another, her foot no longer turned in and she walked normally. Her eyes were also straightened. Talking with her father several years later he said: 'I really can't believe that she was ever cross-eyed or so bumble footed, except for the fact that every now and then

I run across her $600 brace in the back of the cupboard and know I would not have bought it for no reason.'

Several factors can cause eye muscles not to work in a smooth, co-ordinated pattern. Eye muscle dysfunction can become apparent when people are reading, moving their eyes back and forth across the page in an action known as smooth pursuit or tracking. Problems with this movement can be ascertained very simply by holding a finger up in front of a person, about 30 centimetres in front of their face, and asking them to follow it as the finger is moved side to side. The eyes should move smoothly from side to side.

In children with reading problems there will often be difficulty in making their eyes move in slow pursuit. Instead, they will stick and jump. Even where the eyes appear to be moving normally, stress can be detected because after a short time, the subject will start rubbing their eyes, say their eyes are hurting, or the eyes will water. It can actually be so physically uncomfortable for these children that they will stop as soon they can. If your eyes stick and jump, or if it is physically stressful to read, you will not choose to read for very long.

The most common factor causing this sticking and jumping is structural, torquing or twisting of the sphenoid bone.[101] The sphenoid bone is the centre piece of the cranium, forming the posterior of each orbit and locking all the cranial vault bones together with the facial skeleton. Five of the six eye muscles are attached to this bone. Thus slight torquing or twisting of the sphenoid will result in unequal tension on the eye muscles which may result in sticking and jumping of the eyes.

Also the cranial nerve supply to these muscles are unmyelinated which makes them very vulnerable to pressure as they pass through extremely tight knooks and crannies of the cranial system on their path from the brain to the muscle. Any tension or pressure on these nerves due to cranial bone distortion may cause differential muscle response creating loss of co-ordinated eye movement. The most common form of torquing is to have the bone twisted down and to the left, which makes looking up to the left quite painful and often makes co-ordinated eye movement difficult.

There are two approaches to correct the sphenoid bone distortion. One is chiropractic and requires a qualified cranial chiropractor or osteopath to manipulate the cranial bones. This will be most effective if there is lumbar-pelvic stability as the skull and pelvic system are interdependant.[102] These cranial adjustments can be very effective in creating a more balanced skull and cranial membrane system. This is more an 'inside-out' approach.

The other option is to balance the eye muscles and musculature of the cranium to release the sphenoid bone and return it to its proper position or an 'outside-in' approach. This can be done using kinesiology and acupressure techniques to reset the musculature and structure. These procedures require special training and should only be performed by a qualified practitioner.

Deformed palate

The hard palate or maxilla forms the roof of the mouth and can also be out of normal alignment or distorted resulting in a vaulted or arched palate. In extreme cases it is termed a cathedral palate. The hard palate is a most important part of the cranio-facial system. Distortions of the palate are indicative not only of sphenoid bone imbalance, but of the whole cranial and dural membrane system being torqued or misshappen.[103]

A normal palate has an ovoid shape, wider at the canine (dog teeth) and narrowing posteriorly at the 7 and 8 year old molars.[104] It is flatly arched and can accommodate the full width of both thumbs between the upper canine teeth. A vaulted palate indicates that the maxillary and palatine bones have not been allowed to grow and develop in the normal configuration resulting in a deep and lumpy trench in the roof of the mouth.[105] This can be so extreme that some people have difficulty putting one thumb into their palate without touching their canine teeth.

The narrowness of the maxillary bones usually coincides with a torquing of the sphenoid bone and is often observed in people with eye muscle co-ordination problems.[106]

In terms of physiological function, these high palates can have a number of repercussions notably the narrowing of the sinuses and the nasal airway. With this loss of dimension general congestion and blockage are more prone to occur. Thus the allergic rhinitis phenomenon is commonly seen with narrow or vaulted palates. The air passages become restricted and pollens and airborne particles may get stuck in the mucus. Often the space is so congested that the pollen gets stuck between two layers of mucus and can't move. If the pollen stays in place for too long, the constant irritation will inevitably generate an allergic reaction.

People with high arched palates are therefore more prone to have allergies to pollens and other inhalants, and as I have discussed, allergies are a stress

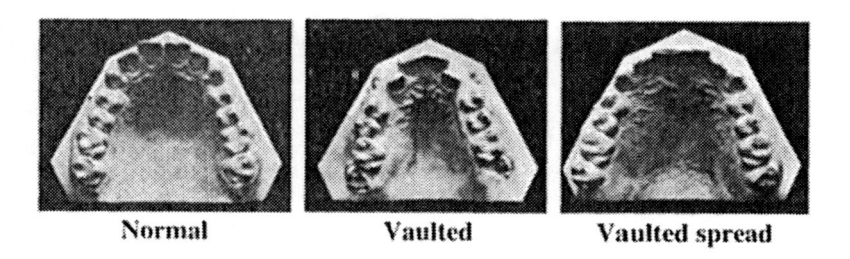

Figure 10.3. A comparison of normal (ovoid) and arched/vaulted palates before and after palate spreading.

that can affect brain function. Also, due to the airway restrictions these people are commonly mouth breathers because if you can't get the air in through your nose you have to get it in through your mouth. This mouth breathing also tends to create a forward head posture and subsequent full body postural distortions such as round shoulders.[107] Physically, these people tend to have long narrow faces and eyes that droop at the corners.

Crowded teeth
People who have vaulted palates always have crowded teeth.[108] If your palate is broad and ovoid, the perimeter of the maxillary bones which contain the upper teeth is quite large and can easily accommodate a full set of teeth. If the palate is vaulted or highly arched, there is a smaller perimeter to accommodate the same number of teeth. The result is crowded teeth.

The shape of the palate impacts on how the lower jaw fits into the cheekbones and has a great deal of effect on occlusion or bite. The lower jaw fits into the upper jaw with upper slightly overlapping. When the palate or upper jaw fails to develop fully then the lower jaw has to move into a compromised position. This can either be in front of or behind the maxilla or upper jaw. Most of the time if there is a narrow upper jaw from an arched or vaulted palate the lower jaw will sit back creating an overbite, and in the extreme the buck teeth effect. In a smaller percentage of cases the bottom jaw will be forced forward and protrude. Aside from the poorer aesthetics created by theses jaw positions there are the on-going functional problems associated with not only the teeth but as mentioned above the whole functional nerve supply of the body including the brain.

For example full body postural problems are usually present when there is an overbite. The jaw bone is pushed back on the temporomandibular joint (TMJ), and since the TMJ is the pivot point for balance of the cranium on the neck, and cervical spine distortion will result which will be compensated for by lumbar or lower back spinal distortion.[109] Weakness of lower limb muscles is also common, especially in cases where there is also a cross-bite, the line between the two front teeth (incisors) of the upper and lower jaw not being in line. This often results in children shuffling their feet rather than lifting them for each step.

In other words, the shape of the palate determines not only the way the teeth fit together, but also will have resonance throughout the whole spinal column and is ultimately a structural stressor that can affect brain integration. TMJ imbalance is very commonly associated with persistent head and neck aches as well as with occlusion or bite problems.[110] Often these headaches are low grade and chronic, which of course, impacts on mental function.

Both these oral factors can be corrected by a qualified 'functional' orthodontist preferably fluent in cranial mechanics of the sphenoid and intracranial dural membrane system and full body postural balance. Their aim is to create a more functional jaw to jaw relationship whilst at the same time improving the function of the cranial and dural membrane system using various types of dental appliances and braces.

Once the shape of the palate and cranial/body balance has been redressed, it is very common for people to be free of allergies and often, they will find they are also able to read more easily. An orthodontist I refer clients to, Dr. Harry Marget, was doing general dentistry and orthodontics. He had a patient with a vaulted palate and crowded teeth who he had been treating for general dental problems.

This patient went to Germany and when he returned several years later, went back to see Harry for a checkup. Harry was amazed to see the man no longer had a vaulted palate or crowded teeth. What had happened? He was told that while in Germany, the patient had seen an orthodontist who had spread his palate and straightened his teeth. But most remarkably, the patient was also suddenly free of the allergies he had had all his life and, most inexplicable of all, could now read fluently. Harry was so impressed by these observations that he flew to Germany to learn the technique and has practiced it for many years.

Another client I referred to Harry was a lady of almost 50, who had such a vaulted palate that she could not get one thumb between the teeth of her upper jaw. She was a mouth breather and had suffered allergies all her life, and had always had difficulty reading as she tended to skip lines, a sign of eye muscle imbalance. She underwent palate-spreading work.

The appliance that was put in to spread the palate has a little ratchet attached to it which is adjusted each day to maintain outward tension on the maxillary bones. This small but constant tension causes the maxillary bones to slowly move outward and as they move outward the palate will drop.

Her palate spread over time, and after several weeks, she was startled one morning to find that for the first time in her life, the air rushed in through her nose. She said it sounded like a freight train and it took her some time to get used to the sound of her own breathing. Once the palate was fully spread, her allergies abated and she was no longer exclusively a mouth breather, which significantly improved her appearance. As a bonus, her reading became dramatically easier and more fluent.

In my clinical work I see many of these structural problems and usually as a package in children with learning problems. In adults, they can present as neck and lower back pain and chronic headaches, all of which may affect our abilities to think clearly. A recent study of people suffering from 'whiplash' injury, but with no overt neurological damage, displayed significantly reduced speed of information processing and performance on tests for divided attention. It was suggested that reduced working memory may account for the more global cognitive problems observed.[111]

In this chapter I have illustrated just how integrated a human being is. Our brain integration is not just a function of mental activity, but rather the sum result of our physiological, energetic and structural integrity. The brain is therefore the focus of a delicately balanced, amazingly complex and interconnected system that goes well beyond the grey matter traditionally considered to be our 'brains'.

In the final chapters, I will discuss a model of reality that lays a foundation for understanding the energetic effects I have discussed so far in the book. I will also take a quantum leap into the uncertain world of mind and consciousness.

PART THREE

The big picture

The most beautiful and most profound emotion we can experience is the sensation of the mystical. It is the sower of all true science.

He to whom this emotion is a stranger, who can no longer wonder and stand rapt in awe, is as good as dead.

To know what is impenetrable to us really exists, manifesting itself as the highest wisdom and the most radiant beauty which our dull faculties can comprehend only in the most primitive form—this knowledge, this feeling is at the centre of all true religiousness.

The cosmic religious experience is the strongest and oldest mainspring of scientific research.

My religion consists of a humble admiration of the illimitable, superior spirit who manifests himself in the slight details we are able to perceive with our minds.

That deeply emotional conviction of the presence of a superior reasoning power, which is revealed in the incomprehensible universe forms my idea of God.

Albert Einstein quoted in Ajit Mookerjee, Yoga Art.

Chapter Eleven

AN ALL ENCOMPASSING REALITY

THE NATURE OF REALITY

To provide a view of reality which encompasses the amazing interplay of the faculties of the human brain, the final part of this book will be a journey into the nature of mind and consciousness.

But we must prepare for that journey. Understanding how the subtle energy flows of acupuncture or Ch'i could have such profound effects on brain function requires us to construct a framework of reality that embraces both the physical and the metaphysical. Without such a framework, from the standpoint of orthodox science, many of the things I have discussed in this book would seem improbable at best and impossible at worst.

Much of this chapter is speculative: it is based on models that are internally consistent but which, generally, cannot yet be fully tested. In this chapter we will therefore be asking you to step beyond your normal perceptions of what seems real in order to appreciate that there may be an even greater reality that lies beyond.

The model of reality that will be presented here is a synthesis of my personal experience, my extensive reading in both eastern and western esoteric literature and a theoretical model developed by Dr William Tiller, Professor Emeritus of Material Science at Stanford University. Professor Tiller's theory was further elaborated by Dr Richard Gerber in his seminal book, *Vibrational Medicine*, which considers the role of subtle energy in healing.[1]

Gerber's book gave me a scientific explanation of the more esoteric experiences that had occurred in my life. Finally, I had a model for astral travel and out-of-body experiences; for the etheric realms I accessed during deep meditation and for the phenomenal ability of acupressure stimulation to heal.

TWO DIVERGENT MODELS OF REALITY

THE WESTERN PHYSICAL MODEL

The orthodox western scientific view of reality is primarily built on the foundations laid down by the Greek philosopher Democritus (460 -370 BC), who was famous for his atomic theory, the essence of which holds that the only ultimate reality are atoms: minute, solid, invisible and indestructible particles that make up all matter. All that exists in this theory is either matter or void (space).[2]

Following the lead of Isaac Newton, modern science held to the premise that the world is a physical structure consisting only of particulate matter and space. Newton elaborated the laws by which the matter in this physical world interacts and in the centuries since the Newtonian Revolution, these principles have been refined and tested.

Part of the process of science is the systematic investigation by experimentation to test the prediction of hypotheses. Many of these experiments generate results that did not make sense in the Newtonian paradigm. At this point, Albert Einstein developed his Theories of Relativity which showed that Newton's Laws of Gravity are only correct when applied in a particular context: that is, from the perspective of a stationary individual on the earth and at velocities well below the speed of light.

As we view matter from other perspectives relative to observer and movement, and at speeds approaching the speed of light, Newtonian physics fails to predict the outcomes and hence in such contexts is no longer a valid theory. But in these contexts Einstein's theories correctly predict the outcome.

Likewise, when we move to the subatomic level, the principles of Newtonian physics also fail and need to be replaced by a body of experimental knowledge and theories called quantum mechanics. This is the mechanics of quantum systems. Quantum refers to the sub atomic level.

Western science is clearly based upon 'objective' observation, but only in certain contexts. Subjective observation is rejected as not being reproducible and hence, not dependable. But there is a failure to understand that an observer is always making a subjective observation as he is using sensory data processed by his brain, which interprets this data based on his unique life experience. To surmount this problem, science now attempts to let machines and electronic instruments do as much measurement as possible (but still a human mind must interpret the meaning of the data). Science is clearly then limited to the contexts of that which can be measured with these instruments.

To quote Richard Cytowic from his book *The Man Who Tasted Shapes*, 'it is a truism that science tells us how the physical universe 'really is', but its rejection of direct experience leads to a distorted view of it (the world) ... Science simplifies reality by leaving out whatever fails to fit the conceptual framework within which it is working at the moment.'[3]

This is the basis of all controlled experiments. In such experiments, there is an attempt to eliminate all factors that may affect the outcome of the experiment, except for the factor which is under investigation. Many scientists do not understand this and perceive what they are doing as a representation of reality, not a reduced piece of reality.

Aldous Huxley expressed this misunderstanding beautifully as early as 1946 when he wrote: 'The scientific picture of the world is inadequate for the simple reason that science deals only with certain aspects of experience in certain contexts. All this is quite clearly understood by the more philosophically-minded men of science. But most others tend to accept the world picture implicit in the theories of science as a complete and exhaustive account of reality.'[4]

Michael Katz states this another way. 'Science strives to reduce our experience to symbols. Experiences are colorful, multi-faceted, and fuzzy along the edges; symbols are bland, one-dimensional, and precisely-bounded. Real world observations can be bulky and ill-shaped and can have both strong and tenuous ties with a myriad of other real world observations; abstractions are built of simple, smooth-faced elements, uncoupled from other constructs ... Scientifically, we give up the shifting and elusive mystery of the world, but, in exchange, we gain the standardised and reproducible abstractions from which we can build determinate explanations.'[5]

While most people in the West believe that 'science' does provide them with a total picture of reality (albeit a picture of a physical universe in which only physical matter exists), this has not always been the case. Earlier schools of western scientific thought perceived reality to be not only physical, but to also contain vital forces that were not perceptible by the five senses. And yet, these vital forces were recognised as being instrumental in creating and maintaining the structure of the physical universe.[6]

This same holistic view was also applied to the human body which was seen by the early scientific philosophers not only to be physical, but to also contain subtle, unseen energies that organised and maintained its structure. The school of thought that proposed that the body is more than merely physical, rests on principles first ascribed to the eastern classic, the Huang-di-Nei-Ching or the *Inner Classic of the Yellow Emperor* which was compiled by unknown authors in China starting as early as 2500 BC and written down between the first century BC and the early first century AD. In the West Hippocrates proposed a similar concept of vital energy in about 400 BC. Both these philosophic traditions assume that the 'natural' state of things is order and harmony, and that there exists within 'nature' a force which attempts to preserve a perfect equilibrium and reestablish order and harmony whenever it has been perturbed.

The Hippocratic School called these natural adaptive powers the physis. In Hippocratic thought the physis was perceived as a 'healing power' or 'self-adjusting power', within the body that 'though untaught and uninstructed, it does what is proper to preserve a perfect equilibrium'. Physis is also the root of the word physician, and in Hippocrates' view, as a guardian of the physis, the physician clearly had a supporting role: 'Not as a ruler or a violator of nature ... he stands ready to aid the healing power that is inherent.'[7]

This holistic view prevailed in the West until English lawyer and philosopher Sir Francis Bacon (1561–1626) established the primacy of the scientific method based on objective observation. Despite the almost wholesale takeover by the physical view of the human body, small schools of holistic medicine persisted, particularly in northern and eastern Europe.

THE EASTERN ENERGETIC MODEL

In contrast to the blinkered views of western science, eastern sages practicing the science of yoga and various healing arts, viewed the subtle energy bodies to be the origin of matter, with mind the mechanism by which consciousness invests order into life.[8] In this model, the subtle energy flows of the acupuncture and chakra systems provide an energetic template upon which matter is organised.[9]

Since the energy systems in eastern science are based on the flows of these subtle energies, which are currently beyond the measurement of scientific instruments, they are said to be metaphysical or beyond the physical. The challenge is to create a nexus between these two streams of thought and to bring the physical and metaphysical together into one integrated system.

Modern physics is once again beginning to acknowledge the existence of more subtle levels of physical matter. In quantum mechanics and particle physics, it is recognised that the world that we see is not the world that exists. What looks like solid matter, we now know is made up of sub-atomic particles which themselves are made up of even smaller particles, which, in turn, appear to be more energy than matter. What to the human eye appears to be a static world full of solid physical objects is in reality, nothing but a sea of subatomic particles in constant motion, with many of these particles constantly blinking into and out of existence.[10]

In fact, these particles are not measured in units of mass but rather in electron volts, a measurement of energetic force. As well, there are quantum mechanical properties of matter that seem improbable and are difficult to comprehend. One of these is that electrons can appear as either particles (matter) or as wave forms (pure energy). How they appear depends not upon their essential nature, but rather upon how the observer chooses to measure them.[11]

Another bizarre property of the quantum world is called non-locality, a concept that really stretches the imagination. If a stream of electrons is split by a beam splitter, so that two electrons are travelling apart at approximately twice the speed of light (600,000 kms per second), and the observer chooses to observe one as a particle, the other immediately becomes a particle, even if it is on the other side of the universe. As improbable as this sounds it has been scientifically demonstrated to be true.[12]

AN INTEGRATED MODEL OF REALITY

For the past three decades Professor Tiller has been working to provide scientific models that explain certain subtle energetic phenomenon such as the flow of Ch'i and various psychic phenomenon such as telepathy, clairvoyance and distance or remote healing. He has created a model of reality that finally succeeds in incorporating the physical domain of the West and the metaphysical domain of the East.

Richard Gerber termed this model the 'Tiller-Einstein Model of Negative-Positive-Space/Time' because its insights are derived from the Einstein equation that relates energy to matter: $E = mc^2$. Einstein's equation suggests that energy and matter are interconvertible and interconnected, with subatomic matter considered as a packet of frozen energy. The release of energy from its frozen form is the massive power behind the atomic bomb.

While we normally think of reality as having only three dimensions, Einstein's equations have led to the concept of Space/Time, which is the fourth dimension in which we exist. If you feel this is a difficult concept to grasp, be comforted by the fact that even the physicist Stephen Hawking, in his book *A Brief History of Time*, conceded that he too had problems wrapping his mind around the idea of this fourth dimension.[13]

ASPECTS OF POSITIVE AND NEGATIVE-SPACE/TIME

In this new model, reality can be considered to consist of at least two domains: Positive-Space/Time and Negative-Space/Time. Each has its own unique properties and is governed by its own particular principles. Although in Tiller's multi-dimensional model, he specifies five important and uniquely different domains, four of them are sub structures of the 'vacuum' so, for the purposes of this chapter, we will refer to all of them as the Negative-Space/Time domain. For a broader and more detailed understanding, the reader is referred to Professor Tiller's seminal new book, *Science and Human Transformation: Subtle Energies, Intentionality and Consciousness*.[14]

POSITIVE-SPACE/TIME. PHYSICAL REALITY

This is the physical domain based on visible matter. Originally, it was only observable via the five senses of sight, sound, smell, taste and touch. With the naked eye, there is a physical world of appearances that is quite different to the world that can be perceived with other spectral wavelengths.

Humans are limited to the visible spectrum of the rainbow which runs from red to violet. This is only a tiny slice of wavelengths, less than 1/1000th of a metre long, which is in the middle of the electromagnetic spectrum. In this spectrum, wavelengths stretch from less than a quadrillionth of a metre, to more than a million metres in length (see Fig. 11.1).

This ultra-thin visible slice of a very long and continually expanding spectrum of electromagnetic energy was taken to be all of reality for millennia. It is only within the last century and the advent of electronic instrumentation that many of the once invisible aspects of this domain have become known. These invisible wavelengths include infrared, ultraviolet, radiowaves, microwaves, x-rays and gamma rays.

Using this new instrumentation, scientists were surprised to find that some animals 'see' into parts of the light spectrum which are beyond human perception. For example, bees see deep into ultraviolet wavelengths. Flowers 'know' this and produce groups of strongly UV absorbing pigments called 'flavanols', which present patterns to the bee's eyes in order to lure them directly to the nectarium containing the sweet nectar.

Similarly, the group of snakes called pit vipers, of which rattlesnakes are a common example, have infrared sensors in a row of pits above the upper lip and under their eyes. Just as soldiers can use special infrared sensitive binoculars to see the enemy moving at night, the rattlesnakes can 'see' mice and other warm-blooded mammals moving in complete darkness.

Properties and Principles of Positive-Space/Time

The major property of Positive-Space/Time is that it is electromagnetic in nature. Electromagnetism is the interconnection of a flow of electrons (electricity) and magnetism such that whenever there is a flow of electrons along a conductor, a magnetic field is created perpendicular to this flow (see Fig. 11.2). Likewise, whenever a magnetic field is fluxed (passed) across a conductor, a flow of electrons is created.

This is exactly how the generator in your car generates electricity. Attached to the central shaft of the generator are a set of strong magnets, surrounded by thousands of coils of fine copper wire. As the fan belt turns the pulley of the central shaft, the magnets are spun around inside the coils of copper. As the magnetic flux is pulled across the copper, a flow of electrons is created, powering the lights, ignition and firing the spark plugs. It also charges the battery.

In Positive-Space/Time, the physical domain, matter is associated with the

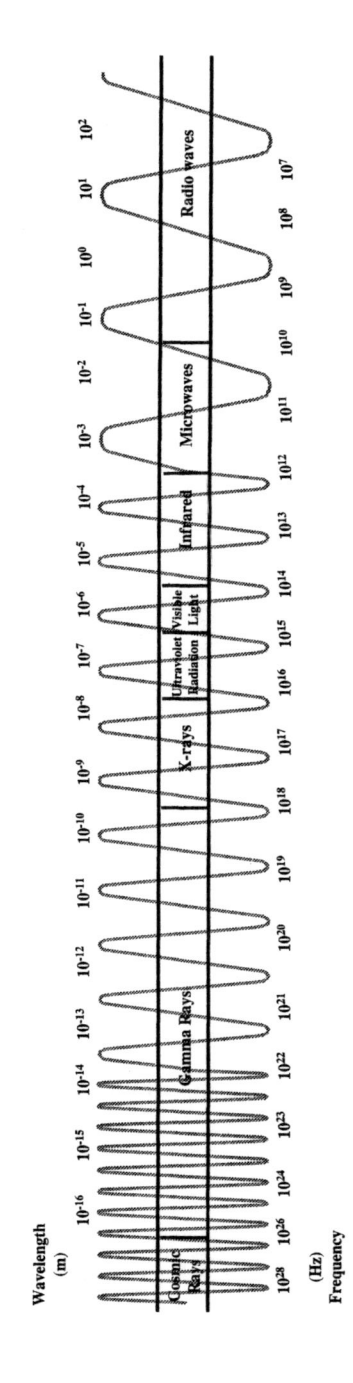

Figure 11.1. Graphic of electromagnetic spectrum. Note that our physical senses only allow us to be consciously aware of the thin slice, visible light, of this limitless electromagnetic spectrum.

force of electricity and electromagnetic radiation (see Fig. 11.4).

The first principle of Positive-Space/Time is governed in accordance with the rules of relativity which say that matter cannot exceed the speed of light. So matter in this domain is restricted to velocities which are less than 300,000 kilometres per second. The reason this is true is that when you look at Figure 11.3, as velocity increases towards the speed of light, mass increases exponentially. In short, it requires more and more energy to make an object move faster and faster and soon the energy required to increase speed at all is beyond that which is available.

The second principle of Positive-Space/Time is the principle of entropy, which states that there is an inherent tendency toward a decrease in free energy, expressed as disorder or chaos. Stated another way, it says that energy

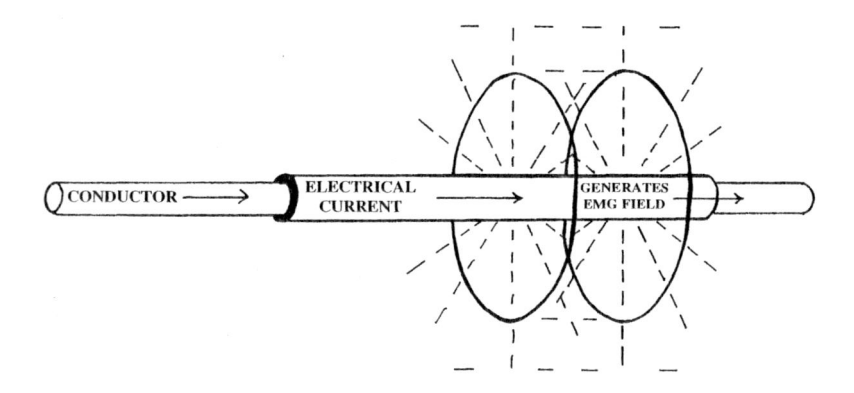

Figure 11.2 EMG field. A magnetic field is always generated perpendicular to the flow of electricity as in the schematic diagram above.

runs downhill. This is why, in the physical world, things tend to decay and deteriorate over time.

The third principle of Positive-Space/Time is the law that opposites attract. A positive always attracts a negative and a negative always attracts a positive—but likes repel. We are all familiar with what happens when you bring two strong magnets together. If opposite poles are brought together they strongly attract (in fact, you'd better watch out for your fingers!) but like poles will repel each other.

NEGATIVE-SPACE/TIME. METAPHYSICAL REALITY
This is the domain of metaphysical reality. These are the subtle energy flows that are non-material at the physical level but which underlie the material

world. These energies are not perceptible at the level of the five senses nor via electronic instrumentation. These energies are currently only knowable via the mind, although instrumentation bordering on the ability to image these energies in a scientifically testable way, is getting closer to reality each year.[15]

Knowledge and understanding of these subtle energy flows has been best developed by eastern sages, although they are recognised as aspects of mystical experiences in all parts of the world. The Chinese acupuncture meridian system and the chakra and nadi system of the Indian yogis are two of the better documented of these etheric energy systems.

These traditions hold that it is possible, at certain levels of conscious development, to use the mind as an organ of psychic perception. Chakras, which will be discussed in more detail later in this chapter, are centres of subtle energy influx that bring universal or cosmic energy into our energy being. When consciousness has reached a certain degree of development, the chakras also become organs of psychic perception enabling those who have higher realisations to directly observe the flow of subtle energies.[16] Clairvoyance is

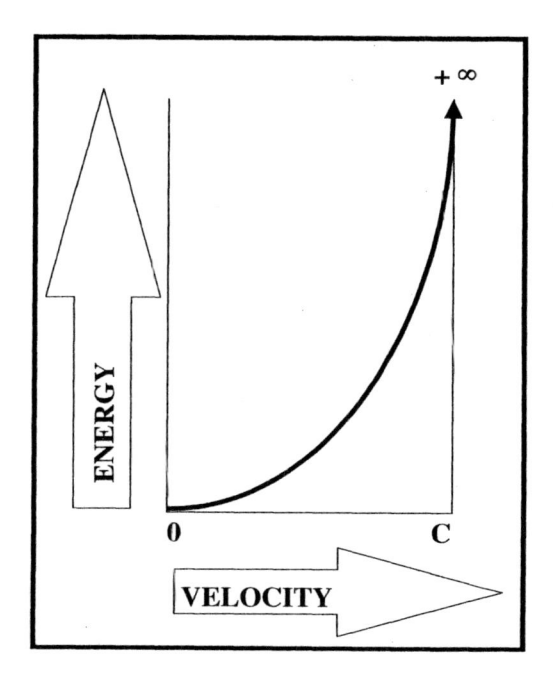

Figure 11.3. Physical Matter is limited to the Speed of Light. According to Einstein's equation $E = mc^2$ as matter approaches the speed of light it increases in mass requiring more energy to move it faster.

324 *A Revolutionary Way of Thinking*

the ability to see auras and to see beyond the immediate physical reality. Clairvoyance means 'clear vision.'

Once conscious perception of these subtle energy flows has been developed, the rules and principles by which they operate can also be known. It is precisely in this way that knowledge of the chakra and the meridian systems developed so many thousands of years ago.

Properties and Principles of Negative-Space/Time
While the major property of Positive-Space/Time is associated with electricity, the major property of Negative-Space/Time is associated with magnetism and a force Professor Tiller describes as 'magnetoelectric' radiation. In Negative-Space/Time it is predominantly the magnetic, rather than the electric

PHYSICAL *positive space/time*

Properties of Positive Space/Time
- Realm of physical matter
- Physical world
- Electricity primary force
- Electromagnetic fields
- Positive entropy - tendency towards disorder
- Velocity of matter limited to Speed of Light (300,000km/sec)
- Opposites attract

VELOCITY

Properties of Negative Space/Time
- Realm of subtle matter/spirit
- Metaphysical world (eg. thoughts & emotions)
- Magnetism primary force
- Magnetoelectric fields
- Negative entropy - tendency toward order
- Velocity in excess of Speed of Light not only possible but general
- Likes attract

ETHERIC *negative space/time*

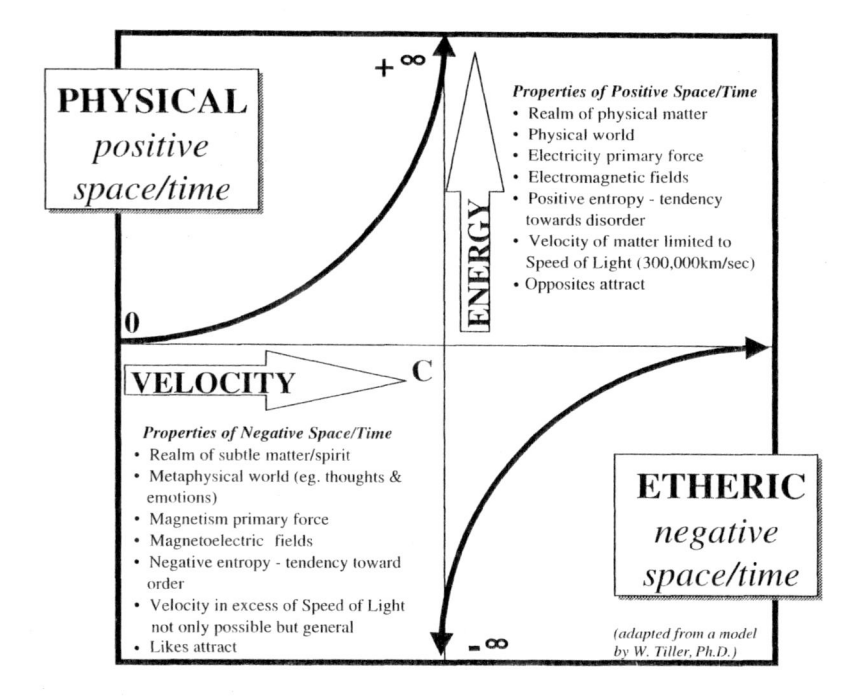

(adapted from a model by W. Tiller, Ph.D.)

Figure 11.4. Model of Positive and Negative-Space/Time. Physical and metaphysical reality are both predictable from Einstein's equations demonstrating that matter and energy are interconnected. While physical reality is known to our physical senses and can be investigated with electrical instrumentation, metaphysical reality at this time remains theoretical and can only be known to our psychic senses as we do not yet possess the instrumentation capable of interacting with this realm.

component that dominates. It is the weak coupling between these two domains that leads to electro-magentism (see Fig. 11.4).

One of the major components involved in hands-on healing appears to be magnetic in nature. As Dr Gerber noted, 'early studies with magnetic detectors were unable to register any significant magnetic fields around a healer's hands . . . (However) utilising an ultra-sensitive magnetic-field detector called a SQUID (super-conducting quantum interference device) has demonstrated significant increases in the magnetic fields emitted by healer's hands.'[17]

In Negative-Space/Time—the metaphysical domain, subtle matter (negative mass particles) is associated with magnetism and can move faster than the speed of light.

The first principle of Negative-Space/Time therefore, is that velocities greater than the speed of light are not only possible but are general. Inspection of the lower right hand quadrant in Figure 11.4, shows that as you approach the large values on the horizontal axis, you are moving toward infinite velocity which means, to quote Professor Tiller, 'we approach a condition in which we can be everywhere in no time, which means we are approaching omnipresence'.[18]

This is the domain of mind. Just one of the discriminated subtle domains in Tiller's new model.

The second principle of Negative-Space/Time is the metaphysical principle of negative entropy, which is a tendency towards order. Taken to its logical extreme of perfect order it could be considered God or cosmic consciousness. Cosmos means 'order.'

The third principle of Negative-Space/Time is the law that like attracts like. This is the factor that underlies the practice of homeopathy in which the energetic pattern of a substance that produces illness will cure that illness when manifest at the physical level.[19] For example, Feverfew is a herb that when eaten will produce the symptoms of fever. When Feverfew has been homoeopathically prepared by serial dilution to immeasurably small amounts, when taken, the energetic pattern of the homeopathic solution will serve to combat fever.

THE PARADOX OF LIFE

In the material world, Positive-Space/Time is apparent everywhere and entropy rules. All things tend to decay. Monuments, even of stone, will degrade and over thousands of years, return to the sands of time.

Nature provides one exception: The paradox of life itself. There are trees, like the Sequoias of California and the Huon pines of Tasmania, that live for thousands of years continually renewing themselves. Life itself displays properties of negative entropy, a tendency towards order.

From randomly distributed minerals and molecules, plants construct highly organised structures that persist over time. From two cells, an egg and a sperm, animals create highly complex organisms by feeding on plants. Many of these animals may live for many decades, all the time maintaining the integrity of a complex and highly organised physical body.

The life force appears to be associated with the negative entropic character of self organisation which totally contravenes the law of positive entropy. It does so by the constant input of energy, but by using this energy to organise matter according to the energetic template. But once the organism dies, the physical matter does indeed follow the rules of decay or positive entropy.

But what is it that causes atoms and molecules to organise themselves into complex living organisms in the first place? In the West it is said to be the result of the genetic patterns contained within the DNA molecule. It is clear that the molecular physical structure is indeed dependent upon the genetic programming of the organism, and the repair of DNA is essential for the maintenance and health of the organism.

Is this all there is?

What is interesting to note is that from the instant of fertilisation of the ovum by the sperm, for the first 10 days of foetal development, the organising factors remain obscure. After 10 days, various chemical markers and gradients begin to guide the development of the foetus and biochemistry takes over. At the moment of fertilisation, however, an electric field is generated with an axis that later becomes the spinal axis and it appears that this organisation is somehow related to the axis of energy which acts as an energetic template during these initial stages.[20]

In the East, it is said that the energetic template of the etheric (energetic) body is what provides the directions for the organisation of physical matter. And once that matter has been organised, the maintenance of its on-going structure is dependent upon a constant flow of subtle, nutritive energy coming from the energetic systems of the organisms. In fact, in this model it is believed that the physical form cannot be maintained without the energising nourishment and spatial guidance provided by the etheric template.[21]

The energetic template is an expression of negative entropy, or a tendency toward order. The wellspring of the force organising matter into life. This is the very life force that is the basis of holistic healing. But at death, the inflow of subtle energy ceases and the energetic template begins to disintegrate, leading to the decay of the physical being.

At the same point, the West perceives only a loss of biochemical and physical energy.

His Holiness the Dalai Lama, in a recent address, told the story of the death of his teacher, a passing that he personally witnessed. The teacher's body did not decay for seven days but remained radiant even though it was summer and the day-time temperatures were high. The Dalai Lama also told of another saint who had remained in this radiant state for 15 days following his death in India.[22] How do we account for this lack of decay in the bodies of these highly-realised beings?

Whatever the answer, the big question is: What is the difference in the physical body a second before death and a second after death, apart from the absence of organising energy? In the East, death is described as a withdrawal of the etheric or subtle energy, which is then followed by the cessation of chemical and physical activity. It could be hypothesised that the saints had achieved such energetic harmony at such subtle levels that it took far longer for this process of biochemical decay to set in.

In summary, from an energetic perspective, the nature of the body is first and primarily a negative entropic energy structure around which physical matter becomes organised. What we consider to be 'life' is actually negative entropy in action.

We realise that what has been outlined here may seem a lot to grasp, but it lays the essential foundations for understanding the discussion of the multi-dimensional human being.

THE MULTI-DIMENSIONAL BEING

Once we incorporate the subtle bodies of man into his physical body, we begin to see a multi-dimensional being. While the physical body is the only body currently recognised in western thought, in the East, the subtle bodies associated with this physical body have been very well defined.

In the East it is generally recognised that humans have a physical body which is surrounded and interpenetrated by at least four other subtle bodies.[23] These other bodies exist at different frequencies of subtle vibration. For instance, as electromagnetic radiation exists over a spectrum of frequencies—from microwaves to gamma rays, the magnetoelectric radiation also exists over a frequency range of vibrations, from lowest vibrations of the etheric to highest vibrations of the causal or spiritual body.

Figure 11.5 illustrates the four primary subtle bodies beyond the physical. It should be recognised that this is a highly simplified presentation in that each of the subtle bodies may have a number of layers, each with its own unique properties.

The Physical Body

This is the body you see touch and feel. The body that is made up of blood, muscle and bone. This is the body that hurts when it is injured; that gets hungry every few hours and that feels the tightened gut of anxiety. This is also the body from which we can derive the joy of physical pleasure. This is the body we know the best. It is the body with the lowest vibrational frequency, a frequency which fortunately for us, falls within the range of the visible spectrum.

The Etheric Body
Interpenetrating and surrounding the physical body like a glove on a hand, is the most dense of all the subtle bodies. The etheric body is the realm of the acupuncture meridian system and also the subtle body that most directly interfaces with the physical body. In fact it is within the acupuncture system that the magneto-electric energy flows such as Ch'i are transduced (changed in form) into the electromagnetic energy of the physical body. This forms a primary interface between the electromagnetic flows of the physical body and

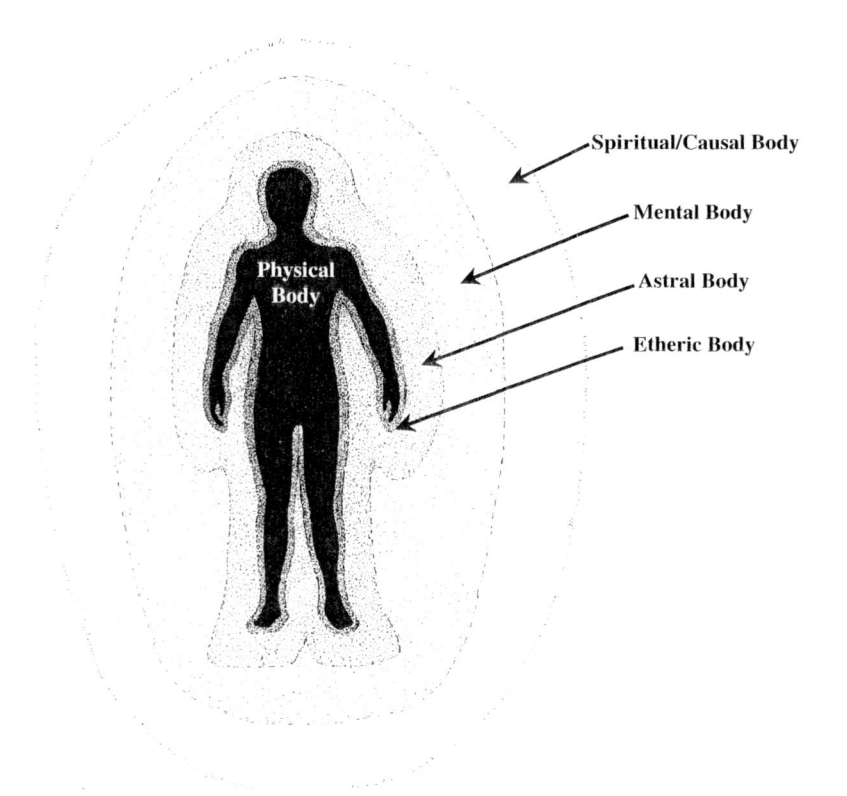

Figure 11.5. The Multi Dimensional Body. Interpenetrating and extending beyond the physical body of the subtle bodies of Man. The etheric body fits the physical body like a glove fits a hand while the astral body has a more amorphous shape and the mental and spiritual bodies become egg-shaped.

the subtle energy flows of the other subtle bodies. While acupoints have electrical properties, they are also the portals and controllers for the flow of vital Ch'i in the etheric body.

The Astral Body

Interpenetrating the physical body and extending beyond the etheric body is the astral body, which is the realm of the emotions. The subtle matter of the astral body is at a higher frequency than the etheric body and very magnetic in the Negative-Space/Time sense, in that like attracts like. Have you ever noticed that when you are angry it attracts more anger and that when you are joyful, you are likely to notice more joy around you. This emotionally magnetic tendency is the basis of many truisms including, 'misery loves company', 'everybody loves a lover' and 'like minds attract.' Opposites only attract at the physical level.

At the level of astral matter, emotions exist as a vibration pattern which then probably interface with the brain via transduction to electromagnetic-electrochemical energy of nerve conduction in the amygdala or pineal gland. This is because the amygdala is the emotional centre of our subconscious processing, and the pineal gland secretes hormones which control our moods.[24]

These emotions then become physical feelings via nerve signals from the amygdala to the hypothalamus which controls the autonomic nervous system and the pituitary, the master gland of the endocrine system. In other words, feelings are the physical body's way of experiencing what is really a subtle body vibrational pattern.

The Mental Body

Interpenetrating the physical and extending beyond the astral body and consisting of even higher and more subtle vibrational energies is the mental body, the realm of thoughts. This is the vehicle in which Self manifests and where our concrete intellect is expressed. Intellect is the ability to draw abstractions about physical reality and to make decisions. The word itself means 'choice'.

Like the other subtle bodies, the mental body itself has several layers. The lower mental body dwells upon mental images obtained from direct sensory experience, and analytically reasons about purely concrete objects. The higher mental body is concerned with more abstract things and concepts, often relating to other thoughts. Higher abstract reasoning is a property of this realm.

While the astral body generates emotions, the mental body generates thoughts as vibrational patterns which can be called thought-forms. These thought-forms can create patterns within the astral body which may then be transduced in to neural activity which is experienced as feelings. 'I just had a very pleasurable thought.' Similarly, unpleasant thoughts can create unpleasant feelings.

Thus thought-forms are the means by which the mental body can create and transmit concrete ideas to the brain for expression and manifestation. These ideas may then be turned into action as the areas of the brain controlling movement are activated by conscious intent.

The Causal or Spiritual Body
Interpenetrating the physical body and extending beyond the mental body, and consisting of the highest subtle vibrational energies, is the causal body. This is the realm of spirit, of higher Self and of your connection to God, whatever you conceive him or her to be. This body deals with the essence of things and the true causes that lie behind the illusion of appearance. This is the site of transcending consciousness.

It is also the realm from which *will* originates and provides us with the power to achieve goals in our life. In the esoteric traditions, will is said to originate within a very high level within the causal body. When activated, it causes transduction to thought forms—of action; which the mind then uses to activate the physical body. 'Thy will be done.'

Have you ever watched an Olympic athlete going for the gold? This is willpower in action, the force that allows a true champion to push beyond his or her previous physical limitations.

It is also the realm of devotion, of establishing a connection with the universal consciousness that some call God. At the level of the mental body, the Self is manifest. At the level of the causal body, the Soul is manifest and the limitations of physical time and space cease.

Clearly the causal body is in the domain of Negative-Space/Time in which, as Professor Tiller so sagely noted, 'we can be everywhere in no time.' This is the timeless space of Zen where All is One and the appearance of separation disappears.

CHAKRAS—SPINNING WHEELS OF LIGHT

The chakra system is the other primary subtle energy system. Chakras are energy centres that are perceived as whirling vortices or whirlpools of subtle energy to which clairvoyants and yogis have ascribed various colors.[25]

In structure and when viewed from the front, they are held to appear as spinning wheels or discs of light. Chakra is a Sanskrit word that signifies a wheel, and because chakras are perceived to be spinning discs of light they could be considered to be a 'spinning wheel of light'. From the side they are said to appear as cones of light which project outward from a point on the skin.

The chakra system consists of seven primary chakras and many minor chakras. In fact, each joint has a minor chakra associated with it, and there may be more than 360 individual chakras in the human body.[26]

The primary chakras are the crown chakra, located at the top of the head and projecting upwards; the brow chakra, projecting forward from the point between the eyebrows; the throat chakra, projecting forward from the notch of the throat. The heart chakra projects forward from the bottom of the sternum. The naval chakra projects forward from the naval. The sacral or sexual chakra projects forward from just above the pubis, and the root chakra which projects downward at about an 80 degree angle forward from the perineum. Smaller chakra cones also project from the back of the body at a point opposite the site of the major frontal cones.[27] (see Figure 11.6)

Chakras, which penetrate all levels of the subtle body from the causal to the etheric, act to transduce the magnetoelectric energies of the subtle bodies into electromagnetic energy for use at the physical level. This transduction of negative entropic, ordering energy is one of the primary mechanisms that maintains the coherence of the etheric template, which in turn, maintains the functions of the physical body.

Chakras act as subtle energy step-down transformers, stepping down the higher frequency vibrations of the causal to the mental body; the mental frequencies to the lower vibrations of the astral body and the emotional vibrations of the astral body to the densest subtle energy of the etheric body[28]. Each energetic vibration can affect the body above or below it and the chakras are the integrating sites of the subtle bodies.

At the level of the etheric body, the chakra and acupuncture systems interact and together create the energetic template that then manifest as the physical body.

Via the chakras, subtle energy changes in any of the subtle bodies can become manifest as physiological events at the cellular level. In this way the various subtle bodies interact with, and affect the structure and function of the physical body.

In order to understand how the complex interaction of subtle bodies with the physical body via the chakras is manifest in everyday life, consider the following scenario:

You have your heart set on winning a particular job. The strong desire or will for this job had originated at the level of the causal body. Motivated by this desire you apply for the job and give it your best shot at the interview.

When you receive the letter from the personnel department, the information contained in it is decoded by the intellect of the mental body and the horrible thought occurs, 'My God, I didn't get the job!' This thought-form may then create the vibrational pattern of 'rejection' at the astral level. The emotion of rejection will then cause a distortion at the etheric level which, when transduced via the etheric-physical interface at the amygdala, it becomes a stream of neural impulses to the hypothalamus whose output is the *feeling* that is finally experienced at the physical level.

Suddenly, there is a change in your posture: shoulders slump, head droops and you feel heavy, all physical feelings accompanying the emotion of rejection. What you physically experience is thus only at the end of a long chain of events that take place at many levels of your being.

While the higher subtle levels actually initiated the eventual physical response, all you were consciously aware of was the physical response, which is one of the reasons why it has been so easy to ignore the existence of these subtle bodies for so long in the paradigm of western science.

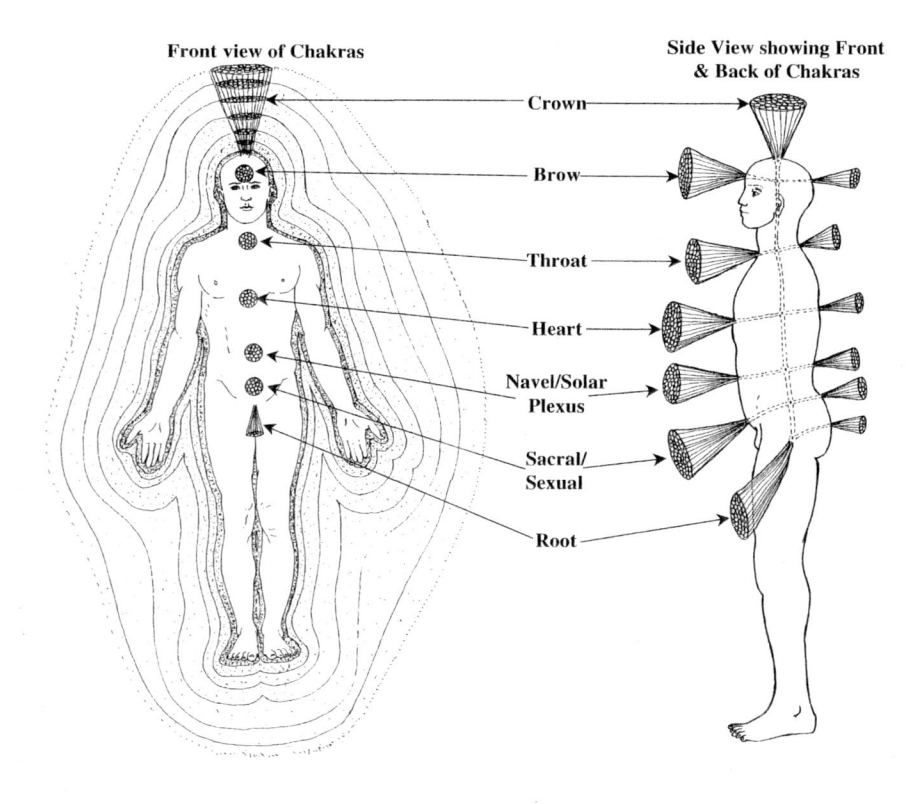

Figure 11.6. Location of the Major Chakras. Note that there is a central psychic channel that connects the crown with the root chakra and to which all the other chakras are connected. The primary cone of each chakra is made up of many smaller cones. Each primary chakra cone projects from the front and the back of the body with the front cone being the larger of the two. Note also that each primary chakra penetrates all layers of the human body from the physical to the spiritual.

CHAKRAS AND PHYSIOLOGY

The yogis say chakras have their physiological effects predominantly by their connection to the endocrine glands and various autonomic nerve plexuses. Each chakra is associated with a particular endocrine gland and a specific nerve plexus at the level of their location within the physical body.[29] (See Figure 11.7).

Table 11.1 Endocrine and Autonomic Nervous System Plexuses and Physiological System associated with each Chakra.

CHAKRA	ENDOCRINE SYSTEM	NERVE PLEXUS	PHYSIOLOGICAL SYSTEM
ROOT	Gonads	Sacral-Coccygeal Plexus	Reproductive
SACRAL	Leydig Cells	Sacral Plexus	Genitourinary
NAVEL	Adrenal Glands	Solar Plexus	Digestive
HEART	Thymus Gland	Heart Plexus	Circulatory
THROAT	Thyroid Gland	Cervical Ganglia Medulla	Respiratory
THIRD EYE	Pituitary Gland	Hypothalamus Pituitary	Autonomic Nervous System
CROWN	Pineal Gland	Cerebral Cortex Pineal	CNS Central Control

Homeostasis of the body is predominantly maintained via the autonomic nervous system and its connections to the hypothalamus and the endocrine system. The autonomic nervous system consists of two branches; the parasympathetic nervous system and the sympathetic nervous system. The parasympathetic nervous system is involved with energy conservation and storage and generally calms your physiology down. The sympathetic nervous system is involved with energy use and activity and is the origin of the fight or flight response.

Located deep in the base of the brain, just above the roof of the mouth, the hypothalamus contains various sensors or groups of cells that are sensitive to various physiological parameters such as temperature, blood viscosity and hormonal levels. In addition, the hypothalamus receives the output from the visceral sensory receptors in the internal organs that relay information about their state of function to the brain. For instance, when your stomach begins to stretch because you have eaten a big meal, visceral receptors in the wall of the stomach send signals to stimulate one of the nuclei in the hypothalamus.

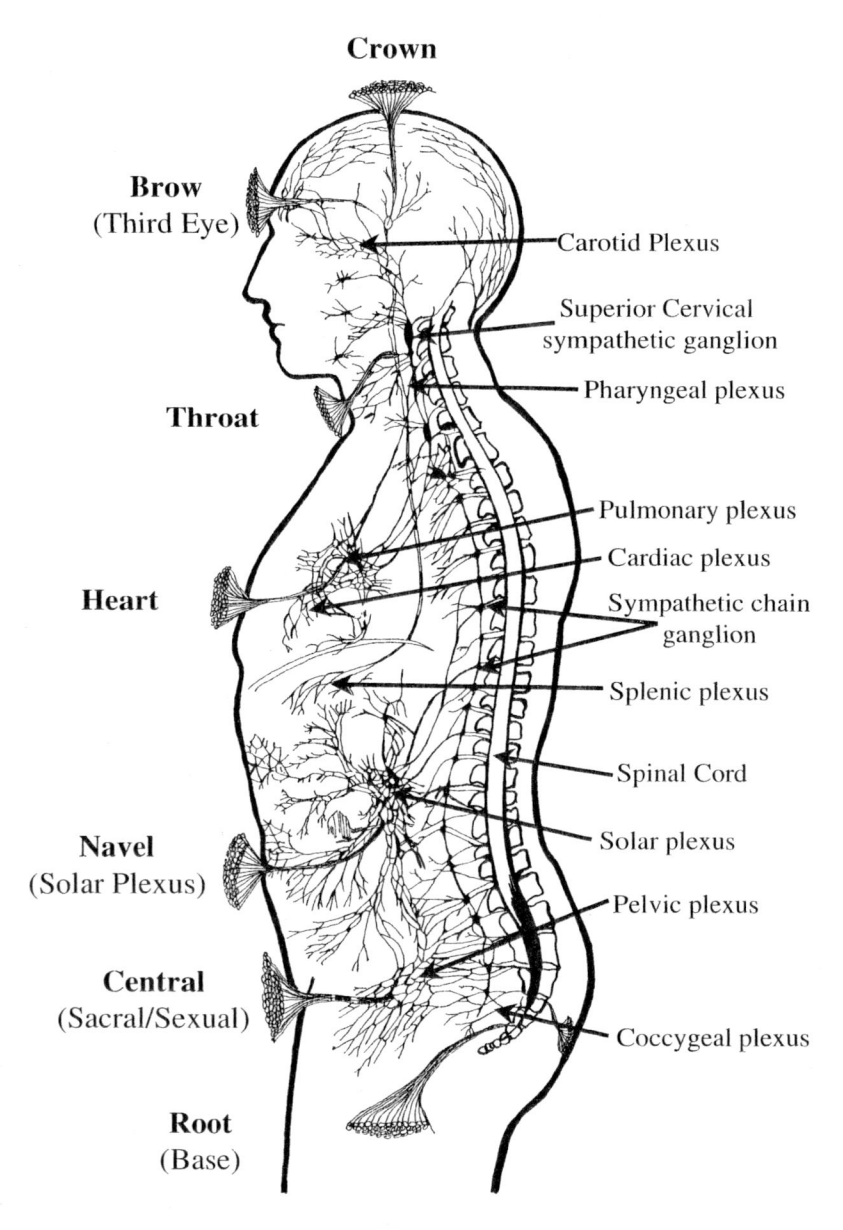

Figure 11.7. Chakra and Nerve Plexuses Locations. Each of the major chakras is associated with a major nerve plexus within the body.

This then initiates the sensation of satiety, eliciting a feeling of being full, hence you stop eating.

Other visceral receptors relay information to the hypothalamus about the oxygen and carbon dioxide levels in your blood and the pressure in your arteries and this information is integrated by the hypothalamus. The hypothalamus then sends out messages via the autonomic nervous system to normalise these functions and maintain homeostasis.[30] In both the parasympathetic and sympathetic nervous systems, there are collections of nerves that anastomose (form a network) at certain locations within your body. These are called the autonomic nerve plexuses. For example, the solar plexus is situated just below the centre of the rib cage, slightly to the left hand side, the cardiac plexus is located just behind the heart and the coccygeal plexus sits just in front of the coccyx or tail bone.

As nerve conduction is relatively rapid, the autonomic nervous system provides the body with a means of rapid adaptation to changes within the internal and external environment that affect its homeostasis. If the perturbation is only momentary, this rapid adaptation is all that is required to maintain a physiological balance. If, however, the perturbation is on-going, a longer-term adaptation is necessary. This is the role of the endocrine system.

The endocrine system is composed of a series of ductless glands that secrete hormones. The master gland of the system is the pituitary gland because the hormones it secretes regulate all the other endocrine glands of the body. As an example, when this master gland secretes thyroid stimulating hormone (TSH), it causes the release of thyroxin from the thyroid gland which then controls your basal metabolic rate.

The master gland, however, is really more an overseer than a master because it only does what the hypothalamus tells it to do. When the hypothalamus, which is monitoring the temperature of the blood, observes a decrease in body temperature, it releases thyroid stimulating hormone releasing factor into the blood vessels that connect directly to the pituitary gland. The pituitary, you will recall, hangs off the bottom of the hypothalamus (Chapter 3, Figures 3.17 and 3.20).

This pituitary releasing factor causes the pituitary to release TSH, which in turn, causes the release of thyroxine from the thyroid gland. The thyroxine then causes all the cells in the body to metabolise more rapidly in order to raise the body temperature. The hypothalamic temperature sensors then register that the body is getting too warm, which then shuts off the release of thyroid stimulating releasing factor, ceasing the release of TSH from the pituitary, which stops the release of thyroxine from the thyroid gland. Again, the body temperature begins to decrease.

This bio-feedback cycle occurs throughout the day and allows your body to maintain a constant temperature. If your body had to make all these adjustments by constant autonomic nervous system activity, the physiological cost would be extremely high in terms of energy expenditure. Instead, it uses an energetically inexpensive method of the production of a few molecules of hormone to achieve the same end.

On the other hand, if you find yourself momentarily in an environment that is too cold and your core temperature begins to decrease, you do not have time to wait for the endocrine system to act. Instead, via the sympathetic nervous system, a series of impulses is sent to the muscles to cause you to shiver, and by this physical activity, your temperature is maintained.

What we have outlined here, shows the critical interplay of the autonomic and endocrine systems in the maintenance of your body's homeostasis. But what do chakras have to do with these physiological systems?

The simple answer is that the chakras translate the energy of the higher dimensions of the subtle bodies into physiological response via their connections to these two dynamic physiological systems. To more fully understand how these apparently separate and ethereal energy structures can have such profound affects on our physical being, we need to know more about the structure of the chakra system.

THE CHAKRAS AND THE NADI SYSTEM

Just as the brain is connected to disparate parts of the body via the fine network of the nervous system, the chakras are likewise connected to each other and to specific parts of the physical-cellular structure via subtle energetic channels called 'nadis'.[31] Knowledge of the nadi system has again come down to us from the eastern sages who had achieved a high level of conscious development which enabled them to use their psychic organs of perception to investigate the non-physical, energetic structure of the human body.[32]

In the same way it took western science hundreds of years to understand the function of the finer physical structure of the human body, so too over very long periods the yogis were able to decipher the intricacies of the subtle energy channels called the nadi system. Nadis can be considered fine threads or minute channels of subtle energetic matter which are similar to the meridians of the acupuncture meridian system. Like the meridian system, there are bigger and smaller nadi channels associated with physiological structures within the body[33] (see Fig. 11.8).

Various sources have described up to 72,000 nadis that are interwoven within the physical body, particularly the nervous system. Some of these nadis connect to the endocrine glands while others are interconnected with the autonomic nervous system.[34] In this way it becomes apparent how the chakras may affect the function of these physiological structures.

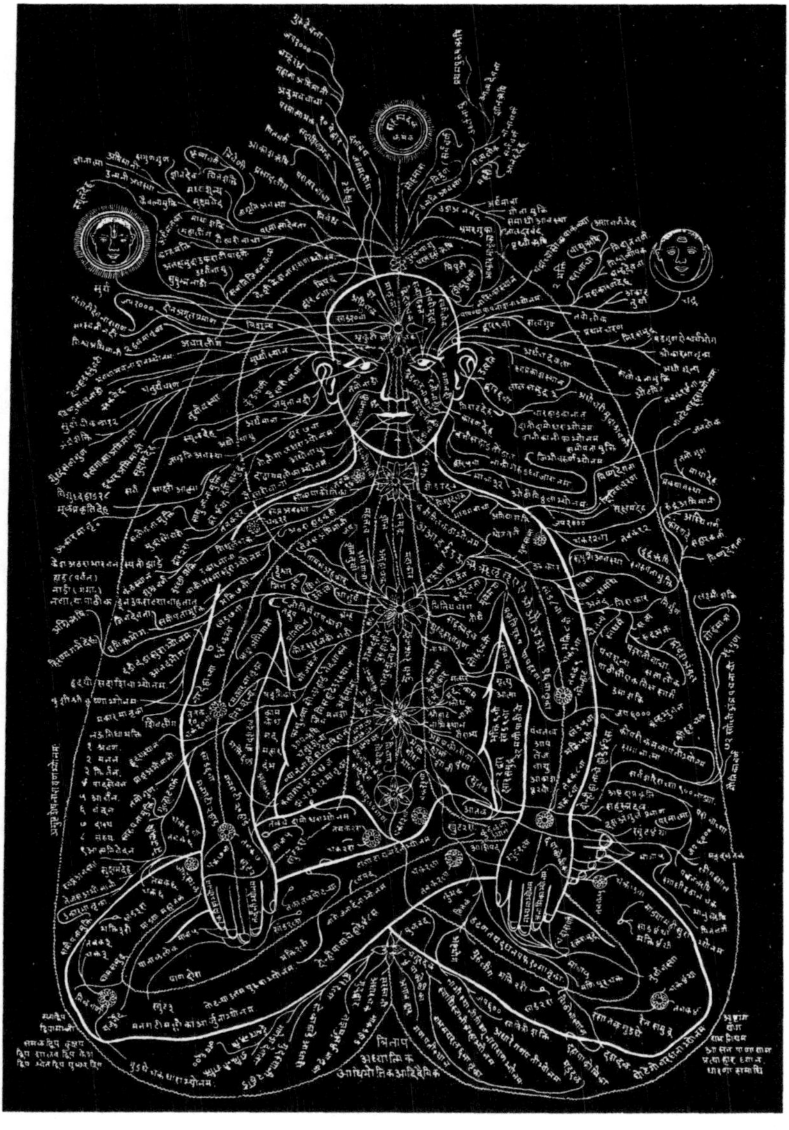

Figure 11.8. Original drawing of chakras from the Yogic literature showing many of the nadi channels.

It is said that the chakras provide an influx of cosmic energies that the yogis term 'Prana', which was their way of describing the manifestation of the life force or 'elan vital'. Prana is said to originate as cosmic energy or free energy of the universe that is conducted into the body via the chakra cones. This could be termed the 'primary outpouring'. Once it enters the chakra cones, Prana is then distributed to the associated endocrine organs and nerve plexuses via the nadi system.[35]

When this pranic energy is stepped down to the level of the etheric, it then can activate the etheric-physical interface causing physiological change. The yogis observed that the pranic energy provided a nutritive source of negative entropic—or self-organising energy that maintains the etheric template. And it is the etheric template, you will recall, that ultimately sustains physiological function (see Fig. 11.9).

As an analogy, western scientists have come to understand that plants can transduce the subtle energy of sunlight into physical matter. In a similar way, chakras transduce subtle cosmic energy into physiological function. In a sense, human beings are able to synthesise cosmic energy into human function just as plants are able to photosynthesise photons of light into cellular matter.

CHAKRAS AND THE SUBTLE BODIES

The yogis say that each chakra has a predominant colour or frequency vibration. The crown chakra appears as white light, which is all colours together. The brow chakra appears as indigo or violet; the throat chakra appears as blue; the heart chakra as green; the naval chakra as yellow; the sacral or sexual chakra as orange and the root chakra as red.[36]

While these colours are not present at visible wavelengths (if they were we would be able to both see and photograph them), they appear to be subtle energy vibrational frequencies that are 'supra-harmonics' of these colours. That is as high C is a harmonic of middle C, the same musical note, just at a higher vibrational frequency, the chakra colours may be a harmonic of visible light colours, but just at vibrational frequencies far above those in the visible light spectrum.

The subtle energies producing the colour of the chakras appear to occupy an extended frequency range of magnetoelectric radiation, like the colour spectrum of visible light in the electromagnetic spectrum. Because they are magnetoelectric in nature, they are not, as yet, able to be recorded with scientific instrumentation.

Not only is each chakra 'tuned' to a specific colour, each appears to be tuned to a specific subtle body, or a layer of a subtle body. The root chakra (red) appears to be tuned to the lowest levels of the etheric body—those most intimately

An All Encompassing Reality 339

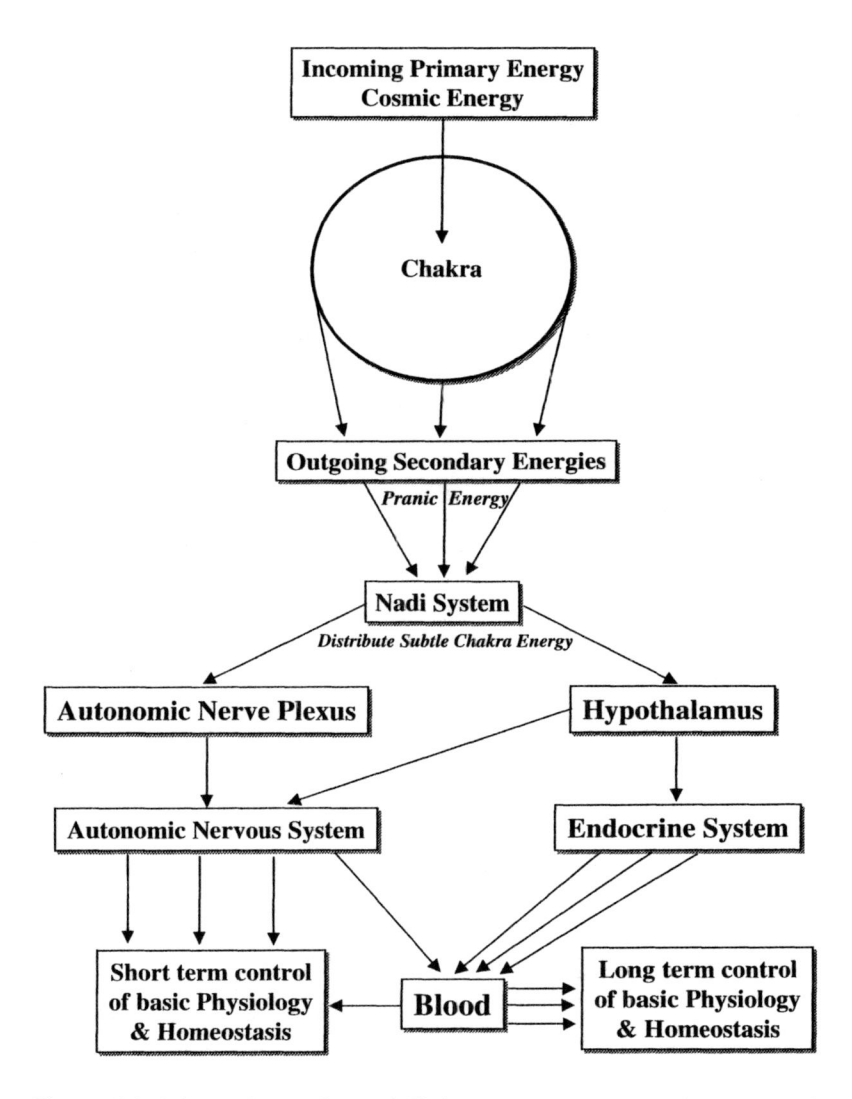

```
        ┌─────────────────────────┐
        │ Incoming Primary Energy │
        │     Cosmic Energy       │
        └─────────────────────────┘
                     │
                     ▼
                 ╱───────╲
                │ Chakra  │
                 ╲───────╱
                     │
                     ▼
        ┌─────────────────────────┐
        │ Outgoing Secondary Energies │
        └─────────────────────────┘
                 Pranic Energy
                     │
                     ▼
              ┌──────────────┐
              │  Nadi System │
              └──────────────┘
          Distribute Subtle Chakra Energy
            ↙                        ↘
┌────────────────────────┐   ┌──────────────┐
│ Autonomic Nerve Plexus │   │ Hypothalamus │
└────────────────────────┘   └──────────────┘
            │                        │
            ▼                        ▼
┌──────────────────────┐   ┌──────────────────┐
│ Autonomic Nervous    │   │ Endocrine System │
│      System          │   │                  │
└──────────────────────┘   └──────────────────┘
    │   │   │                        │
    ▼   ▼   ▼                        ▼
┌──────────────┐  ┌───────┐  ┌──────────────┐
│ Short term   │  │       │  │ Long term    │
│ control of   │◄─│ Blood │─►│ control of   │
│ basic Physi- │  │       │  │ basic Physi- │
│ ology &      │  │       │  │ ology &      │
│ Homeostasis  │  │       │  │ Homeostasis  │
└──────────────┘  └───────┘  └──────────────┘
```

Figure 11.9. Primary Outpouring and Chakras. Cosmic(pranic) energy entering the chakras is transduced via the nadi system from magnetoelectric subtle energy to electromagnetic physiologic energy in the hypothalamus and at the autonomic nerve plexuses. In this way chakras exert control over basic homeostasis of the body.

involved in our physiological homeostasis. Hence it is tuned to the most earthly aspects of human function which is the physical survival of the individual.

The sacral or sexual chakra (orange) is, as its name implies, is strongly linked to the next level of the etheric body which is involved with reproduction and maintenance of the species. The naval chakra (yellow) is tuned to the higher levels of the etheric body and the lower frequencies of the astral body. It is involved with issues of power, both on a physical plane and on the level of physical feelings.

The heart chakra (green) is tuned to the higher levels of the astral body involved with the higher emotions of love and compassion. The throat chakra (blue) is tuned to the lower mental body and is concerned more with interpretation and expression of sensory experience. The brow, or third-eye chakra (violet) is tuned to the frequencies of the higher mental body, the realm of abstract ideas, reasoning and insight. The crown chakra (white) is tuned to the highest vibrational frequencies of the causal body and hence, is our connection to higher consciousness.

At normal levels of awareness, we operate only at the level of physical consciousness. Aware only of the physical world, and ideas and concepts which relate to that world. At this level of consciousness, the chakras operate predominantly as subtle organs maintaining our physiological function.

When the chakras are operating only in their physiological capacity, they are said to be 'closed'. As the level of consciousness rises above the physical level, the chakras become organs of psychic perception and are said to 'open'. As each chakra opens, the person may gain a particular type of psychic perception. While the types of perceptions ascribed to each chakra can appear fanciful when viewed from the level of physical consciousness, each has been extensively described throughout the millennia by those who have managed to achieve the highest levels of consciousness.[37]

When consciousness rises and the root chakra opens, the person may gain the ability to levitate astrally. That is, the sense of floating upward in space, leaving the physical body behind. If consciousness rises higher again, and the sacral or sexual chakra opens, it is said that the person may now perceive the presence of subtle beings. If the consciousness rises further and opens the navel chakra, it is said that the person may develop the ability to see the perfection of the process; that things are indeed perfect just as they are.

Once consciousness has risen to the point where the heart chakra opens, the person may become omnisentient which means they are able to access the feelings of the people around them, and they are said to be able to develop unconditional love and total compassion. Upon the opening of the throat chakra, it is said that the person has the potential to gain clairaudience which means the ability to hear others' thoughts, otherwise known as telepathy.

When consciousness rises to open the brow chakra, it is said that the person may gain clairvoyance or the ability to see beyond the illusions of physical appearance. When the brow chakra is open, people can usually see the subtle energy emanations of other human beings, and it is in this way that knowledge of the subtle energy systems of the chakras and meridians have been described. Clairvoyants can also develop the ability for 'remote viewing,' or the facility to describe distant places and events without having to actually go there.[38]

While this process may proceed in as orderly a fashion as we have described, with the consecutive opening of each chakra and its attendant psychic abilities, it is far more common for these psychic phenomenon to occur individually or in combination. For instance, with the opening of the root chakra, a person can sometimes experience other psychic experiences other that astral levitation. These can include clairvoyance and clairaudience.

Likewise with the opening of the third eye or brow chakra, various types of extra sensory perception become manifest according to a person's spiritual and emotional history or mental tendencies. Such psychic perceptions are often of short duration usually occurring immediately after the initial opening of the chakra.

But when finally, consciousness reaches its zenith and the crown chakra opens, it is said the person can gain supra or cosmic consciousness, which is the realisation of your true nature and of your connection to God. Your true nature, in this context, is that you are not separate from others, or from the universe, but are one with all and one with God. This is said to be the state of true bliss or enlightenment.[39]

The nature of our organ of both conscious awareness and psychic perception, our mind is the topic of the next chapter.

Chapter Twelve

REALMS OF CONSCIOUSNESS

DEFINING THE MIND

What allowed me to heal myself so I could walk again was my mind. But what do we mean when I talk about mind?

The word 'mind' is used in many different contexts. Some references are only to the function of the physical entity: the brain. Others refer to the most esoteric aspects of our mental ability. The word itself is applied in so many different situations to mean so many different things - witness the column space it takes up in every dictionary. It is essential, therefore, at the outset of this chapter to define exactly what I mean when I talk about 'mind'.

The way I will use the word mind refers to the properties of the mental body, both the lower mental aspects of intellect and the higher aspects of conceptualisation. I am talking about the mind's ability to think and to deal with the interpretation of sensory experience, as well as its ability to realise higher abstractions and connections that give it the extraordinary facility to channel energy.

My personal interest in understanding the mind arose from what my accident forced me to address, both within my physical body and within my mental being. Before my accident, I now understand, I had only been using my lower mental body, the intellect, which allowed me to investigate and understand the physical world, the world around me that I could see, touch and feel. In the quest to regain my physical function I was forced inside and found I had to use all my inner resources. In the process I discovered parts of my mind that had heretofore been unknown to me.

During years of practicing martial arts I had developed the ability to use my mind to direct the subtle energy of Ch'i through my physical body. Using this mind-directed Ch'i, I could break boards and tiles with my bare hands.

But even though I could do this and I realised that it was not my physical hand that was smashing the boards, but the energy I projected through my hand with my mind, I did not understand how this could be. I just did it.

So martial arts provided the portal for me to develop the higher aspects of mind that control the flow of subtle energies within the body. Now, when confronted with a dysfunctional body, I had the tools I needed to heal myself. I was able to use several levels of my mind to achieve the healing that I was determined was going to take place. Though I did not, at that stage, know that will originated from my higher spiritual body, I was still able to bring this power into play by using my mind as the channel for this energy from my higher Self.

I was also able to use the lower levels of my mental body, my intellect, which held in its memory the exact maps of the nerve pathways that ran from my brain to my paralysed legs. I had the will, I had the ability to direct subtle energy with my mind and I had the anatomical knowledge of exactly where I needed to send the mind's energy.

Now, having delved more deeply into the nature of human experience, both through exploring esoteric literature and through extensive meditation, I fully comprehend how it was possible to reactivate my paralysed limbs by using the power of my mind. In essence, the will of my spiritual body was being transduced via my crown and brow chakras into the etheric energy of Ch'i, which I was then directing along the nerve pathways into the muscles in my legs. The organising negative entropic energy of Ch'i was then able to manifest coherence in the physiological function of my damaged nerves. In time, I was able to walk again.

I also now understand that my will to heal was not only for myself to walk again but also to allow me to realise my path in life; in the Buddhist system, my Dharma. From the perspective of my higher Self, it was not an accident but the call to redirect my life.

MIND — SUBTLE STRUCTURE AND FUNCTION

The subtle structure of the mind, from my perspective, is contained within the mental bodies of the subtle being. As I have intimated, the mental body can be subdivided into a number of different layers, each of which has different mental properties.

Lower mental bodies are the precinct of the intellect and intellectualisation and are the seat of our individual ego, the part of us that believes 'I' is all that exists. The higher mental bodies are the realm of the higher Self, in which the 'I' of ego begins to give way to the recognition that 'I' am part of something far greater than my individual Self. (See Fig. 12.1).

In this model of consciousness, the physical body occupies only the densest, lowest three layers of the physical-etheric body, which is only the lowest, densest of the energy bodies of man. Above the physical-etheric is the domain of the emotions, layer 6; the domain of thought, layer 5; and the domains of spirit, layers 4 to 1.

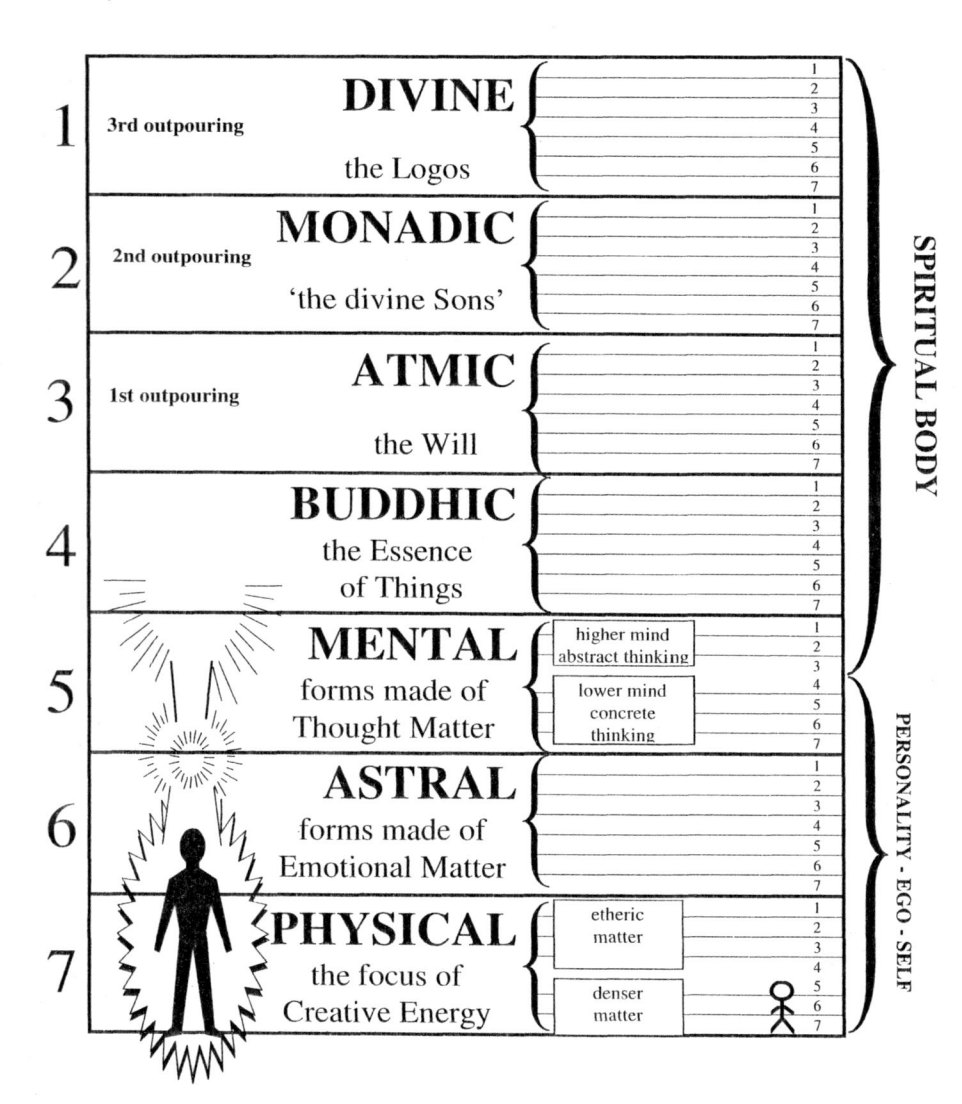

1	3rd outpouring	**DIVINE** the Logos	1,2,3,4,5,6,7
2	2nd outpouring	**MONADIC** 'the divine Sons'	1,2,3,4,5,6,7
3	1st outpouring	**ATMIC** the Will	1,2,3,4,5,6,7
4		**BUDDHIC** the Essence of Things	1,2,3,4,5,6,7
5		**MENTAL** forms made of Thought Matter	higher mind abstract thinking / lower mind concrete thinking
6		**ASTRAL** forms made of Emotional Matter	1,2,3,4,5,6,7
7		**PHYSICAL** the focus of Creative Energy	etheric matter / denser matter

Layers 1–4: SPIRITUAL BODY
Layers 5–7: PERSONALITY · EGO · SELF

Figure 12.1. The Layers of Mind.

Note that the domain of mind is divided into the higher mind, the interface with spirit and will, while the lower mind is the interface with our emotions and the world of our physical senses. Depending upon what level of mind you are operating from, the mind can be an instrument of either ego or spirit/soul. The greater part of us is thus non material subtle energies, emotion, thought and spirit which animate the denser etheric energies manifest as physical form.[1] Likewise, when will is transduced from the higher spiritual Atmic body, it may be used as an instrument of ego or spirit/soul.

Just as the etheric body is the interface where the magnetoelectric energy is transduced for physiological function, the mind or mental body, is the interface where the higher magnetoelectric energies of emotion, thought and spiritual direction are transduced for mental function. The non-material mind then, is the interface that activates the mental functions of the structure that is the physical brain.

How this might occur is purely speculation on my part, however it does provide a conceptual framework within which mental functions can have an effect at the level of the physical body. How can a thought, which is a subtle energy vibration—a thought-form—then create feelings, sensations or actions within the physical body?

Consider for a moment that the power behind a thought originates within your spiritual body. The thought-form then generated within the mental body can cause a specific pattern in astral matter which is the energetic aspect of emotion. This astral-emotional pattern then interfaces with the etheric body creating a reciprocal etheric pattern. It is then transduced to a specific pattern of neural activity within the physical brain.

Depending on the nature of the original thought-form and the force behind it, the astral emotional pattern will cause a greater or a lesser intensity of neural activity. This would manifest as specific patterns of neuronal firing in the brain. This neural activity may then also activate other neurons that lead to physiological responses that we call feelings, sensations or even physical action.

MIND—THE NEUROLOGICAL SUBSTRATE

I would like to contrast my proposition on the nature of mind with the currently theorised scientific understanding of mind. Until the last two decades, there was little understanding of how the brain worked. But in the past 20 years or so, and particularly in the last 10 years, with the use of powerful devices such as functional Magnetic Resonance Imagining (fMRI), and Positive Emission Tomography (PET) scanners, it has become possible to probe the mysteries of this most complex of all structures, and the neural correlates of mental activity are becoming rapidly known.

In fact, progress in this area has been so rapid that many scientists are beginning to make sweeping statements about science now being in the position to understand the exact nature of mind and consciousness.[2] In my opinion, the mistake that is being made here is to think that the Positive-Space/Time events that occur within the nerves of the brain, are themselves the source of thought and consciousness. Neuroscientists are currently talking of 'understanding the mind', because they now understand some of the neural correlates within the brain that occur when the mind is used.[3]

It is my strong belief that all that can be known from the use of the scientific instrumentation available at this time, as sophisticated as it appears to be, is the neurological activity that takes place in Positive-Space/Time which is actually elicited by mental processes that occur in the mental body in Negative-Space/Time.

While many neuroscientists feel they are on the threshold of understanding consciousness itself, all they are really on the threshold of comprehending is the neurological activity generated by consciousness.

WHAT IS CONSCIOUSNESS?

Consciousness is another term that has been used to mean many things to many different people. It has been used to describe any state, from merely being sentient or capable of having a reaction to stimuli, to the highest states of human experience.

From my perspective, consciousness denotes a level of mental and spiritual self awareness. In this definition the key word is 'awareness' and it means being aware of your thoughts and the source of those thoughts. In such a context you cannot have emotional awareness, rather you are aware of your emotions at mental and spiritual levels. Likewise you are aware of your physical vehicle, the body and its sensations as an extension of your consciousness.

Human conscious experience may be derived from two different sources: sensory experience and mental/spiritual events. If I should push a pin into your hand, you would have consciousness of the acute sensory experience of a pin-prick. You would be clearly aware that the source of this conscious event was a physical, sensory stimulus. This is known as 'bottom-up' processing.

In contrast, you may have a thought that originates within your mind that had no antecedent sensory experience. In fact, you can have a thought about something you have never experienced nor are ever likely to experience. Yet, you are conscious of these thoughts and indeed, may even use these thoughts to commit conscious acts. Creative writing, designing and composing are examples of purely mental events or activities of pure consciousness. This is known as 'top-down' processing.

While current neurological theory is beginning to explain many of the neural events involved in bottom-up processing, it still provides no clues as to how top-down processing might be achieved. No one can yet identify the source of an original thought. Neither can anyone explain the well-spring of inspiration.

Chalmers, in his fascinating book, *The Conscious Mind*, has called the 'bottom-up' concept of consciousness, the 'easy problem' because it is ultimately solvable with the mechanistic approaches of neuroscience.[4] There has been real progress in recent years of the understanding of the mechanisms and neural substrates involved in sensory processing and integration within the brain and the behaviours arising from this processing.

Yet, even when the last neuron involved in a sensory experience and its interconnections are fully understood, it still leaves what Chalmers calls the 'hard problem'—the mystery of subjective experience. Why should the processes in the brain produce subjective experience at all?[5]

The subjective experiential aspects of conscious experience of our world are called qualia, the essence of the subjective experience, the intrinsic qualities of, say for instance, the colour purple or the fragrance of a rose. These are sensory-derived qualia, but then there are qualia of mind devoid of sensory origin—introspection of our thoughts, watching our own brain activity. These 'top-down' processes producing the qualia of our subjective mental existence, are less easily explained, if they can be explained at all, by mechanistic models.

There have been models constructed to suggest that top-down processing may originate within the brain via reciprocal and recurrent neural networks.[6] But what is it that initiates activity in these networks? I feel this begs the question.

There are areas of human consciousness that lie far beyond normal waking awareness. Among these, are experiences in which the person is aware that their consciousness has become separated from their vehicle of their physical body. Two common examples are near-death experiences and out-of-body experiences, otherwise known as astral travel.

NEAR-DEATH EXPERIENCES

It is a well documented phenomenon that millions of people have 'died' but lived to tell the tale. The physiological signs all indicated death: the heart stopped, breathing ceased and in many cases, brain activity disappeared, sometimes for up to 45 minutes. Yet the person came back to life. These people have reported experiences during the time that they were 'dead' in which they were still conscious, and were even aware of observing their dead body and the events occurring around it.[7]

Elisabeth Kubler-Ross, an acknowledged expert on near-death experiences, having studied 25,000 cases, notes several commonalties. One is that the people often report seeing or meeting people whom they have loved in their life, but who are now dead. The second is that there is an absence of physical sensation, particularly pain. The third is that people experiencing near-death perceive themselves to be whole and complete even though they may be 'looking down' on a body with amputated limbs. They also report that there is no negative judgment, only dispassionate observation. The fourth is that the people can return from a near-death experience with intact memory of the events that occurred during the time they were 'dead'.[8]

A particularly remarkable aspect of the experience of meeting loved ones during the period of 'death' is that in no case has anyone ever reported conversing with, or seeing someone who is currently alive. In her book *On Life After Death*, Kubler-Ross writes that even though she has questioned thousands of children about whom they saw, spoke to, or interacted with when they were 'dead', never had they seen or talked with anyone who is still alive.

Dr Kubler-Ross gives a fascinating example. A young girl reported that she had seen her mother 'just before she came back'. As it happened, the girl's mother had died in another operating room in the same hospital minutes before her daughter had 'returned'. Kubler-Ross wondered why, if this were all merely hallucinatory or wishful thinking, no child ever mentioned a living parent, sibling or friend?[9] It's a telling point.

Another commonly reported phenomenon was for the 'dead' person to observe a tunnel of light that appeared to lead onto another plane of existence, one that is often described as being 'blissful and incredibly peaceful'. At this juncture these people say that there was a choice they had to make between remaining in this light-filled plane or returning to their physical body.[10] The instant they decided to return to their physical body, they found themselves looking once more out of their physical eyes. Many of these people may have been in a state of coma during the time that they reported being out of their body, but the coma ended with the return of consciousness to their body.

I would like to share the story of a middle-aged woman I met one evening. When she found out that I worked in esoteric areas, she related the following story to me: She said 'I don't tell this to many people because they usually laugh at me or think that I'm crazy. But I want to know what happened to me.'

She told me that when she was in her 20s, she had a horrible car accident in which she lost control of her car on a wet road, in a construction zone. The guard rail on the edge of the road had not been finished and her car ran directly into the end of the rail.

The guard rail penetrated the front of the car, the engine compartment and into the cabin where it peeled the muscles off her right leg, from her knee to her hip. At the same time the steering wheel was driven into her chest. Many ribs were broken and she also suffered a fractured skull when her head collided with the windscreen. She described an horrendous accident.

The woman told me that at the instant of the accident, she had felt her consciousness leave her body. As she watched the muscles being flayed from her femur and her skull break, she experienced no pain. She merely watched. She remained in this disembodied consciousness, looking down on her mangled body from above. She said, 'I was there observing the firemen using the jaws of life to cut my body out of the wreck. When my body was moved into the ambulance, I still hovered above it, calmly watching, as not once but twice I 'died' on the way to the hospital and my heart was restarted with a defibrillator.

'After emergency surgery, I was in a coma for almost six months. All this time I hovered above my body, watching the comings and goings of the nurses and doctors and my concerned family. I listened to what they were talking about and watched what they did. At the end of this period of coma, suddenly a tunnel of light appeared before me and I knew I had to make a choice whether to go or to stay. For reasons that I'm still unable to explain to myself, I made the decision to stay. The instant I made that decision, I was suddenly looking out of my eyes at the ceiling where I had once hovered. I had regained consciousness.'

What this woman meant to say is that she had regained physical consciousness because she had, in fact, been conscious throughout the entire experience. She had left her physical body and with it her physical consciousness at the instant of the accident. Her consciousness persisted or existed within subtle bodies throughout the long months of the coma.

In the state of coma the body is run via the lower brain centres of the medulla and the brainstem with almost no cortical activity. Hence the person is living on vegetative functions alone: the heart beats, they breathe and intestinal peristalsis continues. In this state, only the etheric and physical bodies are functioning. The higher subtle bodies are separated from the physical being. It has been observed by people who have experienced this state that the subtle bodies are usually not far away from the physical body. This has also been reported by clairvoyant individuals who have observed people in this state.

Further observations made by this woman were that she had memory of events that had occurred when she was 'out-of-her-body' and that these memories were later confirmed by people who were present during that time. For example, she was able to tell her family that she had died twice on the way to the hospital and indeed the hospital records confirmed this to be true. She could also tell her family about the conversations that had taken place both between themselves and with her, while she had been in coma. More remarkably, she was also able to tell them about what she had 'seen' them do during their visits with her in the hospital.

Although it may have, as with implicit memory experiments with anaesthetised people, been possible for her brain to record auditory events while she was unconscious, what is harder to explain is how she could 'see' what was happening in her room when her eyes were bandaged as a result of the skull fracture.

Many doctors and scientists would like to dismiss such observations as simply projections, illusions or hallucinations. Kubler-Ross carefully questioned several totally blind people about their near-death experience. In spite of their physical blindness, they were not only able to tell who worked on them during the resuscitation, but gave intimate details of the attire and clothing of all the people present.[11]

Observations like these must have an explanation but none is forthcoming from the realm of western science and physical consciousness. From this perspective, events of this nature are clearly impossible. In fact, as Dr Kubler-Ross pointed out after her first encounter with a patient who had undergone a near-death experience, 'my students were shocked that I did not call this hallucination and illusion, or a feeling of depersonalisation. They had a desperate need to give it a label—something they could identify—and then put it aside and not have to deal with it.'[12]

There is a framework for dealing with this but it requires you to move beyond the limitation that consciousness is merely physical and to step into the realms of the subtle bodies where such occurrences become perfectly understandable.

OUT-OF-BODY EXPERIENCES

Out-of-body experiences are another form of human experience that fall outside rational scientific explanation. The tendency is also to denigrate these as illusions or hallucinations which are not 'real'. But to the individuals who have had these experiences they know them to have been real occurrences in their lives. Millions of people have experienced such events, but again, whenever they report them, they are told they are fantasising, deluded or just plain crazy. But could there be an explanation for these apparently bizarre encounters with another realm of consciousness?

From the perspective of the subtle bodies, this is quite understandable and even quite predictable. The etheric body is not only the interface to the physical body, but is so tightly interwoven with the physical that it cannot be easily separated from it. It is said that when you die, your astral, mental and spiritual bodies are separated from your etheric and physical bodies. It is the higher subtle bodies which may be considered the vehicle of your soul, and which are in a sense 'immortal', because they persist after your death.[13]

The etheric body, on the other hand, is said to disintegrate as your physical body decays. This indicates that the higher mental bodies can be separated from the etheric and physical bodies. While this does not normally occur while a person is in ordinary waking physical consciousness, it may occur as a result of traumatic physical injury as in near-death experiences, or, as a result of altered states of consciousness.

Something we all experience every day is the transition from the waking consciousness to the altered state of consciousness that we call sleep. Some individuals, during this transition or after the physical body enters the sleeping state, suddenly find themselves conscious of being out of their body. In this state, they may travel, often covering great distances and making observations of the world around them. When this happens, most people wake and may not be able to recall the details of the experiences or, perhaps even the experience itself. In other cases, individuals remain fully conscious of 'astral travelling' and can easily recall what they observed, did and heard. Indeed some astral travellers are even able to report on real geographic locations that they have never actually visited in their waking state or with their physical body.[14]

An example of this type of out-of-body experience was related to me by a close friend who is also a doctor. In his teens, he was an exchange student in the United States. His American friends were taking him to a movie theatre in a town some distance from where he was living, a town he had never seen before.

His two friends were in the front of the car and he was dozing in the back seat. He heard them say that they had become lost and didn't know how to get to the theatre. At that instant, he found his consciousness out of his body and above the car. This disembodied consciousness raced ahead of the car over the town and 'saw' the theatre. He then returned to his body, opened his eyes and said to his friends, 'You just have to go two blocks straight ahead to the park, turn right, go two blocks and then turn left at the traffic lights. The theatre is on your right.'

They said, 'How do you know? You've never been here before. And besides, you were asleep.' My friend replied, 'Just do it!' As the car approached the park, my friend realised that he was looking at the same park he had just seen a moment before but now from the perspective of the ground and not the air. The theatre was precisely where he had 'seen' it to be.

Two other mechanisms are capable of producing altered states of consciousness: The first is the use of psychedelic or hallucinogenic drugs and the second is deep meditational states. While the use of psychedelic or hallucinogenic drugs may produce a separation of the higher subtle bodies from the etheric and physical bodies, it is uncontrolled and usually only of a short duration. Also, from the perspective of those who can access these altered states from the entry point of higher consciousness, drug-induced experiences are said to be only a faint illusion of the real experience.

Through meditation many individuals have also had out-of-body experiences. In these states, it is commonly reported that they observe their physical body and may then leave it to travel to other places. While on these astral journeys, they report seeing and hearing as if they had physical eyes and physical ears. They also remember what they saw and heard as if they had a physical brain. At the instant of returning, they report once again looking out through their physical eyes.[15]

Most of those who doubt that such experiences can take place, have never had one. And such doubters are usually very strongly tied to rational thought and physical consciousness. I, for one, have had out-of-body experiences, both induced by drugs and meditation, and this was despite the fact that at the time I was a hyper-rational research scientist who doubted the reality of these experiences. I had no model in which to place them.

I will have to admit that these out-of-body experiences did create much consternation in my normal consciousness as I tried to understand the observations that I had made during them. Even though they seemed implausible, I also knew them to be as real as the waking consciousness I was currently experiencing. Because science is based on observation, what was I to do with the observations that did not fit within my rational paradigm of that time? What I did is what most people do with these experiences. I swept them under the carpet and chose to ignore them.

As I was a child of the 1960s, my first out-of-body experience was prompted by psychedelic drugs: LSD and mescaline. One evening, after having LSD, I was quietly sitting listening to music in the living room of a house that belonged to a close friend. I was the only person in the room. Suddenly, I found my consciousness out of my body and near the ceiling of the room. From that vantage point, my consciousness was looking down on my body. My first thought was, 'Hey, that's Charles' body'. To my consciousness Charles' body appeared to be asleep on the couch. Then I became aware of the voices of my friends who were talking in the room next door.

In a way I still do not comprehend, I willed my consciousness to enter the other room. It seemed to pass right through the wall. 'I', as my consciousness, began to observe with marked fascination, my friends' conversation; what they were doing, and that I had an awareness of my disembodied presence in the room. At that instant I got scared. The thought that crossed my 'mind' was, 'If I was here in this room, who was in my body in the other room?' In a flash, my eyes opened and I was looking out at the room in which my body was sitting. For a few moments, I thought, 'that must have been a dream ... or an hallucination.' But it seemed so totally real.

So I decided to go into the other room and interrogate my friends who were not on drugs. Always the scientist, I was looking for validation of the observations and had the presence of mind to carefully frame the right questions. I did not say, 'What did you say and what did you do?' Had I done so, what they told me may have contaminated my actual observations as I may have attempted to make my memories fit their story. Instead I said, 'A few minutes ago, did you say such and such to Peter? And did Peter reply such and such to you? And did Peter get up, walk around the table and look over your shoulder at what you were doing?' I was that specific about my observations. My friends could then either confirm or disprove what I reported. Much to my surprise, they confirmed that everything I had heard and seen was true. In fact, their response was, 'How the hell did you know that?'

This experience left me totally confused. On the one hand, I knew it had happened, and independent observation had confirmed it. But on the other hand, it was physically impossible for such an experience to have taken place. Wasn't it?

Following the drug experience, I became very interested in meditation because it seemed to offer a way of investigating such states of consciousness in a more conscious way. In a number of deep meditations, I have also found myself out of my body as disembodied consciousness. As I was not on drugs and fully conscious, these events could not merely be explained as a consequence of some chemically induced state.

During one of these meditations I found myself out of my body, racing above the ground over a desert area that I had never seen before. The colours and the detail of the desert were complete. I could see the cacti, the texture of the sand and some amazing rock outcrops. I was totally aware that it was only my mind that was travelling and that I had no physical body. This was confirmed by my 'return' to my physical body which was in fact enduring a cold New England winter.

It was only years later when, for the first time I travelled through Arizona, that I realised the rock outcrops directly ahead of me where the same rock outcrops I had seen in that meditation. In fact, my recall of that out-of-body experience was so acute I could predict what was behind the outcrops before I even arrived there. The only difference was one of perspective. I was now looking at the outcrops from the highway whereas in the meditational state, I had been looking at them from a height of 10 metres up.

Now while this is all very interesting, what does it mean for consciousness?

LESSONS FROM NEAR-DEATH AND OUT-OF-BODY EXPERIENCES

The reason for presenting these esoteric experiences is for the lessons they provide about the nature of consciousness. You will have noticed in all of the examples above that the individuals involved always identified the 'I' of their Self with their disembodied consciousness and not with their physical body. If consciousness was a property of the brain alone, how could you ever have conscious experiences outside of the physical body? This is true of all individuals who have had such experiences. They all identify the 'I' with the consciousness that is doing the observation and not their physical, structural being.[16] This phenomenon cannot be explained in the current western paradigm which allows only the physical and denies the existence of the metaphysical.

But science demands an explanation! Science is about observation and creating models to explain those observations. When your model cannot explain a valid observation it says that the model is either wrong or more likely, incomplete. Because millions of people have had these types of out-of-body experiences, many of which have been validated by external observers, science must provide an explanation.

In reality, all western scientists can say is not that the metaphysical does not exist, but rather that they are ignorant of its existence. Absence of proof is not proof of absence. If you cannot measure something, all you can say is that you are ignorant of the presence of that which you cannot measure, not that what you cannot measure does not exist.

To support this statement from my scientific experience, in 1969, I was working in a research laboratory analysing for polychlorinated biphenyls (PCBs), which at the time were suspected of being potential environmental pollutants. Our instrumentation could measure PCB concentrations to the low parts-per-million, and we had analysed many samples from all over the North Atlantic ocean and the north-eastern coast of the United States. We did not find PCBs in any sample, except those at points of discharge. Our conclusion therefore, was that PCBs did not represent a significant environmental pollutant.

In the last half of 1969, a scientist perfected the electron-capture detector for the gas chromatograph, the instrument we use to measure PCBs. This new detector increased our detection range by a factor of one million, which meant we could now measure PCBs in the parts-per-trillion range. Guess what? When the same samples were reanalysed, PCBs were everywhere but just in the part-per-billion range below our original level of detection. Even more importantly, subsequent toxicological research revealed that PCBs at the parts-per-billion level, had significant sub-lethal effects on the reproduction of many bird and marine species. They were definitely a major environmental pollutant.

Just because we could not measure PCBs did not mean they were not there, it just meant that we could not measure them. They were there, and in concentrations that were significant but we were ignorant of their existence. Based on that ignorance we were wrong in our assessment of the initial danger of PCBs.

It would appear that the Western scientific paradigm may indeed provide an incomplete model of human experience. In addition to the electrical and electromagnetic fields involved with the physical world of Positive-Space/Time, there appear to be other types of frequencies that remain undetectable to instruments that operate only in Positive-Space/Time. Therefore, these instruments cannot provide any information about the existence of subtle energies that have frequencies in another frequency domain. The domain of Negative-Space/Time. Instruments capable of measurement in the Negative-Space/Time domain are currently being developed.[17]

Currently the only instrument that exists to investigate the subtle energy vibrations of Negative-Space/Time, is the human mind, but a human mind that is operating at a higher level than physical consciousness.

MIND: THE INSTRUMENT OF CONSCIOUSNESS

To be conscious is to be aware of your current reality. Physical consciousness is limited to that which the physical receptors can detect. Your physical reality is dominated by sensory input. Since we have millions upon millions of sensory receptors (the eyes and ears alone are sending millions of impulses per second to the brain), a river of sensory input into our nervous system, our consciousness is swamped by this unending sensory input. As a result our consciousness is almost wholly focused on sensory experience as our reality.

Yet we are also aware that our consciousness is multi-tiered. When we are having a physical experience, we can at the same time, be conscious of that experience and be conscious of being conscious of that experience. This is the bizarre and astounding conundrum of consciousness. Even more remarkable, we are conscious of being conscious of being conscious of the experience. This hall of mirrors, the multifaceted awareness of our own consciousness, is sometimes referred to as 'the observer within.'

What makes mind the instrument of consciousness is, that like any other instrument, it can be focused. But unlike other instruments, it is not what it is focused on that determines the observational experience, it is rather the *level* of consciousness that is being focused *through* it that determines our experience.

Here is a simpler analogy: If we were to look at a petrie dish of pond water with the naked eye, we would see a petrie dish of pond water. When we look at the same water through a microscope, using visible light, the wee beasties of the microworld dance before our eyes. Were we to look at the same scene through a microscope using infrared light, a pageant of shimmering luminescence would denote areas of heat and cold. The physical wee beasties disappear.

Were we to view the same petrie dish of beasties with an electron microscope our focus would reveal monsters of horrible dimensions. Viewing exactly the same scene through an electron force microscope, we would see only piles of atoms. In all of this the scene, the petrie dish of pond water, has remained the same. What has changed is the frequency domain of which we are conscious. But to be aware of these different conscious domains, we needed to use different instruments.

With consciousness, the instrument—the mind—remains the same. It is just the level of consciousness through which our world is perceived that changes. Normally, thought directs our consciousness or at least, our conscious attention. Depending on what we are attending to, we may perceive either a physical or a metaphysical world. Once you move into the realm of thoughts and emotions the physical world is left behind. When you are in a state of mental concentration, the physical ceases to exist.

How many times do you find yourself 'coming back' from being deep in thought? How many times have you driven down the road contemplating an issue in your life and suddenly found yourself well past where you were meant to turn and realised you hadn't been attending to the physical world at all, even though your physical eyes had been processing millions upon millions of pieces of sensory data every second?

What kind of consciousness can account for this duality of action? Of being able to process physical sensory data; making decisions on the basis of that data (driving the car), but at the same time being unaware of this real-time data processing because another level of your consciousness is processing abstract data and making decisions on the basis of what is occupying your thoughts?

This remarkable capacity for dual mental processing most likely relies upon the dual sensory perceptual systems within the brain. While the amygdala-limbic system is guiding your survival, getting the car safely from point A to point B and beyond, the hippocampal-cortical system was fully occupied with abstract thoughts. These are, however, still only describing the neural correlates of mind.

But the neural correlates, the sequence and patterns of nerve firing in various parts of the brain, are not the mind. While our limbic brain is capable of running our physical body in the physical reality of real time to maintain our physical survival, the higher cortical centres appear to be able to generate thought that is not only non-survival oriented but free from physical substrate. Indeed it appears to be the latter type of consciousness that allows us to escape the bounds of our physical body in out-of-body and near-death experiences.

When out of body there is no consciousness of our physical being. The survival centres appear to be left behind and inactive but (here's the rub) conscious observation, thought, and memory are retained. What a piece of work is man!

This higher level of consciousness also has the capacity to override the lower level of physical survival-oriented consciousness. For instance, you see a child drowning in a raging torrent and without a moment's hesitation dive in to save them. Clearly, your physical survival centres would be screaming, 'Don't jump in the water. It's very dangerous. You could die!' But from some higher centre within, comes the conscious thought, 'I must save this child!' And this thought is followed by the action that saves the child.

When people who perform such altruistic acts are asked what motivated their bravery, most often they reply, 'I didn't think of the danger to me. All I could see was a child in danger of drowning.' We know that the amygdala would have perceived the danger but a higher will overrode the survival instinct.

FOCUSING THE MIND

Left to its own devices, the mind tends to pay attention and to focus on the sensory experiences at hand. It can be totally preoccupied by a single sensory experience such as an itch that you can't reach. The itch will soon dominate your whole experience of reality. But if someone should suddenly yell 'Fire!' the itch would instantly disappear. In fact, the itch signals remain, but your attention has been shifted elsewhere to a stimulus of more immediate concern.

Or, someone may merely say to you, 'Have you seen that latest movie with Mel Gibson?' Again, the itch will disappear, or rather, your attention has again been shifted, only this time to a matter of interest rather than of survival. As your friend walks away, you might find your attention involved in a fantasy starring Mel Gibson. What happened to the itch?

Consciousness has shifted like a bee going from flower to flower; from the itch as a physical experience (sensory), to the fire as a threatening experience (emotional), to the movie as an interesting experience (concrete thought), to the fantasy as a fulfilling experience, albeit abstract at this stage. The focus of the mind thus determines what we pay attention to and the nature of our conscious experience.

The above describes the consciousness of undirected mind. The Tibetan Lamas say that left to itself, the mind tends to focus on negative physical, emotional and mental states.[18] This tendency is probably related to the fact that negative physical and emotional experiences have greater survival value and leave a stronger imprint in our undirected consciousness.

However there are specific techniques to focus the mind. The term meditation can be applied to describe various techniques that allow you to focus the instrument of the mind beyond mundane concerns and sensory experience. It is interesting to note that in the western definition of meditation, the word alludes to 'dwelling in thought', or 'engaging in a state of contemplation', or to 'practising religious contemplation'. The focus here is still totally on the intellect and intellectualization.

From the eastern concept, meditation is exactly the opposite. In eastern meditative traditions, the techniques you learn are to free yourself from thoughts, not to focus on thoughts; to allow yourself to experience consciousness, without thought. But in this sense, 'focus' is not what we understand as intense concentration directed by intellect. Rather the intellect moves aside so that the essential consciousness of all that you are can be experienced.

This is one of the greatest challenges of meditation to western minds, to let go of thoughts and to be 'conscious'. This is also true of other eastern techniques such as martial arts. One of the hardest things to develop as a western practitioner of martial arts is 'focus' which means that you do not focus on any one thing, but on all things simultaneously.

The first thing you become aware of as a karate beginner, a white belt, is how fast the brown and black belts are. They seem to know what you are going to do before you do. But as you achieve higher levels of training and begin to learn the technique of karate focus, the white belts whom you spar with appear to become slower. I contemplated this experience from both sides and realised that what was happening was, as I let go of my concentrated focus on objects, and allowed that focus to expand to include the whole, I too could 'know' what my opponent was going to do the instant they started an action.

For instance, if my opponent was going to kick to my head, just by the bodily tensions that were developing and the subtle shifting of weight; the initial movement of the foot before it left the floor had already signaled to me the entire movement that was to follow. Since I knew this, I had plenty of time to decide what counter and counter attack I was going to use. It looked to me like the person was moving in slow motion.

In a sense what I found martial arts to be was a moving meditation, which is why we always began and ended our karate classes with meditation allowing us to focus our minds, not on the specific, but rather on the whole.

If meditational techniques are diligently practised, it becomes possible to know the world from the point of view of consciousness, rather than mind.

THE POWER OF WILL

The ability to focus is determined by our will. In this context we are defining will as that force or energy from a higher spiritual plane (Figure 12.1) that empowers our thoughts. Thus 'will-power'.

It can be directed by any level of our consciousness: I can focus my physical action towards a physical goal such as winning a race by using my will to win. Likewise I can focus my emotional will to compassionate ends such as feeling empathy for a friend in difficult circumstances. I can focus my mental will to solve a difficult problem. Or, through prayer or invocation, I may focus my spiritual will to achieve contact with God.

Thus is appears that energy follows thought and if the power behind thought is will, then it is will that truly directs your energy. But the end to which that energy will be put is determined entirely by your conscious focus. Consciousness and will both use the vehicle of mind as the instrument of their expression.

If you are an athlete, the focus is physical. Any athlete achieving their personal best draws not only on their physical strength but on the will to win. Champions are basically those athletes who are able to focus their will and hence to increase the energy they have to achieve their goal. In fact, they often seem to transcend their physical limitations. But this is still grounded at the physical level of consciousness.

Will can also be used to drive etheric energies. Hence when a martial arts expert breaks a board with his fist he does this by directing the Ch'i through the physical vehicle of his arm into the board. It is the will-directed Ch'i that breaks the board not the fist. The proof of this is that if you punch the same board with all your physical might, but without the focus of mind to direct Ch'i, all you will achieve is a bloodied fist.

The Qi Chong masters have developed the ability to take this to an even higher degree when they demonstrate such powerful mind focus that without moving a muscle, they can project their Ch'i to knock another person to the ground.

MIND TO MIND

Throughout the book we have alluded to the ability of energy directed by the mind to affect the physical. But it also appears that one mind can directly affect another. As hard as the mind affecting the physical body is to explain, it becomes even more obtuse to explain how one human mind may be able to directly affect another human mind.

Some recent experiments which use sophisticated coupled multi-channelled

Electrocardiograms (ECG), which measure heart activity, and Electroencephalograms (EEG) which measure brainwave patterns, have given us proof that minds do communicate or transmit physiologically observable energy.

The heart is a dynamic energy generating system and it produces the largest electromagnetic energy signal in the body, the ECG. In fact, the electromagnetic energy generated by the heart is distributed throughout the body with the ECG signal of the heart being observable in every cell.[19] As well, the EEG brainwaves ride on top of the ECG signal if one electrode is attached above the head and one below the heart.[20]

Within the individual, the ECG pattern within the EEG brainwaves appears most strongly in the occipital lobes at the back of the skull, with very little signal registering in the frontal lobes.

What is even more remarkable is that if two people sit facing each other at a distance of approximately two metres with their eyes closed, and if one, the sender, simply focuses his or her mind on sending compassionate thoughts to the other person, the ECG signal from the sender appears in the EEG brainwave pattern in the frontal lobes of the other person.[21] In other words what is being measured here is the direct transference of a pattern of thought to another person and this thought is creating in the other person a measurable physiological resonance between the two people.

This experiment provides us with the first tangible evidence of the interconnection of minds. When this experiment was repeated with men who had taken part in a 35 year longitudinal study which looked into the effects of caring and uncaring parents on their adult health status. In this study researchers used the term 'caring' rather than 'love' because caring is a many faceted term that includes the positive perceptions of love, understanding, empathy and justice, as well as other positive and responsible parental role attributes.[22]

Examples of positive words that the men used to describe caring parents were: 'loving, lovable, friendly, warm, open, understanding, kind, sympathetic, sensitive, sincere, just, fair, considerate, patient, hard-working, intelligent, discerning, respectful, strong, sense of humor, cheerful and secure'.

Examples of negative words used to describe uncaring parents were: 'quick-tempered, not affectionate, cold, intolerant, no self discipline, inflexible, impatient, egotistical, authoritarian and opinionated'—all attributes based in insecurity.

One of the most remarkable discoveries was that 87 percent of the men who rated their mothers and father low on parental love and caring, had diseases diagnosed in mid-life, whereas only 25 percent of the subjects who rated both parents high on parental love and caring had diseases diagnosed in mid-life. Unequivocally this demonstrates the power of love.[23]

When the same researchers sent compassion and loving thoughts to participants in the study, there were two quite different outcomes. The ECG signal of the sender was clearly registered in the frontal lobes of the men with caring parents. In contrast, the ECG signal of the sender was greatly diminished and out of phase in the men who had experienced an upbringing with uncaring parents. It is as if these men could not receive the transmission of human caring.

In order for this transference of the ECG signal from one person to another to take place, it was essential that the person transmitting the signal focused their mind and intent on compassion. If they just sat there thinking random thoughts, the transference was greatly diminished or eliminated.

What is the difference in energy transmission between the person focusing their mind on true compassion or just having random thoughts? The answer seems to be what happens within the sender when they focus on compassion. In a recent study by Professor William Tiller and others, it was discovered that when people performed what they defined as 'the heart focus technique', it activated a little-studied nerve pathway that runs from the heart to the old reptilian brain.[24] Basically this technique is a matter of focusing your mind on feelings of compassion and love for your fellow man.

This heart-generated signal created an entrained brainwave pattern. In concert with this entrained brainwave pattern, the pattern of breathing and heart rate also appeared to 'lock' into a very stable state. Thus the very act of focusing the mind on compassion generates activity within the heart that elicits a very stable ECG signal.

How in the western scientific paradigm can you explain the transference of the compassion generated ECG signal from one person into the physiology of another person with whom they are not in physical contact? In short, at the present time and in the present paradigm, there is no way to explain it.

The model presented in the previous chapter, however, provides a rational explanation. The subtle energy of the mind-directed thought of compassion (a Negative/Space-Time event), appears to be transduced into the Positive/Space-Time electromagnetic and physiological ECG signal of the sender. This stable ECG signal then generates a Negative/Space-Time magnetoelectric resonance pattern which is transmitted to the other individual. This magnetoelectric resonance pattern is then again transduced into the electromagnetic ECG signal that appears within the EEG brainwaves of the other person.

THE HEART AND MIND IN HEALING

Hands-on healing is an interesting misnomer because in many cases this form of healing requires no touch at all. What it does require is that the person doing the healing needs to focus their mind on compassion and love for the one being healed. The biophysical energy of the hand contains much heart energy with a strong ECG component.[25] Obviously this would generate a strong magnetoelectric resonance which could be transmitted from healer to patient in much the same way as the ECG signals were transmitted from the sender into the brain of the receiver.

It appears that in many cases of hands-on healing it is the transfer of subtle energies of compassion and love directed by the mind of the healer that effects the healing. For instance in a clinical trial designed to investigate the effects of laying on of hands, 44 otherwise healthy males agreed to a have a surgical biopsy or small wound, created in their upper arm.

The patients were then placed in individual, isolated rooms and instructed once a day for the next 16 days to place their wounded arm through a sleeve which was fitted to an opening through the wall. In the other room their wound was either treated by a healer, using non-contact techniques (laying on of hands), or received no treatment at all.

By the eighth day of the experiment the treated group had an average wound size which measured 10 times smaller than the untreated group. By the 16th day, 13 of the 23 treated subjects were completely healed. None of the untreated group displayed complete healing at the conclusion of the study.[26]

The transference of magnetoelectric energy utilizing the Negative/Space-Time property which negates distance as a factor, may also account for the efficacy of distance healing such as prayer. The person doing the praying is always separated by some distance, and often considerable distances from the person who is the object of their prayers. Yet prayer has been shown to have very powerful effects in healing.[27]

In a 10 month randomised prospective, double blind study to investigate the clinical effects of prayer, a computer assigned 393 patients receiving standard medical care in a coronary unit either to a group that was prayed for by volunteer prayer groups from Roman Catholic and Protestant churches, or to a group who were not specifically remembered in prayer. The results were striking: the prayed for group was five times less likely to require antibiotics, three times less likely to develop pulmonary oedema, none required breathing tubes and fewer died. As the cardiologist and former professor at the University of California, Dr Randolph Byrd stated, 'If this was a new drug or surgical procedure, it would have been heralded as a medical breakthrough in the treatment of coronary conditions'.[28]

One conclusion that can be drawn from these results is that by a person transmitting their love and compassion to another via the medium of prayer, the harmonising and balancing nature of these mind-generated subtle energy states may be the mechanism by which physical dis-ease is healed or eased.

A group in the United States known as Spindrift has been further quantifying the effects of various kinds of prayer. They have observed that the more stressed an organism or person is, the better the results of prayer;

the more often prayer is used, the better the results; all parts of a body system are affected equally and, it is important that the person doing the praying know who and what is being prayed for. This last element in particular suggests how vital it is that the person doing the praying is able to focus specifically on the object of their prayer.[29]

When I care for someone or something, be it another human being or a pet, by focusing my thoughts on love and compassion I simultaneously generate within myself a greater state of physiological harmony and peace as witnessed by the effects of the 'heart focus' technique discussed above.

This may be the basis for the value of an older person owning a pet because it gives them something to care for, thus entraining a state of harmony and compassion within themselves. It is well known that the health of elderly people who are given an animal to take care of is significantly improved compared to those who are bereft of a love object. Just introducing dogs into nursing homes for the elderly people to pet has been shown to improve the health status of the residents.

BEYOND MIND. HIGHER CONSCIOUSNESS

The American psychologist William James in his 1901 book *The Varieties of Religious Experience* spoke of the state of ecstasy and its four qualities: ineffability, passivity, noetic quality and transience. Noetic is a word derived from the Greek 'nous', which means intellect or understanding. It is also the root of our word knowledge but defines knowledge which is experienced directly, and which is accompanied by a sense of certitude. It is a knowing experience.[30]

In the West, we equate experience of pure consciousness, such as the knowing of God, to the realm of religion. We set it apart from our normal experience of reality. In the East, these noetic qualities involving experiences of pure consciousness are well known and have many different terms to describe them. In fact, it is recognised that higher consciousness is a state of pure consciousness that can be attained by anyone who diligently follows a prescribed set of meditative and spiritual practices.

The difference between our normal waking consciousness and higher consciousness is that the first is the result of mental processing using the interface of the human brain, while the second is based in pure knowing. States of pure knowing have this ineffable quality that we are not able to express in words. They are beyond the intellect, beyond the mind.

To quote William James again, describing religious experience, he says, 'The subject says that it defies expression, that no adequate report of its content can be given in words. It follows from this that its quality must be directly experienced. It can not be imparted or transferred to others.' To those who experience them, mystical states are also states of knowledge providing insight into truths unknown to the discursive intellect. Although inarticulate, they remain illuminations and revelations that carry a sense of authority and certitude.[31]

A common state of higher consciousness described in the eastern literature is termed Samadhi. According to Swami Sivananda, Samadhi is 'inner Divine experience which is beyond the reach of speech and mind. There is no language or means to give expression to it. The state of Samadhi is all bliss, joy and peace. All mental activities cease now. There is no difference between subject and object.' Oneness.[32]

The Yogis call the practice of yoga, 'the science of yoga' because they say that the rules and principles of consciousness are every bit as rigorous as the rules and principles that apply to western science. By the application of diligent meditative practise and discipline, it is held to be inevitable that your consciousness will rise beyond the mundane level of the physical.

The rules and means of achieving higher levels of consciousness are well known to the masters of all esoteric traditions who have achieved enlightenment, cosmic or super consciousness. These individuals can and do direct others in the methods of how to move beyond the constraints of the physical world. The masters promise that with perseverance and by following the prescribed methods, it is possible for anyone to achieve higher conscious experience.

> *'Beyond the senses are the objects,*
> *beyond the objects is the mind,*
> *beyond the mind, the intellect,*
> *beyond the intellect, the Atman,*
> *beyond the Atman, the non-manifest,*
> *beyond the non-manifest, the Spirit,*
> *beyond the Spirit there is nothing,*
> *this is the end, the Pure Consciousness'.*
> Katha Upanishad, Ajit Mookerjee, Yoga Art

REFERENCES

Chapter 2
1. Legg, A.T., Physical therapy in infantile paralysis. In: *Principle of Practice of Physical Therapy*, Vol II. Mocked, W.F. Prior Co. Inc., Hagerstown, MD, p.45, 1932.
2. Kendall, H.O. & Kendall, F.P. *Muscle Testing and Function.* Williams & Williams, Baltimore, MD, 1949.
   Kendall, H.O. & Kendall, F.P. Case during recovery period of paralytic polio myelitis. U.S. Public Health Bulletin No.242, April, 1938
   Kendall, H.O. & Kendall, F.P. Physical Therapy for Lower Extremity Amputation. War Department Technical Manual, Washington, DC. U.S. Government Printing Office, p.8–293, 1946.
3. Goodheart, G.J. Jr. *You'll Be Better. The story of Applied Kinesiology.* A.K. Printing, Geneva, Ohio, Chapter 1, p.2, 1986.
   Walther, D.S. *Applied Kinesiology.* Synopsis. Systems D.C., Pueblo, CO, p.2, 1988.
4. Guyton, A.C. *Textbook of Medical Physiology.* 8th Ed. W.B. Saunders & Co., Philadelphia: PA, pp.170–184; 1991.
5. Owen, C. An endocrine interpretation of Chapman's reflexes. Based on Chapman and Owen's research at the Kirlesville College of Osteopathy and Surgery. Privately published, 1937.
   Walther, D.S. *Applied Kinesiology. Vol I. Basic Procedure and Muscle Testing.* Systems D.C., Pueblo, CO, pp.220-223, 1981.
6. Bennett, J. Dynamics of correction of abnormal function. From Terence Bennet Lectures, ed. by R.J. Martin, Sienna Madre, CA, privately published, R.J. Martin, DC, 1977.
7. Goodheart, G.J. Jr. *Applied Kinesiology.* 4th ed., Detroit, MI, privately published, 1967.
   Walther, D.S. *Applied Kinesiology.* Vol I. pp.234–239, 1981.
8. Mann, F. Acupuncture, *The Ancient Chinese Art of Healing and How It Works Scientifically.* Random House Inc, New York, NY, 1962.
9. Goodheart, G.J. Jr. Chinese lessons for chiropractic. Chiro. Econ., Vol 8(5), March/April, 1966.
10. Chang, S.T. *The Complete book of Acupuncture.* Celestial Arts, Berkeley, CA, p.3, 1976.
    Xinnong, Cheng (chief ed) *Chinese Acupuncture and Moxibustion.* Foreign Language Press, Beijing, China, p.1–2, 1987.
11. The 20th Century French scholar/diplomat George Soulié de Morant studied

acupuncture in China with Chinese masters between 1901–1917. Upon his return to France, he taught clinical applications of acupuncture to French physicians and introduced acupuncture theory of the classical texts to the French and European medical community through his truly monumental three volume text L'Acupuncture Chinoise (Chinese Acupuncture) in 1939, 1941 & 1955. It was Soulié de Morant that introduced the terms 'meridian' and 'energy' to the West from his translation of the terms 'Jing' and 'Ch'i' or 'Qi' from traditional Chinese texts.

12. Niboyet, J-E-H. Nouvelles constalations un les propriet's 'lectrique des points chinois. Bulletin de la Soci't' de'Acupuncture, Vol.4 (30), 1938.

    Roppel, R.M. & Mitchell, F. Jr. Skin points of anomalously low electric resistance: current voltage characteristics and relationships to peripheral stimulation therapies. J. Am. Osteopathic Assoc., 746:877–878, 1975.

    Hyvarien, J. & Karlson, M. Low resistance skin points that may coincide with acupuncture locations. Medical Biology 55:88–94, 1977.

13. Bossey, J & Sambuc, P. Acupuncture et systeme nerveux: les acquis. Acupuncture et M'decine Traditionnelle Chinois, Paris. Encyclopedic des M'decine Naturelles, 1B-1, 1989.

    Helms, J.M. *Acupuncture Energetics. A Clinical Approach for Physicians.* Medical Acupuncture Publishers, Berkeley, CA, pp.26–27, 1995.

14. Senelar, R. & Auziech, O. Histophysiologie du point d'acupuncture. Acupuncture et M'decine Traditionnelle Chinois, Paris. Encyclopedic des M'decine Naturelles, 1B-2C, 1989.

15. Niboyet, J.E.H. La Moindre Resistance à l'Electricite de surfaces punctiformes et de trajets catanes concordant avec les points et meridiens, bases de l'Acupuncture, Marseille. Thése de Sciences, 1963.

    Reichmanis, M. et al. Electrical correlates of acupuncture points. IEEE Trans, Biomed, Eng. BME 22.533–535, 1975

    Helms, J.M. *Acupuncture Energetics.* pp.20–21, 1995.

16. Kaptchuk, T.J. *Chinese Medicine. The Web that has no Weaver.* Ryder, London, p.80, 1983 (see also the table on page 110.)

    Anonomous, The Location of Acupoints. Foreign Language Press, Beijing, 1990.

    Kaptchuk, T.J. Ibid p.343–357, 1983.

17. Maciocia, G. *The Foundations of Chinese Medicine.* Churchill Livingstone, London, pp.15–34, 1989.

    Xinnong, Cheng (chief ed) *Chinese Acupuncture and Moxibustion.* pp.18–24, 1987.

    Porkert, M. *The Theoretical Foundations of Chinese Medicine.* The MIT Press, Cambridge, MA, p.43–76, 1974.

18. Kaptchuk, T.J. *Chinese Medicine.* pp.1–33, 1983

19. Porkert, M. *The Theoretical Foundations of Chinese Medicine.* p.46, 1974.

20. Kaptchuk, T.J. *Chinese Medicine.* pp.77–114, 1983

    Gerber, R. *Vibrational Medicine.* Bear & Company, Santa Fe, New Mexico, pp.176–177, 1988.

Xinnong, Cheng (chief ed) *Chinese Acupuncture and Moxibustion.* pp.22–24, 1987.
21. Connelly, D.M. *Traditional Acupuncture. The Law of the Five Elements.* The Centre for Traditional Acupuncture, Inc, Columbia, Maryland, p.15, 1975.
22. Needham, J. Science and Civilisation in China. Vol. 5, part 2, Cambridge University Press, Cambridge, p.92, 1974.
23. Kaptchuk, T.J. *Chinese Medicine.* pp.34–49, 1983
    Gerber, R. *Vibrational Medicine.* Bear & Company, Santa Fe, New Mexico, pp.188–189, 1988.
24. Rogers, C. *An Introduction to the study of Acupuncture. The Five Keys.* Acupuncture College Publishing, Sydney, p.6, 1986.
25. Kaptchuk, T.J. *Chinese Medicine.* pp.7–15, 1983
26. Rogers, C. *An Introduction to the study of Acupuncture* p.7–8, 1986.
    Gerber, R. *Vibrational Medicine* p.176, 1988.
27. Xinnong, Cheng (chief ed) *Chinese Acupuncture and Moxibustion.* pp.15–18, 1987.
    Maciocia, G. *The Foundations of Chinese Medicine.* p.7, 1989.
28. Xinnong, Cheng (chief ed.), Ibid, pp.108–244, 1987
29. Thie, J.F. *Touch for Health.* De Vorss & Company, Marina del Rey, Ca, 1979.
30. Levy, S.L. & Lehr, C. *Your Body Can Talk. The Art and Application of Clinical Kinesiology.* Hohm Press, Prescott, Az, pp.4–5, 1996.
31. Beardall, A.G. Differentiating the muscles of the lower back and abdomen. Selected Paper of the International College of Applied Kinesiology. Lawrence, K.S. International College of Applied Kinesiology, 1980.
32. Beardall, A.G. *Clinical Kinesiology, Vols. I, II, III, IV, V.* Beardall, DC. Inc., Lake Oswego, Or, 1980, 1981, 1982, 1983, 1985.
33. Beardall, A.G. *Clinical Kinsiology, Volume III. TMJ, Hyoid Muscles & other Cervical Muscles including Cranial Manipulation.* Beardall D.C. Inc. Lake Oswego, Or, pp.2–4, 1982.
34. Levy, S.L. & Lehr, C. *Your Body Can Talk* pp.5–6, 1996.
    Dickson, G.J. *What is Kinesiology?* IHK Publishing, Buddina, Qld, p.44, 1990.
35. Dickson, G.J. Ibid., p.58, 1990
    Utt, R. *Stress the Nature of the Beast.* Applied Physiology Publishing, Tucson, Az, pp.43–44, 1997.
36. Beardall, A.G. *Clinical Kinsiology, Volume III.* pp.2-4, 1982.
    Dickson, G.J. *What is Kinesiology?* p.58–60 1990
37. Walther, S. *Applied Kinesiology. Vol 1 Basic Procedure and Muscle Testing,* Systems DC, Pueblo, Co. pp.1–5, 1981
    Utt, R. *Stress the Nature of the Beast.* pp.23–28, 1997
38. Krebs, C.T. The Emotional Control of Muscle Response. Why your arm goes weak when you think a negative thought. In: Proceedings of the 4th International Kinesiology Conference, Zurich, Switzerland, October 14–18, pp.57–63, 1997.
39. Barton, J. *Encyclopedia of Mind and Body Volumes I, II, III, IV, V, VI, VII,* Biokinesiology Institute, Shade Cove, Or, 1981.

40. Parker, A. & Cutler-Stuart, J. *Switch on your Brain.* Hale & Ironmonger, Petersham, NSW, 1986.
    Hannaford, C. *Smart Moves,* Great Ocean Publishers, Arlington, VA., 1995.
41. Dennison, P. & Dennison, G.E. *Brain Gym, Teachers Edition, Revised.* Edu-Kinesthetics, Inc., 1994.
    Hannaford, C. *Ibid.,* pp.108–129, 1995.
42. Stokes, G. & Whiteside, D. *One Brain. Dyslexia Learning Connection and Brain Integration.* Three in One Concepts, Inc. Burbank, Ca., 1984
    Stokes, G. & Whiteside D. *Structural Neurology.* Three in One Concepts Inc., Burbank Ca, 1985
43. Utt, R. *The Law of Five Elements,* International Institute of Applied Physiology, Tuscon, Az. 1989
44. Renee, Weber. The Enfolding—Unfolding Universe: A conversation with David Bohm. In *The Holographic Paradigm,* Ed. Ken Wilber, New Science Library, pp.68–79, 1982.
    Talbot, M. *The Holographic Universe.* Grafton Books, London, 1991.
45. Guyton, A.C. *Textbook of Medical Physiology.* 8th ed. p.646, 1991.
    Kosslyn, N.M. et al. Visual imagery activates topographically organized visual cortex: PET investigations. J. Cognitive Neurosci. 5:263–287, 1993.
    Damasio, H. et al. Visual recall with the eyes closed and covered activates early visual cortices. Soc. Neurosci. Abstracts, 19:1603, 1993.
46. Noback, C.R. Strominger, M.L., & Demarst R.J. *The Human Nervous System,* 4th Ed., Lea & Fibiger, Philadelphia, Pa, pp.375–395, 1991.
    Krebs, C.T. The Emotional Control of Muscle Response. In Press.
47. Dickson, G.J. *What is Kinesiology?* 1990
    Holdway, A. *Health Essentials: Kinesiology.* Elements, Dorset, 1995
    Levy, S.L. & Lehr, C. *Your Body can Talk.* 1996
    Scott, J. & Goss, K. *Clear your Allergies in Minutes.* Health Kinesiology Publishing, San Francisco, Ca, 1988
    Barton, J. *Allergies—How to Find and Conquer.* 3rd ed. Biokinesiology Institute, Shady Cove, Or, 1983.
    Stokes, G. & Whiteside, D. *Structural Neurology,* Three In One Concepts Inc., Burbank, Ca, 1985.
    Dewe, B.A.J., & Dewe, J.R. *Professional Kinesiology Practice Volumes I, II, III & IV,* Professional Health Publications International, Auckland, NZ, 1990, 1990, 1991, 1992.
48. Levy, S.L. & Lehr, C. *Your Body can Talk.* 1996.

Chapter 3

1. Hannaford, C. *Smart Moves,* Great Ocean Publishers, Arlington, VA., p.18, 1995.
2. Hannaford, C. Ibid., p.20, 1995
3. Steven, C.F. The neuron. Sci. Am. 241(3): 49, 1979.

4. Lichtman, J.W. et al. Seeing Synapses: new ways to study nerves. American Association for the Advancement of Science, Annual Meeting, San Francisco, Feb, 1994.
   Hannaford, C. *Smart Moves.* p.24, 1994.
   Jessell, T.M. Neuronal survival and synapse function. In *Principles of Neural Science.* 3rd ed, Kandel, E.R., Schwartz, J.H. & Jessell, T.M. (Eds), Appleton & Lange, Norwalk, CN. pp. 942–943, 1991.
5. Concar, D. Brain boosters. New Scientist (Feb 8, 1997): 32–36, 1997.
6. McLean, P.D. *The Truine Brain in Evolution, Role in Paleocerebral Functions.* Plenum Press, New York, NY, 1990.
7. McLean, P.D. Ibid., pp.228–244, 1990.
8. Kupferman, I. Learning and memory. In *Principles of Neural Science.* 3rd ed. pp. 1005–1006, 1991.
9. Kolb, B., & Whishaw, I.Q. *Fundamentals of Human Neuropsychology.* 3rd ed. W.H. Freeman & Company, New York, NY, pp.412–501, 1990.
   Tortora, G.J., Grabowski, S.R. *Principles of Anatomy and Physiology.* 8th ed. Harpers Collins College Publishers, New York, NY, pp.406–408, 1996.
10. Kandel, E.R. Brain and behaviour. In *Principles of Neural Science.* 3rd ed. p.10, 1991
    Tortora, G.J. & Grabowski, S.R. *Principles of Anatomy and Physiology.* 8th ed. pp.411–413, 1996.
11. Kandel, E.R. & Jessell, T.M. Touch. In *Principle of Neural Science.* 3rd ed. pp.370–374, 1991.
12. Penfield, W. & Rasmussen, T. 1950. *The Cerebral Cortex of Man: A Clinical Study of Localisation of Function.* Macmillan Press, New York, NY, 1950.
    Geshwind, N. Specialisations of the human brain, Sci. Am., 241:158–171, 1979.
    Tortora, G.J. & Grabowski, S.R. *Principles of Anatomy and Physiology.* 8th ed. pp.438–440, 1996.
13. Walsh, K. *Neuropsychology. A Clinical Approach.* 2nd ed. Churchill Livingstone, Melbourne, 1987.
14. Kupfermann, I. Localisation of higher cognitive and affective functions: the association cortices. In: *Principles of Neural Science.* 3rd ed. pp.823–826, 1991.
15. Damasio, A.R. *Descartes' Error. Emotion, Reason & the Human Brain.* G.P. Putman & Sons, New York, NY, pp.134–143, 1994.
16. Kandel, E.R. Brain and behaviour. In: *Essentials of Neural Science and Behaviour.* Kandel, E.R., Schwartz, J.H. & Jessell, T.M. (eds), Appleton & Lange, Norwalk, CN, pp.11–13, 1995.
17. Kandel, E.R. Brain and behaviour. Ibid. pp.12–15, 1995.
18. Kandel, E.R. Perception of motion, depth and form. In: *Principles of Neural Science*, 3rd ed. pp.445–447, 1995.
19. Noback, C.R., Strominger, N.L. & Demarest, R.J. *The Human Nervous System.* 4th ed., Lea & Febiger, London, pp.398–401, 1991.

20. Kolb, B & Whishaw, I.Q. *Fundamentals of Human Neuropsychology.* 3rd ed. pp.185–189, 1990.
21. Kolb, B. & Whishaw, I.Q. *Fundamentals of Human Neuropsychology.* 3rd ed. p.504, 1990.
22. Guyton, A.C. *Textbook of Medical Physiology*, 8th ed., W.B. Saunders Company, Sydney p.642, 1991.
23. Côté, L. Crutchen, M.D. The basal ganglia. In: *Principles of Neural Science.* 3rd ed. pp.649–653, 1991.
24. Noback, C.R., Strominger, N.L. & Demarest, R.J. Ibid., pp.378–391, 1991.
25. Noback, C.R., Strominger, N.L. & Demarest, R.J. Ibid., pp.385–388, 1991.
26. Tortora, G.J. & Grabowski, R.S. *Principles of Anatomy and Physiology.* p.430, 1996.
27. Noback, C.R., Strominger, N.L. & Demarest, R.J. Ibid., pp.368–371, 1991.
28. Kolb, B. & Whishaw, I.Q. *Fundamentals of Human Neuropsychology.* 3rd ed. p.13, 1990.
    Guyton, A.C. *Textbook of Medical Physiology.* 8th ed., p.652, 1991.
29. Kupfermann, I. Hypothalamus and limbic system: peptidengic neurons, homeostasis, and emotional behaviour. In: *Principles of Neural Science*, 3rd ed. pp. 746–747, 1991.
30. Olds, T. & Milner, P. Positive reinforcement provided by electrical stimulation of septal area and other regions of cat brain. J. Comp. Physiol. & Psychiatry 47: 419–427, 1954.
    Wise, R.A., Bauco, P., Carlezon, W.A. Jr. & Trojnian, W. Self stimulation and drug reward mechanisms. Annals NY Acad. Science. 654:192–198, 1992.
31. Guyton, A.C. *Textbook of Medical Physiology*, 8th ed., pp.652–658, 1991.
    Kupfermann, I. Hypothalamus and limbic system: peptidengic neurons, homeostasis, and emotional behavior. In: *Principles of Neural Science*, 3rd ed. p.737, 1991.
    McClelland, J.L., McNaughton, B.L. & O'Reilly, R.C. Why there are two complementary learning systems in the hippocampus and neocortex. Insights from successes and failures of connectionists models of learning and memory. Psychol. Rev. 102(3):423–425, 1995.
32. Damasio, A.R. *Descartes' Error.* pp.71–75, 1994.
33. Guyton, A.C. *Textbook of Medical Physiology*, 8th ed., pp.656–658, 1991.
34. Kupfermann, I. Hypothalamus and limbic system: peptidengic neurons, homeostasis, and emotional behaviour. In: *Principles of Neural Science*, 3rd ed. pp. 737–740, 1991.
35. Kandel, E.R. & Kupfermann, I. Emotional states. In: *Essentials of Neural Science and Behaviour.* pp.606–608, 1995.
36. Guyton, A.C. *Textbook of Medical Physiology*, 8th ed., p.656, 1991.
37. Guyton, A.C. Ibid., pp.651–658, 1991.
38. Le Doux, J. *The Emotional Brain. The Mysterious Underpinnings of Emotional Life.* Simon & Schuster, New York, NY, 1996.

39. Milner, B. Memory and the human brain. In: *How We Know*. Shaffo, M, Harper & Row, San Francisco, CA, 1985.
    Kolb, B. & Whishaw, I.Q. *Fundamentals of Human Neuropsychology*, 3rd ed. pp.539–541, 1990.
40. Kolb, B. & Whishaw, I.Q. Ibid., pp.544–546, 1990.
    Kupfermann, I. Localisation of higher cognitive and affective functions: the association cortices. In: *Principles of Neural Science*, 3rd ed. pp.830–831, 1991.
41. McLean, P.D. *The Truine Brain in Evolution*. 1990.
42. Monis, J.S. et al. A differential neural response in human amygdala to fearful and happy facial expressions. Nature 383:812–814, 1996.
43. Adolphs, R. et al. Impaired recognition in facial expressions following bilateral damage to the human amygdala. Nature 372:669–672, 1994.

Chapter 4

1. Tulving, E. Organisation of Memory: Quo Vadis? In *The Cognitive Neurosciences*, M.S. Gazzaniga (ed in chief) The MIT Press, Cambridge, MA, p.839, 1995
2. Guyton, A.C. *Textbook of Medical Physiology*, 8th ed., W.B. Saunders Company, Philadelphia, PA, p.655, 1991.
3. McClelland, J.L., McNaughton, N.L. & O'Reilly, R.C. Why are there complementary learning systems in the hippocampus and neocortex: Insights from the successes and failures of connectionists' models of learning and memory Psych. Rev.102(3):419–457, 1995.
4. McClelland, J.L. et al. Why are there complementary learning systems. p.420, 1995.
   Squire, L.R. & Knowlton, B.J. Memory, hippocampus and brain systems. In: *The Cognitive Neurosciences* M.S. Gazzaniga (ed in chief) The MIT Press, Cambridge, MA, pp.825–837, 1995
5. Kupfermann, I. Hypothalamus and limbic system peptidergic neurons, homeostasis and emotional behaviour. In: Kandel, E.R., Schwartz, J.H. & Jessell, T.M. *Principles of Neural Science*. 3rd ed. Appleton & Lange, Norwalk, CN, pp.736–739, 1991.
6. Barbean et al, Decreased expression of the embryonic form of the neural adhesion molecule in schizophrenic brains. Proc, Natl. Acad. Sci. 92:p.2785, 1995.
7. Kupfermann, I. Hypothalamus and limbic system peptidergic neurons, homeostasis and emotional behaviour. In: *Principles of Neural Science*. 3rd ed. p.737, 1991.
8. Squire, L.R. & Knowlton, B.J. Memory, hippocampus and brain systems. In: *The Cognitive Neurosciences*, M.S. Gazzaniga (ed in chief) The MIT Press, Cambridge, MA, p.834, 1995
   McClelland, J.L. et al. Why are there complementary learning systems. pp. 423–425, 1995.
9. Squire, L.R., Shimamura, A.P. & Amaral, D.G. Memory and the Hippocampus. In: *Neural Models of Plasticity. Experimental & Theoretical Approaches*. Byrne, J.H. & Berry, W.O. (eds), Academic Press, New York, NY, p.227, 1989.

10. Kupfermann, I. Hypothalamus and limbic system peptidergic neurons, homeostasis and emotional behaviour. In: *Principles of Neural Science*. 3rd ed. pp.737–739, 1991.
    McClelland, J.L., et al. Why are there complementary learning systems. pp. 423–425, 1995.
11. Halgren, E. Physiological Integration of the declarative memory system. In: *The Memory System of the Brain*, Delacour, J. (ed.) World Scientific Pub Co., London, pp.69–152, 1994.
    McClelland, J.L., et al. Why are there complementary learning systems. pp. 420–427, 1995.
    Squire, L.R. & Knowlton, B.J. Memory, hippocampus and brain systems. In: *The Cognitive Neurosciences*. pp.825–837, 1995
12. Damasio, A.R. *Descartes' Error. Emotion, Reason and the Human Brain*. G.P. Putman's Son, New York, NY, 1994.
    Davis, M. The role of the amygdala in fear and anxiety. Annual Rev. Neurosci. 15:353–375, 1992.
    Davis, M. 1992. The amygdala and conditional fear. In: *The Amygdala: Neurobiological Aspects of Emotion, Memory and Mental Dysfunction*, Aggleton, J.P. (ed) Wily-Liss, New York, NY, pp.255–305.
13. Guyton, A.C. *Textbook of Medical Physiology*. 8th ed. pp.654–657, 1991
    Noback, C.R., Strominger, N.L. & Demarst, R.J. 1991. *The Human Nervous System. Introduction and Review*. 4th ed., Lea & Febiger, London, pp.358–359.
14. Pert, C.A. & Snyder, S.H. Opiate receptor: demonstration in nervous tissue. Science 1731:1011–1014, 1973.
    Simon, E.J. Opiate receptors: isolation and mechanisms. In: *Alcohol and Opiates, Neurochemistry and Behavioral Mechanisms*. Blum, K. (ed.), Academic Press, New York, pp.253–264, 1977.
15. Hughes, J. et al. Identification of two related pentapeptides from the brain with patient opiate activity. Nature 258:77–80, 1977.
    Jessell, T.M. & Kelly, D.D. Pain and Analgesia. In: *Principles of Neural Science*. 3rd ed. pp.394–396, 1991.
16. Valkow, N. et al. Decreased striatal dopaminergic responsiveness in detoxified cocaine—dependent subjects. Nature 386:830–833, 1997.
    Nash, M. The chemistry of addiction. Time, May 5, p.52, 1997.
17. Rhoades, R. & Pflanger, R. *Human Physiology*. 2nd ed. Saunders College Pub. Philadelphia, PA, p.406, 1992.
    Damasio, A.R. *Descartes' Error*. pp.127–164, 1994.
18. Miller, D. & Blum, K. *Overload. Attention Deficit Disorder and the Addictive Brain*. Andrews & McMeel, Kansas City, MO, pp.55–67, 1996.
19. Miller, D, & Blum, K. *Overload*. p.59, 1996.
20. Valkow, N. et al. Decreased striatal dopaminergic responsiveness in detoxified cocaine—dependent subjects. Nature 386:827–830, 1997.

21. Blum, K. et al. Allelic association of human dopamine D_2 receptor gene in alcoholism. J.Am. Med. Assoc. 263:2055–2060, 1990.
    Miller, D. & Blum, K. *Overload* pp.58–62, 1996.
22. Guyton, A.C. *Textbook of Medical Physiology.* 8th ed. p.655, 1991.
23. Guyton, A.C. Ibid, pp.654–657, 1991
    Noback, C.R., Strominger, N.L. & Demarst, R.J. 1991. *The Human Nervous System.* 4th ed. pp.358–359.
24. LeDoux, J.E. Emotion and the amygdala. In: Davis, M. *The Role of the Amygdala in Fear and Anxiety.* Annual Rev. Neurosci. 15:339–351, 1992.
    Damasio, A.R. *Descartes' Error.* pp.69–74, 1994.
    LeDoux, J.E. Emotion, memory and the brain. Sci. Am. 280(6):50-57, 1994.
    Kandel, E.R. & Kupfermann, I. Emotional States. In: *Essentials of Neuroscience and Behaviour.* pp.608–612, 1995.
25. Bootzin, R.R. et al. *Psychology Today. An Introduction.* 7th ed. McGraw-Hill, New York, NY, pp.210–211, 1991.
    Massaro, D.W. & Loftus, G.R. Sensory and perceptual storage: data and theory. In: *Memory.* Bjork, E.L. & Bjork, R.A. (eds) Academic Press, New York, NY, pp.68–96, 1996.
26. Guyton, A.C. *Textbook of Medical Physiology.* 8th ed. pp.644–645, 1991.
    Kandal, E.R. Cellular mechanisms of learning and the biological basis of individuality. In: *Principles of Neural Science*, 3rd ed. pp.736–739, 1991.
27. Kandal, E.R. Ibid, pp.1014–1024, 1991.
    McClelland, J.L., McNaughton, N.L. & O'Reilly, R.C. Why are there complementary learning systems: Psych. Rev.102(3):426, 1995.
28. McClelland, J.L., et al. Why are there complementary learning systems. Psych. Rev.102(3):419–457, 1995.
29. Roediger, H.L. III & Guyrin, M.J. Retrieval Processes. In: *Memory.* Bjork, E.L. & Bjork, R.A (eds) Academic Press, New York, NY, pp.197–231, 1996.
30. Kandal, E.R. Cellular mechanisms of learning and the biological basis of individuality. In: *Principles of Neural Science.* 3rd ed. pp.1014–1016, 1991.
    McClelland, J.L., et al.. Why are there complementary learning systems: Psych. Rev.102(3):423–427, 1995.
31. Bootzin, R.R. et al. *Psychology Today.* 7th ed. pp.228–230, 1991
    Anderson, M.C. & Neily, J.H. Interference and inhibition in memory retrieval. In: *Memory.* Bjork, E.L. & Bjork, R.A (eds) Academic Press, New York, NY, pp. 237–304, 1996.
32. Miller, G.A., Galanter, E. & Pribham, K.H. *Plans and the Structure of Behaviour.* Holt Pub, New York, NY, 1960.
33. Jones, D. Objects, streams and threads of auditory attention. In: Bradley, A. & Weikraaz (eds), Attention: Selection. Awareness, and Control. A Tribute to Donald Broadbent, Oxford University Press, Oxford, pp.87–104, 1993.
34. Dubois, B. et al. Experimental approach to prefrontal functions in humans. In:

Grafman, J. Holyoak, K.J. & Boller, F (eds), Structure and Functions of the Human Prefrontal Cortex. Annals of N.Y. Acad. Sci: 796:41–70, 1995.

Beardsley, T. The Machinery of Thought. Sci. Am. 277(2):58–63, 1997.

35. Braddely, A. Working Memory. In: Gazzangia, M.S. (ed in chief), *The Cognitive Neurosciences*. 3rd ed. pp.755–764, 1995.

    Logie, R.H. The seven ages of working memory. In: Richardson et al. *Working Memory and Human Cognition*. Oxford University Press, Oxford, pp.31–65, 1996.

36. Lezak, M.D. *Neuropsychological Assessments* (3rd ed). Oxford University Press, New York, NY, 1995.

37. McClelland, J.L., et al. Why are there complementary learning systems. Psych. Rev.102(3):420, 1995.

    Tulving, E. Organisation of Memory: Quo Vadis? In: *The Cognitive Neurosciences*, p.841, 1995

38. Penfield, W. & Perot, P. The brain's record of auditory and visual experience. Brain, 86:595-696, 1963. Kandel, E.R. & Jessell, T.M. Touch. In: *Principles of Neural Science*. 3rd ed. pp.370–374, 1991.

39. Keeton, W.T. *Biological Science* 3rd ed. W.W. Norton & Company, New York, NY, pp.460–461, 1980.

40. Damasio, A.R. & Damasio, H. Brain and Language. Sci. Am. 267(3):62–71, 1992.

41. McClelland, J.L., et al. Why are there complementary learning systems: Psych. Rev.102(3):423–424, 1995.

    Roland, P.E. et al. Positron emission tomography in cognitive neuroscience: methodological constraints, strategies, and examples from learning and memory. In: *The Cognitive Neurosciences*. 3rd ed. pp.781–788, 1995.

42. Damasio, A.R. *Descartes' Error*. pp.84–113, 1994.

    Geary, J, A trip down memory's lanes. Time, May 26, 1997, pp.59–65.

43. Christianson, S.A. Flashbulb memories: Special, but not so special. Memory and Cognition 17:435–443, 1989.

    McGaugh, J.L. Significance and remembrance. The role of neuromodulatory systems. Psych Science 1:15–25, 1990.

    McGaugh et al. Neuromodulatory systems and memory storage: Role of the amygdala. Behav. Brain Res. 58:81–90, 1993.

44. Erdelzi, M.H. Psychoanalysis: Freud's Cognitive Psychology. Freeman, New York, NY, 1985

    LeDoux, J. *The Emotional Brain. The Mysterious Underpinnings of Emotional Life*. Simon & Schuster, New York, NY, pp.210–211, 1996.

    Loftus, E.F. Creating False Memories. Sci. Am. 277(3):50–55, 1997.

45. Holmes, B. When memory plays us false. New Scientist 143(1935):32–35, 1994.

46. Christianson, S.A. Eyewitness memory for stressful events: Methodological quandries and ethical dilemmas. In: Handbook of Emotion and memory: Research and theory. Christianson, S.A. (ed), Erlbaum, Hillsdale, NJ, 1992.

47. Düzel, E. et al. Event-related brain potentials of two states of conscious awareness

in memory. Proc Natl. Acad. Sci. 94:5973–5978, 1997.
Motluk, A. Just remember this. New Scientist, 154(2084):16, 1997.
48. Roediger, H.L. III, McDermott, K.B. & Jacoby, D. Mis-information effects in recall: creating false memories through repeated retrieval. J Memory and Language 35 (April):300–318, 1996.
49. Beardsley, T. As time goes by. You must remember this. Really. Sci Am. 276(5): 18–20, 1997.
50. Graf, P. & Schacter, D.L. Implicit and explicit memory for new associations in normal subjects and amnesic patients. J. Exp. Psychol. (Learn. Mem. Cogn.) 11: 501–518, 1985.
51. Schacter, D.L. Implicit memory: A new frontier of cognitive neuroscience. In: *The Cognitive Neurosciences.* 3rd ed. pp.815–824, 1995
52. Schanks, D. Remembrance of things unconscious. New Scientist, 131(1783):33–36, 1991.
Kelley, C.M. & Lindsay, D.S. Conscious & unconscious forms of memory. In: *Memory.* pp.33–58, 1996.
53. Kihlstrom, J.F. et al. Implicit and explicit memory following surgical anesthesia. Psychol. Sci. 1:303–306, 1990.
Jolicic, M. et al. Implicit memory for words presented during anaesthesia. European J. Cognitive Psychol., 4:71–80, 1992.
54. Squire, L.R. Declarative and nondeclarative memory: multiple brain systems supporting learning and memory. J. Cognitive Neurosci. 99:195–231, 1992.
55. Squire, L.R. & Knowlton, B.J. Memory, hippocampus and brain systems. In: *The Cognitive Neurosciences.* 3rd ed. pp.832–836, 1995
56. Wan, R.Q., Panz, K & Olton, D.S. Hippocampal and amygdaloid involvement in nonspatial and spatial working memory in rats: Effects of delay and interference. Behav. Neurosci. 108(5):866–882, 1994.
57. Freud, S. *Introductory Lectures on Psychoanalysis. Standard Edition*, Strachey, J (ed), Norton, New York, NY, 1968.
58. Jacobs, W.J. & Nadel, L. Stress induced recovery of fears and phobias. Psych Rev 92:512–531, 1985.
LeDoux, J.E. *The Emotional Brain.* p.205, 1996.
59. LeDoux, J.E. Emotion, memory and the brain. Sci. Am. 270(6):32–39, 1994.
60. Davis, M. The role of the amygdala in fear and anxiety. Annual Rev. Neurosci. 15:353–375, 1992.
61. LeDoux, J.E. *The Emotional Brain.* p.163, 1996.
62. LeDoux, J.E. Emotion and the amygdala. In: *The Amygdala. Neurological Aspects of Emotion, Memory and Mental Dysfuction*, Aggleton, J.P. (ed), Wiley-Liss, New York, NY, pp.339–351, 1992.
63. Wan, R.Q., Panz, K & Olton, D.S. Hippocampal and amygdaloid involvement in nonspatial and spatial working memory in rats: Effects of delay and interference. Behav. Neurosci. 108(5):866–882, 1994.

64. LeDoux, J.E., Romanski, L.M. & Xagoris, A.E. Indelibility of subcortical emotional memories. J. Cognitive Neurosci. 1:238–243, 1989.
LeDoux, J.E. *The Emotional Brain.* p.250–252, 1996.
65. Davis, M. The role of the amygdala in fear and anxiety. Annual Rev. Neurosci. 15:353–375, 1992.
LeDoux, J.E. Emotion, memory and the brain. Sci. Am. 270(6):3239, 1994.
66. Restak, R.M. *The Brain.* Bantam Books, London, pp.190–191, 1984.
67. Campbell, S & Jaynes, J. Reinstatement. Psychol. Rev. 73:478–480, 1966.
Dodd, J. & Costellucci, V.F. Smell and taste: the chemical senses. In: *Principles of Neural Science,* p.518, 1991.
68. Jacobs, W.J. & Nadel, L. Stress induced recovery of fears and phobias. Psychol. Rev. 92:512–531, 1985.
LeDoux, J.E. *The Emotional Brain.* pp.250–266, 1996.
69. LeDoux, J.E. Ibid, p. 169, 1996.

Chapter 5

1. Kandel, E.R. Brain and Behavior. In Kandel, E.R., Schwartz, J.H. & Jessell, T.M. (eds) *Principles of Neural Science.* 3rd ed. Appleton & Lange, Norwalk, CN. pp.997–1008, 1991.
Kupfermann, I. Learning and Memory. In Kandel, E.R., Schwartz, J.H. & Jessell, T.M. (eds) *Principles of Neural Science.* 3rd ed. Appleton & Lange, Norwalk, CN. pp.997–1008, 1991.
Damasio, A. *Descartes' Error. Emotion, Reason and the Human Brain.* G.P. Putman & Sons, New York, NY, 1994.
Restak, R.N. *The Modular Brain.* Touchstone Book, New York, NY. 1995.
2. Kolb, B. & Whishaw, I.Q. *Fundamentals of Human Neuropsychology.* 3rd ed. W.H. Freeman & Co., New York, NY, pp.272–281, 1990.
3. Walsh, K. *Neuropsychology. A Clinical Approach.* 2nd ed. Churchill Livingstone, Melbourne, pp.279, 1987.
4. Kupfermann, I. Localisation of higher cognitive and affective functions: the association cortices. In: *Principles of Neural Science.* 3rd ed. p.832, 1991.
Kolb, B. & Whishaw, I.Q. *Fundamentals of Human Neuropsychology.* 3rd ed., pp.387–388, 1991
5. Walsh, K. *Neuropsychology.* 2nd ed. p.279, 1987.
6. Walsh, K. Ibid., p.278–279, 1987.
Kupfermann, I. Localisation of higher cognitive and affective functions: the association cortices. In: *Principles of Neural Science.* 3rd ed. p.832, 1991.
7. Damasio, A.R. & Damasio, H. Brain and Language. Sci. Am. 237(3):62–71, 1992.
Kolb, B. & Whishaw, I.Q. *Fundamentals of Human Neuropsychology.* 3rd ed, pp.589, 1990.
Darby, D.G. Prosody and Extra-linguistic Aspects of Communication, Dysfunction with Unilateral Cerebral Infarction. PhD. Thesis, University of Melbourne, 1990.

8. Gazzangia, M.S. The Bi-sected Brain. Appleton—Century Croft, New York, NY, 1970.
   Gazzangia, M.S. One Brain two minds. Am. Scientist 60:311–317, 1972.
   Walsh, K. *Neuropsychology.* 2nd ed. p.309, 1987.
9. Hannaford, C. *Smart Moves.* Great Ocean Publishing Inc. Arlington, VA, pp. 177–197, 1995.
   Hannaford, C. *The Brain Dominance Factor.* Great Ocean Publishing Inc. Arlington, VA, 1997.
10. Bynum, W.F & Porter, R.(eds.) *Companion Encyclopedia of the History of Medicine.* Vol 1. Routledge, London, pp.281–291, 1993.
    Duffy, J. *From Humors to Medical Science. A History of American Medicine.* University of Illinois Press, Chicago, IL., pp.14–15 & 70–77, 1993.
11. Edwards, C.R.W. et al. (eds.) *Davidson's Principles & Practice of Medicine.* 17th ed. Churchill Livingstone, London, pp.776–778, 1995.
12. Kuhn, T.S. *The Structure of Scientific Revolutions* 2nd ed. The International Encyclopedia of Unified Science, Vol 2, No.2, University of Chicago Press, LTP, London, 1970.
13. Parker, A. & Cutler-Stuart, J. *Switch on Your Brain.* Hale & Ironmonger, Petersham, NSW, 1986.
    Dennison, P. & Dennison, G.E. *Brain Gym, Teachers Edition, Revised.* Edu-Kinesthetics, Inc., 1994.
    Hannaford, C. *Smart Moves.* 1995.
14. Devlin, T. & Williams, H. Hands up those who were happy at school. New Scientist 135(1840):40–43, 1992.
15. Restak, R.M. *The Brain.* Bantam Books Inc, New York, NY, pp.45–47, 1984.
    Jessell, T.M. Cell Migration and Axon Guidance. In Kandel, E.R., Schwartz, J.H. & Jessell, T.M. (eds) *Principles of Neural Science.* 3rd ed. Appleton & Lange, Norwalk, CN, 908–911, 1991.
16. Briggs, G.G., Freeman, R.K. & Yaffe, S.J., (eds), *Drugs in Pregnancy and Lactation.* Williams & Wilkins, Baltimore, MD. 1986
    Tortora, G.J. & Grabowski, S.R. *Principles of Anatomy & Physiology.* 8th ed. Harper Collins College Publishers, New York, NY, p.983, 1996.
17. Walsh, K. *Neuropsychology.* 2nd ed. pp.94–98, 1987
    Kolb, & B. Whishaw, I.Q. *Fundamentals of Human Neuropsychology.* 3rd ed, pp.130–136, 1990.
18. Walsh, K. Ibid., pp.94–98, 1987.
    Kolb, B. & Whishaw, I.Q. *Fundamentals of Human Neuropsychology.* 3rd ed., pp.136–139, 1990.
19. Freud, S. Lectures on Psychoanalysis. Standard Edition, Strachey, J (ed), Norton, New York, NY, Volume 24 Indexes and Bibliography, p.301, 1974.
20. Kolb, & B. Whishaw, I.Q. *Fundamentals of Human Neuropsychology.* 3rd ed pp.361–411, 1990.

21. Levy, R.J. Right brain, left brain: fact and fiction. Psychology Today, May, 1985.

Chapter 6
1. Domasio, A.R. & Domasio, H. Brain and Language. Sci. Am. 237(3):62–71, 1992.
2. Just, M.A. & Carpenter, P.A. *The Psychology of Reading and Language Comprehension.* Allyn & Bacon, Newton, MA, 1987.
   Bootzin, R.R., Bowen, G.A., Crocker, J. & Hall, E. *Psychology Today: An Introduction.* McGraw-Hill, Inc. Sydney, pp.290–291, 1991.
   Crowder, R.G. & Wagner, R.K. *The Psychology of Reading*, 2nd ed. Oxford University Press, New York, NY, 1992.
3. Walsh, K. *Neuropsychology. A Clinical Approach.* 2nd ed. Churchill Livingstone, Melbourne, pp.279–280, 1987.
4. Birdwhistell, R.L. *Kinesics and Context.* Allen Lane, London, 1971.
   Mehrabian, A. *Silent Messages.* Wadworth Publishing, Belmont, CA, 1971.
   Pease, A. Body Language. Carmel Publishing Co., Sydney, 1981.
5. Pease, A. Ibid., pp.9–10, 1981
6. Walsh, K. *Neuropsychology.* 2nd ed. pp.288–289, 1987
   Kupfermann, I. Localization of higher cognitive and affective functions: the association cortices. In Kandel, E.R., Schwartz, J.H. & Jessell, T.M. (eds) Principles of Neural Science. 3rd ed. Appleton & Lange, Norwalk, CN. pp.831–832, 1991.
7. Troup, G. Bradshaw, J.L. & Netttleton, N.C. The lateralization of arithmetic and number processing: A review. International. J. Neurosci. 19:231–242, 1983.
   Darby, D.G. Prosody and Extra-linguistic Aspects of Communication, Dysfunction with Unilateral Cerebral Infarction. PhD. Thesis, University of Melbourne, 1990.
8. Aisbett, N. Recession years hit school skills. The Western Australian, August 21, 1993.

Chapter 7
1. Cytowic, R.E. *The Man who Tasted Shapes.* G.P. Putman & Sons, New York, NY, pp.153–162, 1993.
   Damasio, A.R. *Descartes' Error, Emotion, Reason and the Human Brain.* G.P. Putman & Sons, New York, NY, pp.94–96, 1994
   Nunez, P.L. *Neocortical Dynamics and Human EEG Rhythms.* Oxford University Press, New York, NY, 1995.
2. Agnati, L.F., Bjelke, B & Fuxe, K. Volume transmission in the brain. American Scientist 80(4):362–373, 1992.
3. Damasio, A.R. *Descartes' Error.* pp.84–113, 1994.
4. Damasio, A.R. Ibid., pp.84–164, 1994.
5. Damasio, A.R. Ibid., p.95, 1994.
6. Damasio, A.R. Ibid., pp.101–103, 1994.
7. Damasio, A.R. Ibid.,pp.106–107, 1994.

Chapter 8

1. Helms, J.H. *Acupuncture Energetics. A Clinical Approach for Physicians.* Medical Acupuncture Publishers, Berkeley, CA, p.454, 1995.
2. Maciocia, G. *The Foundations of Clinical Medicine. A Comprehensive text for Acupuncturist and Herbalist,* Churchill Livingstone, Melbourne, p.351, 1989.
3. Zhongfang, L. et al. Effect of electroacupuncture of 'Neiguan: on spontaneous discharges of single units in amydaloid nucleus in rabbits. J. Tradit. Chinese Med. 9(2):144–150, 1989.
4. Abad-Alergria, F., Adelantado, S. & Martinez, T. Changes of cerebral endogenous evoked potentials by acupuncture stimulation: AP-300 study. Am. J. Chinese. Med. Vol XXIII (2):115–119, 1995.
5. Walther, D.S. *Applied Kinesiology. Volume 1. Basic Procedures and Muscle Testing.* Systems DC. Pueblo, CO, pp.134–135, 1981.
6. Restak, R. *The Brain.* Bantom Books, New York, NY, p.76, 1984.
7. Guyton, A.C. *Textbook of Medical Physiology.* 8th ed. W.B. Saunders Co. London, p.626, 1991.
8. Hannaford, C. *Smart Moves. Why Learning is not all in your head.* Great Ocean Pubs. Arlington, VA, pp.29–49, 1995.
9. Hannaford, C. Ibid., pp.101–102, 1995.
10. Guyton, A.C. *Textbook of Medical Physiology.* 8th ed. p.563–566, 1991.
    Hubel, D.H. *Eye, Brain and Vision.* Scientific American Library, New York, NY, p.81, 1988.
11. Schor, R. & Tonko, D. The Vestibular System. In: *Vestibular Autonomic Regulation.* Yates, B.J. & Miller, A.P. (eds.) CRC Press, New York, NY, pp.19–22, 1996.
12. Hannaford, C. *Smart Moves.* p.102, 1995
13. Hannaford, C. Ibid., p.103, 1995
14. Mahoney, M.J. & Avener, M. Psychology of the elite athlete: An exploratory study. Cognitive Therapy & Res. 1:135–141, 1977.
15. Jacobson, E. Electrical measurements of neuromuscular states during mental activities. V. Variation of specific muscles contracting during imagination. Am. J. Physiol. 96:115–121, 1931.
    Hale, B.D. The effects of internal and external imagery on muscular and ocular concomitants. J. Sport Psych. 4:379–387, 1982.
    Decety, J. et al. Vegetative response during imagined movement is proportional to mental effort. Behav. Brain Res. 42:1–5, 1991.
16. Cohen, B.A. Role of eye, and neck proprioception mechanism in body orientation and motor co-ordination. J Neurophysiol. 24:1–11, 1961.
    Peterson, B.W., Richmond, F.J. (eds.) *Control of Head Movement.* Oxford University Press, New York, NY, 1988.
    Ghez, C. Posture. In: Kandel, E.R., Schwartz, J.H. & Jessell, T.M. *Principles of Neural Science,* 3rd ed. Appleton & Lange, Norwalk, CN, pp.596–607, 1991.

17. Schor, R. & Tonko, D. The Vestibular System. In: *Vestibular Autonomic Regulation*. Yates, B.J. & Miller, A.P. (eds.) CRC Press, New York, NY, pp.8–24, 1996.
18. Norback, C.R., Strominger, N.L. Demarst, R.J. *The Human Nervous System. Introduction and Review*. 4th ed., Lea & Febiger, London, pp.350–352, 1991.
    Tortora, G.J. & Grabowski, S.R. *Principles of Anatomy and Physiology*. 8th ed. Harper Collins College Pubs, New York, NY, pp.447—449, 1996.
19. Levinson, H.N. *A Solution to the Riddle of Dyslexia*. Springer-Verlag, New York, NY, pp.73–106, 1980.
    Levinson, H.N. *Turning Around the Upside Down Kids, Helping Dyslexic Kids Overcome their Disorder*. Evens, New York, NY, 1992.
20. Dennison, P.E. & Dennison, G.E. *Brain Gym. Teachers Edition, Revised*. Edu-Kinesthetics Inc. Ventura, CA, 1994.
21. Stokes, G. & Whiteside, D. Basic *One Brain Kinesiology* 2nd ed. Three In One Concepts, Burbank, CA, 1987.
    Stokes, G. & Whiteside, D. *Advanced One Brain Kinesiology*. Three In One Concepts, Burbank, CA, 1986.
22. Swain Satayananda Saraswati, *Kundalini Tantra*. Bihar School of Yoga, Mungar, Bihar, India pp.244–252, 1984.
23. Shannahoff-Khalso, D. Breathing Cycles linked to hemispheric dominance. Brain-Mind Bulletin 8(3)Jan, 1983
24. Ingeber, D. Brain breathing. Science Digest, June, 1981.
25. Swami Satayananda Saraswati. *Asana, Pranayama, Mudra and Bandha*. Bihar School of Yoga, Mungar, Bihar, India, pp.255–258, 1977.
26. Dale, R.A. The micro-meridians of the ear and the role of foot acupuncture systems. Proc. Third World Symposium on Acupuncture and Chinese Medicine. Am. J. Chinese Med. Vol II, (supplement abstract), 1975.
27. Xinnong, C. (chief ed). *Chinese Acupuncture and Moxibustion*. Foreign Language Press, Beijing, pp.491–511, 1987.
    Olsen, T. *Auriculotherapy Manual: Chinese and Western Systems of Ear Acupuncture* 2nd ed. Health Care Alternatives, Los Angeles, CA, 1996.
28. Delacato, C.H. *Diagnosis and Treatment of Speech and Reading Problems*. Charles C. Thomas, Springfield, IL, 1963.
29. Hannaford, C. *Smart Moves*. p.119–120, 1995.
30. Hannaford, C. Ibid., p.119, 1995
31. Hannaford, C.Ibid., p.123–124, 1995
32. Dennison, P.E. & Dennison, G.E. *Brain Gym. Teachers Edition, Revised*. Edu-Kinesthetics Inc. Ventura, CA, 1994.
33. Hannaford, C. *Smart Moves* p.120–121, 1995
34. Bennett, T.J. Dynamics of connection of abnormal function, from Terence J. Bennett Lectures, R.J. Martin, ed. Sierra Madre, CA, privately published, R.J. Martin, 1977.
    Walther, D.S. *Applied Kinesiology, Volume 1*. p.235, 1981.

Chapter 9

1. Utt, R. *Applied Physiology Acupressure Formatting for Brain Physiology.* Applied Physiology Publishing, Tucson, AZ, 1991.
2. Jackson, G. Personal Communication, June 1990–July, 1992.
3. Restak, R. *The Brain*, Bantam Books, New York, NY, p.46, 1984.
   Kolb, B. & Wishaw, I.Q. *Fundamentals of Human Neuropsychology.* 3rd ed. W.H. Freeman & Co., New York, NY, p.682–683, 1990.
4. Silberstein, R.B. Topography and dynamics of the steady state visually evoked potential: A window into brain function? Brain topography 5:64–65, 1992.
5. Silberstein, R.B. et al. Stead-state visually evoked potential topography associated with a visual vigilance task. Brain Topography 3:337–347, 1990.
   Silberstein, R.B., Ciociani, J. & Pipingas, A. Study-state visually evoked potential during the Wisconsin card sorting test. Electro-encephalography and Clin. Neurophysiol. 96:24–35, 1995.
6. Farrow, M. Unpublished data, Swinburne Centre for Applied Neuroscience, Swinburne University, Melbourne, Australia, 1995.
7. McCrossin, S. Changes in SSVEP topography, digit span performance and reading comprehension in response to acupressure treatment. Unpublished research thesis, Swinburne University, Melbourne, Australia, October, 1995.
8. McCrossin, S. Ibid, 1995.
9. Eyseneck, H.J. *The Structure and Measurement of Intelligence.* Springer-Vulag, New York, 1979.
   Murphy, K.R. & Davidshofer, C.O. *Psychological Testing.* 3rd ed. Prentice-Hall, N.J., 1994.
10. Cattell, R.B. Theory of fluid and crystalline intelligence: A critical experiment. J. Educational Psych. 54:1–22, 1963.
11. Lezak, M.D. *Neuropsychological Assessment.* 3rd ed. Oxford University Press, 1995.
12. McCrossin, S. The Effect of Acupressure treatment on standard intelligence test scores for children with learning difficulties. Unpublished honours thesis, School of Biophysical Science and Electrical Engineering, Swinburne University, Melbourne, Australia, Nov, 1996.
13. McCrossin, S. Ibid, 1996.
14. DSM-IV: Diagnostic and Statistical manual of mental disorders, 4th ed. American Psychiatric Association, Washington, DC, 1995.
15. Comings, D.E. *Tourette Syndrome and Human Behaviour.* Hope Press, Duarte, CA, 1995.
16. Bradley, C. The behavior of children receiving benzedrine. Am. J. Psychiatry, 94: 577–585, 1937.
    Bradley, C. Benzedrine and dexedrine in the treatment of children's behavioral disorders. Pediatrics 5:24–37, 1950.
17. Safer, D.J. & Krager, J.M. A survey of medication treatment for hyperactive

inattentive students. J. Am. Med. Assoc. 268(8):1004–1007, 1988.
18. Miller, D. & Blum, K. *Overload: Attention Deficit Disorder and the Addictive Brain.* Andrews & McMeel, Kansas City, MO, pp.38–39, 1996.
19. Miller, D. & Blum, K. Ibid., p.39, 1996
20. Miller, D. & Blum, K. Ibid., pp.55–67, 1996
21. Miller, D. & Blum, K. Ibid., 1996
22. Blum, K. et al. Allelic association of human dopamine D_2 receptor genes in alcoholism. J. Am. Med. Assoc. 263:2055–2060, 1990.
   Miller, D. & Blum, K. *Overload.* p.60–61, 1996
23. Miller, D. & Blum, K.Ibid., p.70–71, 1996
24. Blum, K. et al. Prolonged P300 latency in a neuropsychiatric population with the D_2 dopamine receptor A_1 allele. Phramocogenetics, 4:313–322. 1994.
25. Blum, K. et al. Allelic association of human dopamine D_2 receptor genes in alcoholism. J. Am. Med. Assoc. 263:2055–2060, 1990.
   Miller, D. & Blum, K. *Overload.* p.55–67, 1996
26. Abad-Alergria, F., Adelantado, S. & Martinez, T. Changes of cerebral endogenous evoked potentials by acupuncture stimulation: A P300 study. Am. J. Chinese. Med. Vol XXIII (2):115–119, 1995.
27. Feldman, S., Denhoff, E. Denhoff, J. Attention disorders and related syndromes in adolescence and young adult life in minimal brain dysfunction: A developmental approach. In: Denhoff, E. & Stearn, L. (eds) *Minimal Brain Dysfunction: A Developmental Approach.* Masson Publishing Co, New York, NY, pp.144–148, 1979.
   Hechtman, L. Adolescent outcome of hyperactive children treated with stimulants in childhood: a review. Psychopharmacology Bull. 21(2):178–191, 1985.
28. Blum, K. et al. Allelic association of human dopamine D_2 receptor genes in alcoholism. J. Am. Med. Assoc. 263:2055–2060, 1990.
29. Noble, E.P. et al. Allelic association of the D_2 dopamine receptor gene with cocaine dependence. Drug & Alcohol Dependence, 33:271–285, 1993.
   Uhl, G.R. et al. D_2 receptor gene—the cause or consequence of substance abuse. Trends in Neuroscience, 17:50–51, 1994.
   Comings, D.E. et al. The D_2 gene, a genetic risk factor in substance abuse. Drugs & Alcohol Dependence, 34:175–180, 1994.
30. Comings, D.E. et al. The dopamine D_2 receptor locus as a modifying gene in neuropsychiatric disorders. J. Am. Med. Assoc., 266:1793–1800, 1991.
   Blum, K. et al. Prolonged P300 latency in a neuropsychiatric population with the D_2 dopamine receptor A_1 allele. Phramocogenetics, 4:313–322. 1994.

Chapter 10
1. Tortora, G.J. & Grabowski, S.R. *Principles of Anatomy and Physiology.* 8th Ed. Harper: NY, pp. 892-893., 1996
   Hannaford, C. *Smart Moves. Why Learning is Not All in Your Head.* Great Ocean Publishers, Arlington: VA, p.138. 1995.

2. Williams, X. Hidden causes of memory loss, Australian Wellbeing, No.47:46–48, 1992.
3. Hannaford, C. *Smart Moves*. p.138., 1995
   Guyton, A.C. *Textbook of Medical Physiology*. 8th Ed. W.B. Saunders & Co, Philadelphia: PA, pp.800–801; 837. 1991.
4. Hannaford, C. *Smart Moves*. pp.144., 1995
5. Kupfermann, I & Schwartz, J.H. Emotional states. In Kandel, E.R., Schwartz, J.H. & Jessell, T.M. *Essentials of Neural Science and Behaviour*. Appleton & Lange: Connecticutt, pp.597–602, 1995.
   Guyton, A.C. *Textbook of Medical Physiology*. 8th ed. pp.800–801, 837. 1991.
6. Sali, A. Dietary fibre in health and disease. Australian Family Physician, 19: 315–320, 1990.
   Proposals for Nutritional Guidelines for Health Education in Britian, prepared for the National Advisory Committee on Nutrition Education (NACNE). Health Education Council, London, Sept. 1983.
   Davies, S.A., Stewart, A. *Nutritional Medicine*. Pan Books: London, pp.xxiii–xxiv, 1987.
   Coghlan, A. Simple food guide goes to heart of the matter. New Scientist, 144 (1951):10, 1994
7. Putting Fast Foods to the Test. Choice (April), p.7–9, 1994.
8. Sali, A. Dietary fibre in health and disease. Australian Family Physician 19: 315–320, 1990.
9. Werbach, M. Recent Advances in the Prevention and Treatment of Diseases with Nutrients. Lecture presented in Melbourne, Australia, October 24th 1995.
10. Lonsdale, D. & Shamberger, R. Red Cell transketolase as an indicator of nutritional deficiency. Am. J. Clin. Nutr. 22(2):205–211, 1980
11. Dallman, P.R. et al. Iron Deficiency most common deficiency in children. Am. J. Clin. Nutr. 33:86–118, 1980.
    Pollitt, E. & Leibel, S. *Iron Deficiency: Brain Biochemisty and Behaviour*. Raven Press, New York, 1982.
    Cobiac, L & Baghurst, K. Iron status and dietary iron intakes of Australians. Supplement to Food Australia, pp.510–524, April, 1993.
12. Leibel, R.L., Greenfield, D.B. & Pollitt, E. Iron deficiency behaviour and brain biochemistry. In Winick (ed.) *Nutrition Pre and Post Natal Development*. Plenum Press: NY, pp.383–439, 1979.
    Youdlin, M.B., Ashkenazi, D., Ben-Shachar & Yehuda, S. Brain iron and dopamine receptor function. Adv. Biochem. Psychopharmocol 37: pp.309–321, 1983
    Youdin, M.B., Ben-Shachar, D., Ashkenazi, R. & Yehuda, S. Modulation of dopamine receptor in the striatum by iron. Behavioural and biochemical correlates. Advanced Neurology. 40: pp.161–167, 1984.
13. Black, D. *Diet & Behavior*. Tapestry Press: Utah, pp.4–8. 1989.

Coghlan, A. Simple food guide goes to heart of the matter. New Scientist, 144 (1951):10, 1994
14. The Top 25. The biggest selling items in Australian Supermarkets. Time, June 22, p. 55, 1992.
15. Schoenthaler, S.J. et al. Institutional Nutritional Policies and Criminal Behaviour'. Nutrition Today p.21 May/June, 1985
    Schoenthaler, S.J. et al. Malnutrition and maladaptive behaviour: Two correlational analyses and a double blind placebo controlled challenge in five states. In Essman W.B. (ed.) *Nutrients and Brain Function*. Basil, Switzerland: Karger, p.198–218, 1987.
    Schoenthaler, S.J. et al. The impact of a low food additive and sucrose diet on academic performance in 803 New York City Public schools. Intl.. J. Biosocial Res. 8(2): 185–195, 1986.
16. Schoenthaler, S.J. et al. Ibid, 1986.
17. Schoenthaler, S.J. et al. Ibid, 1986
18. Black, D. *Diet & Behavior*. Tapestry Press: Utah. pp.2, 1989.
19. Schoenthaler, S.J. et al. The impact of a low food additive and sucrose diet. Intl. J. Biosocial Res. 8(2): 185–195, 1986.
20. Beck, D. & Beck, J. *The Pleasure Connection*. Synthesis Press: California, pp. 67–107, 1987.
21. 'Hey bud, ya want some pure Domino? Science News 111 pp.299, (June 7) 1977.
22. Fullerton, D.T. et al. Sugar, Opioids, and Binge Eating. Brain Res. Bull. 14: pp. 673–680, (June) 1980.
23. Tamborlane, W.V. Professor of Pediatrics, Yale School of Medicine, and Jones, T.M., visiting scientist from Australia. Children respond more in blood sugar response than adults. Reported in the New York Times, 1990.
24. Conners, C.K. Not sugar alone but sugar and imbalanced diet low in protein. Reported in Med. Tribune, Jan 9, 1985.
25. Wells, K.C. Laboratory of Behavioural Medicine, Childrens Hopsital, Washington DC. 1985
26. Prinz, R.J. Roberts, W.A. & Hautman, E. Dietary correlates of hyperactive behaviour in children. J. Consult. Clin. Psych. 48: 760–9, 1980
    Schoenthaler, S.J. et al. The impact of a low food additive and sucrose diet. Intl. J. Biosocial Res. 8(2): 207, 1986.
27. Schoenthaler, S.J. et al. Malnutrition and maladaptive behaviour, pp.198–218, 1987.
28. Doraz, W.E. Diet and Delinquency: The Grounding of Four Leading Theories in Human Physiology and Sociology. In Essman, W.B. (ed.) *Nutrients and Brain Function*. Basil, Switzerland: Karger, pp.222, 1987.
29. Munro, N.J. A model of the relationship among energy supply, energy demand and behaviour. In: Essman, W.B. (ed.) *Nutrients and Brain function*: Basel, Switzerland: Karger, pp.231–249, 1987.
    Doraz W.E. Diet and Delinquency: pp.226–227, 1987.

30. Bhagavan, H.N. et al. The effect of pyridoxine hydrochloride on blood serotonin and pyridoxal phosphates contents in hyperactive children. *Pediatrics* 55:437–441, 1975.
31. Coleman, M. et al. A preliminary study of the effect of pyridoxine administration in a subgroup of hyperkinetic children. A double blind crossover comparison with methylphenidate. Biol. Psychiatry 15(5):741–751, 1979.
32. Coleman, M. et al. Ibid, 1979.
33. Reading, C.M. Family Tree connection: How your past can shape your future health. A lesson in orthomolecular medicines. J. Orthomol.Med. 3(3):123–134, 1988.
34. Reading, C.M. Ibid, p.128, 1988.
35. Hoffer, A. Treatment of hyperkinetic children with nicotinamide and pyridoxine. Letter. Can. Med. Assoc. J. 107: 111–112, 1972.
36. Hoffer, A. Ibid, pp.111–112, 1972
    Lonsdale, D. & Shamberger, R. Red Cell transketolase as an indicator of nutritional deficiency. Am. J. Clin. Nutr. 22(2): pp.205–211, 1980
    Thiessen, I. & Mills, L. The use of megavitamin treatment in children with learning disabilities. J. Orthomol. Psychiatry 4(4):228–296, 1975.
37. Zametkin, A.J. et al. Cerebral glucose metabolism in adults with Hyperactivity of Childhood Onset. New England. J. Med. 323(20):1361–1366, 1990.
38. Schoenthaler, S.J. The effects of citrus on the treatment and control of antisocial behaviour: a double blind study of an incarcerated juvenile population. Intl. J. Biosocial Res. 5(2):107–117, 1983.
39. Schauss, A.G. Nutrition and antisocial behaviour. Intl. Clin. Nutr. Rev. 4(4): 172–177, 1984.
40. Schauss, A.G. Ibid, 1984.
41. Walker, S.III. Drugging the American child—We're too cavalier about hyperactivity. J. Learn. Disabil. 8:354, 1975.
42. Durlach, J. Clinical aspects of chronic magnesium deficiency. In: Seelig, M.S.,ed., *Magnesium in Health and Disease*. Spectrum Publications, New York, NY, 1980.
43. Hennotte, J.G. Type A behaviour and magnesium metabolism. Magnesium 5: 201–210, 1986.
44. Pollitt, E. Cognitive effects of iron deficiency anaemia. Letter. Lancet 1:158, 1985
    Lozoff, B. & Brittenham, G.H. Behavioural aspects of iron deficiency. Prog. Hematol. 14:23–53, 1986
    Lozoff, B., Jimenez, E. & Wolf, A.W. Long term developmental outcome of infants with iron deficiency. New England J. Med. 325(10): 687–695, 1991.
45. Soewondo, M.H. & Pollitt, E. Effects of iron deficiency on attention and learning processes in preschool children, Bandung, Indonesia Am. J. Clin. Nutr. 50: 667–674, 1989.
    Pollitt, E., Hathirat, P., Kotchabhakdi, N.J., Missell, L., & Valyasevi, A. Iron deficiency and educational achievement in Thailand. Am. J. Clin. Nutr.. 50:687–697, 1989.

Seshadri, S & Gopaldas, T. Impact of iron supplementation on cognitive functions in preschool and school aged children: the Indian experience. Am. J. Clin. Nutr. 50:675–686, 1989.
46. Youdin, M.B.H., Ben Shachar, D. & Yehuda. Putative biological mechanisms of the effect of iron deficiency on brain biochemistry and behaviour. Am J. Clin. Nutr. 50:607–617, 1989.
47. Mitchell, J. Attention deficit disorder and its treatment. ATOMS, J. Aust. Traditional Med. Soc. pp.15–17. (Summer) 1994/95.
 Sandyle, R. Zinc deficiency in attention deficit hyperactivity disorder. Intl.. J. Neuroscience 52:239–241, 1990.
 Grant, E.C.G. et al. Zinc deficiency in children with dyslexia: concentrations of zinc and other minerals in sweat and hair. British Med. J. 296: 607–609, 1988.
48. Pfeiffer, C.C. *Zinc and Other Micro Nutrients.* Keats Publishing, Connecticut, Chapter 1–18, 1978.
49. Pfeiffer, C.C. Ibid, 1978.
50. Thatcher, R.W. & Lester, M.L. Nutrition, environmental toxins and computerized EEG: A mini-max approach to learning disabilities. J. Learning Disabilities, 18(5): 287–297, 1985.
 Moon, C. et al. Main and interaction effects of metallic pollutants cognitive functioning. J. Learn. Disabil. 18(4): 217–221, 1985.
 Marlowe, M. et al. Hair mineral content as a prediction of learning disabilities. J. Learn. Disabil. 17(7): 418–421, 1984
 Needleman, H.L. & Gatsonis, C.A. Low level lead exposure and the IQ of children. A meta analysis of modern studies. J. Am. Med. Assoc. 263: 673–678, 1990.
51. Colgan, M. & Colgan, L. Do nutrient supplements and dietary changes affect learning and emotional reactions of children with learning difficulties?: A controlled series of 16 cases. Nutritional Health 3:69–77, 1984.
52. Oliver, B. The children who should have been passing, but didn't. J. Orthomol. Psychiatry 12(3): 235–241, 1983.
53. Davies, S. & Stewart, A. *Nutritional Medicine* p.376, 1987.
54. Colquhoun, I. & Bundy, S. A lack of essential fatty acids as a possible cause of hyperactivity in children. Med. Hypotheses 7:673–679, 1981.
 Conner, W.E. & Neuringer, M. The effects of N-3 fatty acid deficiency and repletion upon fatty acid composition and function of brain and retina. In *Biological Membranes: Alteration in Membrane Structure and Function.* Alan R.: Liss Inc. New York, pp.275–294, 1988.
 Stevens, L. et al. Essential fatty acid metabolism in boys with Attention Deficit Hyperactivity Disorder. Am. J. Clin. Nutr. 62. p.761–768, 1995
 Stevens, L. et al. Omega-3 fatty acids in boys with behaviour, learning and health problems. Physiol. & Behav, 59 (415):915–920, 1996.
55. Stordy, J. Benefit of DHA supplement to dark adaptation in dyslexia. J. Clin. Nutr. Lancet, 346:385, 1995.

56. Stordy, J. Dark adaptation motor skills: docosahexaenoic acid and dyslexia. Am. J. Clin. Nutr. Supplement, In Press, 1997.
57. Wurtman, R.J. Control of neurotransmitters synthesis of precursor availability and food consumption. In: Naftolin, R. et al. (eds) *Subcellular Mechanisms in Reproductive Neuroendocrinology.* Elsevier, New York, pp.149–166, 1975.
    Doraz, W.E., Diet and Deliquency: p.277, 1987
    Werbach, M. *Nutritional Influences on Mental Illness:*, pp.10–13; 68–69. 1991.
    Zametkin, A.J. et al. Treatment of hyperactive childen with D-phenylalanine. Am. J. Psychiatry 144(6):792-794, 1987.
58. Davies, S. & Stewart, A. *Nutritional Medicine.* p.20, 1987.
59. Cutter, K. Attention deficit disorder. Australian Wellbeing Magazine No.59:70–72
60. Guyton, A.C. Textbook Medical Physiology. 8th ed pp.377–379, 1991.
61. Buist, R. *Food Chemical Sensitivity. What It is and How to Cope with It.* Harper & Rowe Publishing, Sydney, pp.193–196, 1986.
62. Swain, A.,Truswell, A.S. & Lobbay, R.H. Adverse reactions to food. Food Tech. Aust. 36(10):467–471, 1984
    Werbach, M. *Nutritional Influences on Mental Illness:* pp.70–73 & p.187. 1991.
63. Hannuksela, M. et al. Hypersensitive reactions to food additives. Allergy 42(Nov): 561–575, 1987.
    Salamy, J. et al. Physiological changes in hyperactive children following ingestion of food additives. Intl. J. Neuroscience 16:241–246, 1982.
64. Swain, A., Dutton, S.P. & Truswell, A.S. Salicylates in foods. J. Am Dietetic Assoc. 85(8): 950–960, 1985.
    Swain, A., Soutter, V., Lobloy, R. & Truswell, A.S. Salicylates, oligoantigenic diets and behaviour. Lancet 2:41–42, 1985.
65. Egger, J., Carter, C.M., Graham, P.J., Gumbley, D. & Soothill, J.F. Controlled trial of oligoantigenic treatment in the hyperkinetic syndrome. Lancet 1:540–545, 1985.
    Buist, R. *Food Chemical Sensitivity*, pp.45–55, 1986.
66. David, T.J. Reactions to dietary tartrazine. Arch. Disease Childhood 62:119–122, 1987.
67. Rapp, D. Does diet affect hyperactivity? J. Learn. Disabil. 11 (6). p.383–388, 1978.
68. Egger, J., Carter, C.M., Graham, P.J., Gumbley, D. & Soothill, J.F. Controlled trial of oligoantigenic treatment in the hyperkinetic syndrome. Lancet 1:540–545, 1985
69. Ward, N.I. et al. The influence of the chemical additive tartrazine on the zinc status of hyperactive children—a double blind placebo controlled study. J. Nutr. Med 1: 51–57, 1990.
70. Werbach, M. *Nutritional Influences on Mental Illness*: pp.65–66. 1991.
71. Extracted from: Houssen, M. & Massden, J. *The New Additive Code Breaker.* Lothian Publishing Co., Melbourne, 1989.
72. Gerber, R. *Vibrational Medicine.* Bear & Co., pp.217–223, 1989
73. Wallace, R.A., King, J.L. & Sanders, G.P. Biology. *The Science of Life*, Goodyear Publishing Co. Inc., Santa Monica, California. p.450–454, 1981.

Anderson, K.N., Anderson, L.E. & Glange, W.D. (eds) *Mosby's Medical, Nursing and Allied Health Dictionary.* Mosby, Sydney. p.249–250, 1994.
74. Feldman, D. et al. Steroid hormone systems found in yeast. Science 225:913–914, 1984.
75. Nord C.E. & Edlund, C. Impact of antimicrobial agents on human intestinal microflora. J. Chemotherapy 2(4):218–237, 1990.
76. Crook, W.G. *The Yeast Connection.* Professional Books, Jackson, MI. p.102, 1983.
77. Vayda, W. Systemic yeast infection. Part One. Nature and Health 6(4):72–75, 1985.
78. Wilkin, S.R. Defective immune response in patients with recurrent candidiasis. Infections in Medicine (May-June), 1985.
79. Hannaford, C. *Smart Moves.* p.153. 1995.
80. Crook, W.G. *The Yeast Connection.* p.378, 1983.
   Vayda, W. Systemic yeast infection—Part two. Nature and Health 7(1):69–71, 1986.
81. Vayda, W. Systemic yeast Infection—Part two Nature and Health 7(1):70, 1986.
82. Burgess, D.M. & Streisguth, M.P. Educating students with fetal alcohol sydrom and fetal alcohol effects. Pennsylvania Reporter, 22(Nov):1, 1990.
83. Ohashi & Monte, T. *Reading the Body.* Penguin Books, New York, NY, pp.48–49, 1991.
84. Stokes, G. & Whiteside, D. *Basic One Brain.* Three In One Concepts, Inc., Burbank, CA. Chapters 2–2 to 2–3, 1984.
85. Vayda, W. Systemic Yeast Infection—Part two Nature and Health 7(1):70, 1986.
86. Becker, R.O. *Cross Currents. The Perils of Electropollution. The Promise of Electromedicine.* Jeremy P. Tarcher, Inc. Los Angeles p.174–176, 1990.
87. Becker, R.O. Ibid, p.187, 1990.
88. Becker, R.O. Ibid, p.185–186, 1990
89. Becker, R.O. Ibid, p.187, 1990
90. Leher, E.J. Biological effects of electromagnetic fields. IEEE Spectrum, pp.57–63 (May) 1984.
91. Wertheimer, N. & Leeper, E. First report of relationship between exposure to 60Hz magnetic fields from electric lines and childhood cancer. Am. J. Epidemiology 109:273, 1979.
92. Wertheimer, N.& Leeper, E. Electrical wiring and childhood cancer. Intl.. J. Epidemiology 11:345–355, 1982.
   Tomenius, L. et al. 50Hz electromagnetic environment and incidence of childhood cancer—Stockholm. Bioelectromagnetics 7:191–207, 1986.
93. Coghlan, A. Swedish studies pinpoint power line cancer link. New Scientist, 136 (1845):4, 3, 1992.
94. Edwards, R. Leak links power lines to cancer. New Scientist 148(1998), 4, Oct, 1995
95. Bearsdley, T. Shocking genes. Electromagnetic fields stimulate genetic activity. Sci. Am. 262(7):13 1990.

96. Becker R.O. *Cross Currents.* pp.199–200, 1990.
97. Coghill, R. *Electrohealing. The Medicine of the Future.* Thorsons, London. p.83, 1992.
98. Coghill R. Ibid, pp84–85, 1992.
99. Coghill, R.Ibid,.pp.71–78, 1992.
100. Noback, C.R., Strominger, N.L. & Demarest, R.J. *The Human Nervous System. Introduction and Review.* 4th ed. Lea & Fibiger, London, pp.170 & 264–265, 1991.
101. Ferreri, C. Dyslexia and Learning Disabilities Cured. Digest of Chiropractic Economics, 1983.
    Ferreri, C. & Wainwright, R.B. *Breakthrough for Dyslexia and Learning Disabilities.* Exposition Press of Florida, Pompano Beach, Fl, pp.70–78, 1984.
102. Dejarnette, M.B. Sacro-occipital Research, Society International Publications, Kansas, 1970.
103. Walker, R. Lectures on Cranio-Dental Dysfunction. Presented at the Am. Assoc. of Functional Orthodontics, San Francisco, Ca, 1997.
104. Witzig, J.W. & Sphahl, T. *Clinical Management of Basic Maxillofacial Orthopedic Appliances.* PSG Publishing Company, Littleton, MA, 1989.
105. Enlow, D. H. *Facial Growth.* 3rd ed., Saunders Publishing Company, Sydney, 1990.
106. Krebs, C.T. Clinical observations. Presented at the Proceedings of the SOTO Annual Convention, Melbourne, 1995.
107. Solow, B. Airway adequacy, head posture and cranio-facial morphology. Am. J. Orthodontics 86(3):214–223, 1984.
108. Wiebrecht, A.T. *Crozat Appliances in Interceptive Maxillofacial Orthopedics.* The E.F. Schmidt Company, Milwaukee, Wisconsin, pp.83–137, 1966.
    Wiebrecht, A.T. *Crozat Appliances in Interceptive Maxillofacial Orthopedics,* The E.F. Schmidt Company, Milwaukee, Wisconsin,. pp.10–44, 1969.
109. Walther, D.S. *Applied Kinesiology Volume II. Head, Neck & Jaw Pain and Dysfunction—The Stomatognathic System.* Systems DC, Pueblo, CO, pp.343–375 & 511–515, 1983.
    Goddard, G. TMJ: *The Jaw Connection, the Overlooked Diagnosis.* Aurora Press, Santa Fe, NM, pp.67–74, 1991.
110. Walther, D.S. *Applied Kinesiology Volume II.* p.514, 1983.
    Goddard, G. TMJ: The Jaw Connection, the Overlooked Diagnosis. pp.70 & 113–125, 1991.
111. Radnov, B.P., Dvorak, J. & Valach, L. Cognitive deficits in patients after soft tissue injury of the cervical spine. Spine 17:127–131, 1992.

Chapter 11

1. Gerber, R. *Vibrational Medicine. New Choices for Healing Ourselves.* Bear & Company, Sante Fe, NM, 1988.

2. Castiglioni, A. *A History of Medicine*. Alfred A. Knopf, New York, p. 172, 1958.
   Edwards, P. *Encyclopedia of Philosophy*. The Free Press, New York, Vol 1: p.193–198, 1967.
3. Cytowic, C. E. *The Man who Tasted Shapes. A Bizarre Medical Mystery Offers Revolutionary Insights into Emotions, Reasoning and Consciousness*. G.P. Putman & Sons, New York, 1993
4. Huxley, A. *Science, Liberty and Peace*. Harper & Brothers, New York, p.35–36, 1946.
5. Katz, M.J. *Templates and the Explanation of Complex Patterns*. Cambridge University Press, Cambridge, p.85, 1986.
6. Black, D. *Health at the Crossroads. Exploring the Conflict between Natural Healing and Conventional Medicine*. Tapestry Press, Springville, UT, pp.33–52, 1988.
   Black, D. *Inner Wisdom. The Challenge of Contextual Healing*. Tapestry Press, Springville, UT, pp. 24–38, 1990.
7. Castiglioni, A. *A History of Medicine*. pp.178, 1958.
8. Sri Aurobindo. *The Divine Life*. All India Press, Pondicherry, pp.6–25 & 71–112, 1970.
9. Gerber, R. *Vibrational Medicine* pp.119–226 & 369–401, 1988.
10. Chopra, D. *Quantum Healing. Exploring the Frontiers of Mind/Body Medicine*. Bantam Books, New York, 1989.
11. Chopra, D. Ibid, pp.97–100, 1989.
12. Bell, J. S. *On the Einstein Podolsky Rosen Paradox*. Physics 1: 195, 1964.
    Bohm, D. & Hiley, B J. *The Undivided Universe*. Routledge, London, pp.134–159, 1993.
13. Hawkings, S.H. *A Brief History of Time. From the Big Bang to Black Holes*, Bantam Books, London, p.24, 1988.
14. Tiller, W. A. *Science and Human Transformation. Subtle Energies, Intentionality and Consciousness*. Pavior Publishing, Walnut Creek, CA, 1997.
15. Tiller, W. A. Ibid, pp. 260–272, 1997.
16. Swami Satyananda, Swaraswati. *Kundalini Tantra*. Satyananda Ashram, Gosford, pp. 75–129, 1985.
    Gerber, R. *Vibrational Medicine* pp.119–226 & 369–401, 1988.
17. New technologies detect effects of healers' hands. Brain/Mind Bulletin, 10(16), 1985.
    Gerber, R. *Vibrational Medicine* pp. 149–150, 1988.
18. Tiller, W. A. A Lattice Model of Space. *Phoenix: New directions in the study of man*. Vol 2(2):27–47, 1978.
19. Gerber, R. *Vibrational Medicine* pp.73–77 & 80–89, 1988.
20. Gerber, R. Ibid, pp.49–51, 1988.
21. Gerber, R. Ibid, pp.173–182, 1988.
22. Dalai Lama, Kalachakra Initiation Lectures, Sydney, September, 1996.

23. Gerber, R. *Vibrational Medicine* pp.155–161, 1988.
    Brenman, B.A. *Hands of Light. A Guide to Healing through the Human Energy Field.* Bantam Books, Sydney, pp.29–58, 1987.
    Myss, C. *Anatomy of Spirit. The Seven Stages of Power and Healing.* Crown Publishers, New York, 1996.
    Tiller, W.A. *Science and Human Transformation*, pp.101–129, 1997.
24. Le Doux, J. *The Emotional Brain. The Mysterious Underpinnings of Emotional Life.* Simon & Schuster, New York, 1996.
    Tortora, G J & Grabowski, S R. *Principles of Anatomy and Physiology*, 8th ed. Harper Collins College Publishers, New York, 1996.
    Pert, C.B. *Molecules of Emotion. Why you feel the way you feel.* Scribner, New York, 1997.
25. Leadbeater, C.W. *The Chakras.* The Theosophical Publishing House, London, 1927.
    Swami Satyananda Swaraswati. *Kundalini Tantra* 1985.
    Brennan, B.A. *Hands of Light* 1988.
26. Gerber, R. *Vibrational Medicine* p.130, 1988.
27. Swami Satyananda Swaraswati. *Kundalini Tantra* p.75–129, 1985
    Brennan, B.A. *Hands of Light* 1988.
28. Gerber, R. *Vibrational Medicine* p.128 & 371–373, 1988
29. Gerber, R. *Vibrational Medicine* p.129–132, 1988
    Leadbeater, C.W. *The Chakras* 1927
30. Noback, C.R., Strominger, N L & Demarest, R J. *The Human Nervous System, Introduction and Review*, 4th ed. Lea & Febiger, Philadelphia, pp.323–352, 1991.
31. Swami Satyananda Swaraswati. *Kundalini Tantra* pp.253–258, 1985
    Gerber, R. *Vibrational Medicine* 1988
32. Swami Satyananda Swaraswati. *Kundalini Tantra* 1985
33. Gerber, R. *Vibrational Medicine* pp.131–132, 1988
34. Swami Satyananda Swaraswati. *Kundalini Tantra* pp.12–14, 1985
    Gerber, R. *Vibrational Medicine* pp.128–132, 1988
35. Swami Satyananda Swaraswati. *Kundalini Tantra* pp.253–258, 1985
    Gerber, R. *Vibrational Medicine* pp.276–287 & 371–387, 1988
36. Brennan, B.A. *Hands of Light* 1988.
37. Swami Satyananda Swaraswati. *Kundalini Tantra* pp.84–129, 1985
    Gerber, R. *Vibrational Medicine* 1988
38. Swann, I. *To Kiss the Earth Goodbye.* Dell Publishing Co. Inc, 1975.
    Tiller, W A. *Science and Human Transformation* p.82, 1997.
39. Swami Sivananda. *Spiritual Experiences.* The Divine Life Society, Tehri-Gahwal, India, pp. 62–108, 1995.

Chapter 12

1. Bailey, A.A. *Esoteric Healing. Volume IV, A Treatise on the Seven Rays*. Lucis Press Ltd., London, 1953.
2. Dennett, D. *Consciousness Explained*. Little Brown, Boston, MA, 1991.
   Churchland, P. *The Engine of Reason, the Seat of Soul: A Philosophical Journey into the Brain*. MIT Press, Cambridge, MA, 1995.
   Scott, A. *Stairway to the Mind*. Copernicus Springer Verlag, New York, NY, 1995.
3. Crick, F.H.C. & Koch, C. Towards a neurobiological theory of consciousness. *Seminars in the Neurosciences* 2:263–275, 1990.
   Milner, D & Rugg (eds). *The Neuropsychology of Consciousness*. Academic Press, London, 1992.
   Crick, F.H. *The Astonishing Hypothesis: The Scientific Search for Soul*. Scribner, New York, NY, 1994.
4. Chalmers, D.J. *The Conscious Mind. In Search of a Fundamental Theory*. Oxford University Press, New York, NY, 1996.
5. Chalmers, D.J. The puzzle of conscious experience. *Scientific American* 273 (6), 62–69, 1995.
   Lockwood, M. The Enigma of Sentience. Plenary Presentation, Towards a Science of Consciousness, Tucson, AZ, April 8–13, 1996.
6. Neural Networks and Connectionism. *Consciousness Research Abstracts, Toward a Science of Consciousness*, Tucson, AZ, pp.102–105, April 8–13, 1996.
7. Moody, R. *Life After Life*. Bantam Mockingbird, New York, NY, 1975.
   Ring, K. *Life at Death*. William Morrow Co., New York, NY, 1980.
   Moody, R. *The Light Beyond*. Bantam Mockingbird, New York, NY, 1988.
   Bailey, L.W. & Yates, J. *The Near Death Experience. A Reader*. Routledge, London, 1996.
8. Kubler-Ross, E. *On Death and Dying*. MacMillan, New York, NY, 1969.
   Kubler-Ross, E. *On Life After Death*. Celestial Arts, Berkeley, CA, 1991.
9. Kubler-Ross, E. Ibid., pp.53–59, 1991.
10. Bailey, K.W. & Yates, J. *The Near Death Experience*. Routledge, London, pp. 5–6, 1986.
11. Kubler-Ross, E. *On Life After Death*. p.50, 1991.
12. Kubler-Ross, E. Ibid, p. 47, 1991.
13. Gerber, R. *Vibrational Medicine. New Choices for Healing Ourselves*. Bear & Company, Sante Fe, NM, pp.138–140, 1988.
14. Swann, I. *To Kiss the Earth Goodbye*. Dell Publishing Co. Inc, 1975.
    Monroe, R. *Far Journeys*. Doubleday & Company Inc, Garden City, NY, 1985.
15. Bailey, L.W. & Yates, J. *The Near Death Experience* pp.41–50, 1996.
16. Monroe, R.A. *Far Journeys*, 1985.
    Gerber, R. *Vibrational Medicine* pp.139–142, 1988.
    Bailey, L.W. & Yates, J. *The Near Death Experience*, 1996.

17. Tiller, W.A. *Science and Human Transformation. Subtle Energies Intentionality and Consciousness*, Pavior, Walnut Creek, CA, 1997.
18. Sogyal, Rinpoche. *The Tibetan Book of Living and Dying.* Harper Collins Publishers, New York, NY, 1993.
19. Russek, L.G. & Schwartz, G.E. Energy Cardiology: A dynamical energy systems approach for integrating conventional and alternative medicine. J Mind-Body Health 12(4):4–24, 1996.
20. Russek, L.G. & Schwartz, G.E. Interpersonal heart-brain registration and the perception of parental love: A 42 year follow up of the Harvard master of stress study. Subtle Energies 5(3): 195–208, 1995.
21. Russek, L.G. & Schwartz, G.E. Ibid., Subtle Energies 5(3):201–206, 1995.
22. Russek, L.G. & Schwartz, G.E. Narrative discriptions of parental love and caring predict health status in midlife.: 35 year follow up of the Harvard mastery of stress study. Alternative Therapies 2(6):55–62, 1996.
23. Russek, L.G. & Schwartz, G.E. Ibid. p.60, 1996.
24. Tiller, W.A. McCarthy, R. & Atkinson, M. Toward cardiac coherence: A new non invasive measure of autonomic system order. Alternative Therapies 2(1):1–13, 1996.
25. Russek, L.G. & Schwartz, G.E. Energy Cardiology. J. Mind–Body Health. 12(4): 4–24, 1996.
26. Wirth, D. The Effect of Noncontact Therapeutic Touch on the Healing Rates of Full Thickness Dermal Wounds. Master's Thesis, JFK University, California, 1989.
27. Dossey, L. *Healing Words. The Power of Prayer and Practice of Medicine.* Harpers, San Franscisco, 1993.

    Dossey, L. et al. Special issue on prayer and distant intentionality. Alternative Therapies 3(6):10–107, 1997.
28. Byrd, R.C. Positive therapeutic effects of intercessory prayer in the coronary case unit population. Southern Med. J. 81(7):826–829, 1988.
29. Dossey, L. *Healing Words* pp.97–100, 1993.
30. James, W. *The Varieties of Religious Experience.* Reprinted, 1990, Vintage Books, New York, NY, 1901.
31. James, W. Ibid. p.343, 1901.
32. Swami Sivananda. *Spiritual Experiences.* The Divine Life Society, Tehri-Gahwal, India, pp.62–108, 1995.

SOURCES OF ILLUSTRATIONS

The publishers gratefully acknowledges the artists, authors, and publishers for permission to redraw and adapt these illustrations from the following sources:

Figure 1.1   Photograph courtesy of the *Herald and Weekly Times*, Melbourne, Australia.

Figure 3.4   Hubel, D. 'The Brain'. *Scientific American* Vol. 241(9):41, 1979.

Figure 3.5   Noback, C.R., Strominger, N.L., & Demarest, R.J., *The Human Nervous System. Introduction and Review*, 4th ed., cover drawing, 1991.

Figure 3.9   Gerschwind, N. 'Specializations of the Human Brain'. *Scientific American* Vol. 241(9):160, 1979.

Figure 3.10 Tortora, G.J. & Grabowski, S.R. *Principles of Anatomy and Physiology*, 8th ed., Figure 14.15, 1996.

Figure 3.21 Netter, F.H. *The CIBA Collection of Medical Illustrations, Volume 1, Part I, Section 8*, CIBA Pharmaceutical Company, N.J., Plate 63, p.215, 1983.
Copyright 1983. Novartis. Reprinted with permission from The Ciba Collection of Medical Illustrations, Vol. 1, Part I, illustrated by Frank H. Netter, MD. All rights reserved.

Figure 3.22 Martin, J.H. *Neuroanatomy: Text and Atlas*. Elsevier, New York, Figures 15-1 and 15-2, 1989.

Figure 3.24 Netter, F.H. *The CIBA Collection of medical Illustrations, Volume 1, Part I, Section 8*, CIBA Pharmaceutical Company, N.J., Plate 6, p.28, 1983.
Copyright 1983. Novartis. Reprinted with permission from The Ciba Collection of Medical Illustrations, Vol. 1, Part I, illustrated by Frank H. Netter, MD. All rights reserved.

Figure 4.3	Richardson, J.T.E. et al. *Working Memory and Human Cognition*. Oxford University Press, New York, Figure 2.5, 1996.
Figure 4.5	LeDoux, J.E. 'Emotion, Memory and the Brain'. *Scientific American* Vol. 270(6):38, 1994.
Figure 6.2	Morris, C. Revised diagram developed by LEAP student Christine Morris and used with her kind permission.
Figure 8.3	Tortora, G.J. & Grabowski, S.R. *Principles of Anatomy and Physiology*, 8th ed., Figure 15.9, 1996.
Figure 10.2	Hannaford, C. *Smart Moves. Why Learning Is Not All In Your Head*. Great Ocean Publishers, Arlington, VA, Figure 10.1, 1995.
Figure 10.3	Wiebrecht, A.T. *Crozat Appliances in Interceptive Maxillofacial Orthopedics*. The E.F. Smith Company, Milwaukee, WI, Plate of Occlusal After Treatment from Case No.3, and Plates of Before and After Treatment of Upper Jaw from Case No.18, 1969.
Figure 11.4	Tiller, W.A. A Lattice Model of Space. Phoenix: New Directions in the Study of Man. Vol. II(2):31, 1978.
Figure 11.7	Leadbeater, C. *The Chakras*. The Theosophical Society Publishing House, Wheaton, IL, The Chakras and the Nervous System, pp.40–41, 1927.
Figure 11.8	Ajit Mookerjee. *Yoga Art*. Thames and Hudson Ltd, London, Plate No. 9, 1975.

Appendix A: The Meridian-Muscle-Organ/Gland relations and their associated negative and positive emotions.

Meridian	Muscle	Organ/Gland	Positive Emotion	Negative Emotion
GOVERNING	Teres Major	Spinal Column Brain Stem Cerebral Spinal Fluid	Supported Trust Honesty Truth	Unsupported Distrust Dishonesty
CENTRAL	Supraspinatus	Cerebral Cortex	Self respect Success	Overwhelm Shyness Shame
STOMACH	Pectoralis Major Clavicular	Stomach	Sympathy Empathy Contentment Harmony Reliable	Disappointment Criticism Greed Disgust Unreliable
SPLEEN	Latissimus Dorsi Middle Trapezius	Spleen/Pancreas Spleen	Sympathy Empathy Assurance Confidence Faith in future	Rejected Indifference Anxiety about future
HEART	Subscapularis	Heart	Love Forgiveness Compassion Self worth Self esteem Secure	Hate Anger Unworthy Self doubt Insecure
SMALL INTESTINE	Quadriceps	Small Intestine	Joy Assimilation Nourishing	Sadness Over excited Discouraged
BLADDER	Peroneus Anterior Tibialis	Bladder	Peace/Harmony Patience Courage Resoluteness	Terror/Panic Impatience Fear Restlessness

Meridian	Muscle	Organ/Gland	Positive Emotion	Negative Emotion
KIDNEY	Psoas	Kidney	Courage Decisive	Fear/Anxiety Terror Careless Reckless
PERI-CARDIUM	Gluteus Medius	Pericardium Ovaries/Testes	Calm Responsible Relaxation Tranquillity	Hysteria Gloomy Remorse Jealous
TRIPLE HEATER	Teres Minor Sartorius	Thyroid Gland Adrenal Gland	Balance Elation Lightness Hope	Despair Heaviness Despondent Hopeless
GALL BLADDER	Anterior Deltoid Popliteus	Gall Bladder	Decisiveness Love Righteousness Assertive	Anger Rage/wrath Self righteousness Helpless
LIVER	Pectoralis Major Sternal Rhomboids	Liver	Choice Love Transformation Happiness	No Choice Anger Rage/wrath Resentment
LUNG	Anterior serratus Middle Deltoid	Lung	Cheerful Humility Tolerance Modesty	Grief Depressed Haughty/false pride Intolerance
LARGE INTESTINE	Fascia Lata	Large Intestine	Self worth Letting go Enthusiasm	Guilt Grief Depression

Appendix B

KINESIOLOGY PRACTITIONERS

As stated in Chapter 2, Kinesiology is a developing new health modality with integrated training programs and practitioner registration procedures only just now being set in place. Therefore, individuals calling themselves Kinesiologists vary considerably in their level of training and competence.

The list of organisations below provide at least an entry point for people interested in locating a Kinesiology practitioner in their area. As with any other profession, word of mouth referral is by far the best source for competent practitioners.

LEAP Practitioners

United States

Adam Lehman
19210 Sonoma Hwy
Sonoma, CA 95476
707 328 2838
adam@kinesiohealth.com

Kristina (Tina) Baker
8847 Spectrum Center Boulevard #6306 San Diego, CA 92123
TINZO@aol.com
858 974 9773
858 361 2865 cell

Marge Bowen, EnK, Lmt
Sanctuary for Healing and Integration 860 East 4500 South, Suite 302
Salt Lake City, UT 84107
801 913 6060
marge_bowen@msn. corn

Nancy Crowley
394 East 4750
North Provo, UT 84604
crowley@pxi.net
801 224 7227
801 369 9717 cell

Tami Davis
3738 Belfort Drive
West Valley City, UT 84120
tamidavis@comcast.net
801 969 0558
801 891 6678 cell

Kim Gangwish
Life Enrichment Center
989 W. Princeton Ct.
Louisville, CO 80027
303 717 8860
1 800 537 4478
Ksgangwish@aol.com

Eloise H. Hanby
1062 River Pine Circle
Riverton, UT 84065
Ehanby@aol.com
801 254 4796

Marcia Hart
Box 694
Sun Valley, ID 83353
marciah3 @mindspring. corn
208 726 3586
208 720 3933 cell

W. Steve Hansen
888 W. Smith Lane
Kaysville, UT 84037
steve@dynamicenergies.com
801 444 1309 cell

Mary Huggins
2806 Great Oaks Drive Round
Rock, TX 78681
MaryHuggins@aol.com
www.TouchTheWorld.info
512 255 6489
512 461 4310 cell

Michael A. King
Center for Enhanced Wellness
2681 E. Parley's Way, Suite 203
Salt Lake City, UT 84109
bodyintegrated@hotmail.com
801 259 8909 business

Elaine Lemon
1340 N. Crosswater Way
Eagle, ID 83616
elemonlOlO@aol.com
208 939 3344
208 577 8570 cell

Marie Moon
106 North 19th
Pocatello, ID 83201
mmmarie 1 @msn. corn
201 234 0422

Kate Rupert
2208 E. Little Cloud Circle
Sandy, UT 84093
katerupert@yahoo.com
801 943 3207
801 953 5710 cell

Sharon K. Smith
16730 SW 82 Court
PalmettoBay, FL 33157
Smithsk@BellSouth.net
305 253 3873
305 219 1746 cell

Sandra L. Voge
2454 South 3775 West Ogden, UT 84401
slvoge@hotmail.com
801 731 5086
801 564 8892 cell

Ronald Wayman
Sensory Dynamics Institute
8817 South Redwood Road #C
West Jordan, UT 84088
ronwayman@gmail.com
801 566 6262 office 801 599 3602 cell

KINESIOLOGY ORGANIZATIONS – INTERNATIONAL

Touch For Health Kinesiology Association
PO Box 392 New Carlisle, OH 45344
Tel: 800   466   8342
www.TFHKA.org
admin@tfhka.org

Energy Kinesiology Association
5900 CR 90
Red Rock, Oklahoma 74651
Tel: 580   725   3411
www.energyk.org
info@energyK.org

The U.S. Kinesiology Institute
7121 New Light Trail
Chapel Hill, NC 27516
Tel: 919 933 9299
greentfh@mindspring.com
www.USkinesiology.com

International Institute of Applied Physiology
3014 East Michigan Street, Tucson, Arizona 85714
Tel: 1 520 889 3075
Fax: 1 520 573 3743

International Kinesiology College
Box 2620 Nambour West Old 4560 Australia
Tel: 61 7 5441 3951 Fax 61 7 5476 3343

International Association of Specialised Kinesiologists
www.iask.org

TFH Association of New Zealand
33 Gilshennan Valley, Red Beach, New Zealand.

Tel: 64 9 426 7695

International College of Professional Kinesiology Practice
PO Box 25-162 St Heliers, New Zealand 1130
Tel:6495740077
office@icpkp.com
www.icpkp.com

Edu-K Foundation
Box 3396 Ventura California, 93006-3396, USA
Tel: 1 800 356 2109, Fax: 1 805 650 0524

Three In One Concepts
2001 W. Magnolia Blvd. Burbank, California 91506-1704, USA
Tel: 1 9818 841 4786

TFH Association of Canada
Box 74508 Kitsilano Postal Unit, Vancouver, BC V6K 4P4, Canada
Tel: 1 604 978 6292

Canadian Association of Specialized Kinesiology
Box 621, 1926 Como Lake Avenue
Coquitlam, BC V3J 7X8
Tel: 604 669 8481
Web: www.canask.org
Email: office@canask.org

Energy Kinesiology Awareness Council
www.awarenesscouncil.com
info@awarenesscouncil.corn

The British Kinesiology Federation
PO Box 83, Sheffield, S7 2YN, United Kingdom
Tel/Fax: 44 114 281 4064

Australian Kinesiology Association
PO Box 233 Kerrimuir VIC 3129
0500 50 33 55, Fax: 0500 50 77 55
email: aka@aka-oz.org, website: www.aka-oz.org

Institut Belge de Kinesiologie
Avenue Paul Nicodeme 26, B-1330 Rixensart, Belgium. Tel: 32 2 652 2686, Fax: 32 2 652 1656.

IAK Institut fur Angewandte Kinesiologie GmbH, Freiburg
Eschbachstrasse 5, D-79199 Kirchzarten, Germany Tel: 49 7661 98 71-0, Fax: 49 7661 98 71 49

Kinesiologisch Netwerk Nederland
Rijksweg 14-M, 6267 AG Cadier en Keer, The Netherlands Tel: 31-43.407.80.90 Fax: 31-43.407.80.88
e-mail: ki-net.nl@wxs.nl

Kinesiology Association of Denmark
Hesteskoen 6st th, DK-3000, Helsingor, Denmark Tel:
+45-49 226 970
e-mail KAD83@inet.uni-c.dk

Swedish School of Specialized Kinesiology
Gastrikegatan 11, 113 62 Stockholm, Sweden Tel:
468 339 669, Fax: 468 340 506

The Norwegian Kinesiology Association Herman
Gransvel 17A, N-5034, Lasevag, Norway Tel: 47 553 46
480

TFH Association of Italy
Via F. Ili Blanci 3, 25080 Maderno S/G BS, Italy Tel: 39
365 641 553

Centro de Memoria Celular
Ladislao Martinex 332 1640 MARTINEZ Provincia de Buenos Aires
ARGENTINA
Tel: 54 11 4792 7718
www.memcel.com.ar

Appendix C

BASIC KINESIOLOGY WORKSHOPS FOR STRESS MANAGEMENT AND LEARNING ENHANCEMENT

International: Stress Management

Touch For Health Kinesiology Association
PO Box 392 New Carlisle, Ohio 45344
Tel: 1-800-466-8342
www.TFHKA.org
admin@tfhka.org

The U.S. Kinesiology Institute
7121 New Light Trail Chapel Hill, NC 27516
Tel: 1-919-933-9299
greentfh@mindspring.com
www.USkinesiology.com

International college of Professional Kinesiology Practice
PO Box 25-162 St. Heilers, New Zealand 1740
Tel: 64 9 574 0077
office@icpkp.com
www.icpkp.com

International Institute of Applied Physiology Seven Element Hologram Workshops
3014 East Michigan Street, Tucson, Arizona, 85714. Tel: 1 520 889 3075, Fax: 1 520 573 3743

International Kinesiology College - Konradstrasse
Box 2620 Nambour West Old 4560 Australia
Tel: 61 7 5441 3951 Fax 61 7 5476 3343

Three In One Concepts
2001 W. Magnolia Blvd. Burbank, California 91506-1704, USA Tel: 1 818 841 4786

TFH Association of Canada
Box 74508 Kitsilano Postal Unit, Vancouver, **BC** V6K 4P4, Canada Tel: 1 604 978 6292

Canadian Association of Specialized Kinesiology Box 621,
1926 Como Lake Avenue
Coquitlam, BC V3J 7X8
Tel: 604 669 8481
Web: www.canask.org
Email: office@canask.org

TFH Association of New Zealand
33 Gilshennan Valley, Red Beach, New Zealand. Tel: 64 9 426 7695

The British Kinesiology Federation
PO Box 83, Sheffield, S7 2YN, United Kingdom
Tel/Fax: 44 114 281 4064

IAK Institut fur Angewandte Kinesiologie GmbH, Freiburg
Eschbachstrasse 5, D-79199 Kirchzarten, Germany Tel: 49 7661 98 71-0, Fax: 49 7661 98 71 49

Institut Belge de Kinesiologie
Avenue Paul Nicodeme 26, B-1330 Rixensart, Belgium. Tel: 32 2 652 2686, Fax: 32 2 652 1656.

College Francois de Kinesiologie
Bat Cl, Residence La Plaine, 13127, Vitrolles, France Tel/Fax: 33 42 889 1225

Topping International Institute, Inc/Wellness Kinesiology 2622 Birchwood Avenue, #7, Bellingham, WA 98225, USA Tel/Fax: 1 360 647 2703

Kinesiologisch Netwerk Nederland
Rijksweg 14-M, 6267 AG Cadier en Keer, The Netherlands Tel: 31-43.407.80.90
Fax: 31-43.407.80.88
e-mail: ki-net.nl@wxs.nl

Kinesiology Association of Denmark
Hesteskoen 6st th, DK-3000, Helsingor, Denmark Tel: +45-49 226 970
e-mail KAD83@inet.uni-c.dk

Transformational Kinesiology
Kyndelose, Strandvej 22, 4070 Kirke, Hyllinge, Denmark Tel: +45-46 406 650

Dansk Paedagogist Kinesiologiskole
Kaervangen 14, DK-2820, Gentofte, Denmark Tel: +45-31 673 838
Fax: +45-44 534 306 e-mail: DK_paedkin@post.dk-online.dk

Swedish School of Specialized Kinesiology
Gastrikegatan 11, 113 62 Stockholm, Sweden Tel: 468 339 669, Fax: 468 340 506

The Norwegian Kinesiology Association
Herman Gransvel 17A, N-5034, Lasevag, Norway Tel: 47 553 46 480

TFH Association of Italy
Via F. Ili Blanci 3, 25080 Maderno S/G BS, Italy Tel: 39 365 641 553

South African Association of Specialised Kinesiologists
14 Osborne Road, Claremont Cape 7700m South Africa Tel: 27 21 61 8021

Three In One Concepts: Basic One Brain Kinesiology Workshops
Dominic Burke (Faculty)
PO Box 3 Corinda, Queensland 4075
Tel: (07) 3375 1932

International Learning Enhancement Workshops

Edu-K Foundation
Box 3396 Ventura California, 93006-3396, USA Tel: 1 800 356 2109, Fax: 1 805 650 0524

Three In One Concepts
2001 W. Magnolia Blvd. Burbank, California 91506-1704, USA Tel: 1 818 841 4786

IAK Institut für Angewandte Kinesiologie GmbH, Freiburg
Eschbachstrasse 5, D-79199 Kirchzarten, Germany Tel: 49 7661 98 71-0, Fax: 49 7661 98 71 49

Institut Beige de Kinesiologie
Avenue Paul Nicodeme 26, B-1330 Rixensart, Belgium. Tel: 32 2 652 2686, Fax: 32 2 652 1656.

International College of Kinesiology
Konradstrasse 32, CH-8005, Zurich, Switzerland. Tel: 41 1 440 4268, Fax: 41 1 440 4269

Centro de Memoria Celular
Ladislao Martinex 332 1640 MARTINEZ Provincia de Buenos Aires
ARGENTINA
Tel: 54 11 4792 7718
www.memcel.com.ar

Appendix D

LEAP PRACTITIONERS AND COURSES

The list of centres below can provide referral to qualified LEAP Practitioners. Information on Professional training in the LEAP program is also available from these centres. Melbourne Applied Physiology can provide information on all national and international LEAP practitioners and training.

Australia

Melbourne Applied Physiology
P.O. Box 71, Learmonth, Vic 3352 Australia
Tel: 61 (0)3 5343 2248, Fax: 61 (0)3 5343 2258
email: krebsc@aol.com

USA

Adam Lehman
Insitutute of Bioenergetics Arts & Sciences
19210 Sonoma Hwy   Sonoma, CA 95476
707 328 2838
adam@kinesiohealth.com
LEAP Bl 1

Mr. Ron Wayman
Sensory Dynamics Institute
8817 South Redwood Road #C   West Jordan, UT 84088
ronwayman@gmail.com
801 566 6262 office
801 599 3602 cell
LEAP Bl 1 & 2

Dr. Charles Krebs - author
Will be teaching LEAP Bl 3 & 4 and Advanced LEAP courses.
Contact: Kim Gangwish
Life Enrichment Center
989 W. Princeton Ct.   Louisville, CO 80027
303 717 8860
1 800 537 4478
Ksgangwish@aol.com

Germany

IAK Institute für Angewandte Kinesiologie GmbH, Freiburg
Eschbachstrasse 5, D-79199 Kirchzarten, Germany.
Tel: 49 7661 98 71-0, Fax: 49 7661 98 71 49

Belgium

Institute Belge de Kinesiologie
Avenue Paul Nicodème 26, B-1330 Rixensart, Belgium.
Tel: 32 2 652 2686, Fax: 32 2 652 1656.

INDEX

A

Acupoints, 46, 50, 209–222, 234, 240, 247
Acupressure techniques, 208, 221–231, 241, 268, 307
  auditory integration, 230
  emotional stress, 241
  front-back switching, 228
  right-left switching, 223–5
  top bottom switching, 225–7
  visual integration, 229
Acupuncture Meridian System, 35, 44, 238, 318, 323, 328, 331, 336
Age recession, 30, 58, 65, 201, 258, 292
Ah Shi Points, 209
Akanandana, 26
Alarm points, 66, 209, 298
Alcoholism, 130, 268–9
Allergies/sensitivities, 286–91, 294, 309, 311
  balancing for, 291–3
Amygdala, 97, 102, 111, 114–6, 118–20, 124, 130, 132, 145, 149–51,155–6, 160–1, 195, 199, 210, 329, 331, 356–7
Amygdaloid bodies, 111,
Ansley, 5, 18, 22–3
Anterior cingulate gyrus, 112–3
Anterior commissure, 97, 202
Antibiotics, 293
Anti-oxidants, 285, 291
Applied Physiology, 33, 208, 233, 245–8
Association fibres, 98–9, 228
Association responses, 153–5
Association areas, 90, 114–5, 124, 140, 142, 148, 156, 160
Astral travel, 315, 351–2
Atmic body, 345
Atmospheres, 7, 15

Attention Deficit Disorder (ADD), 130, 180, 182, 238, 262–3, 266, 278
Attention Deficit Hyperactivity Disorder (ADHD), 266–9, 284
Auditory short-term memory, 250–3
Autonomic nervous system, 108, 115, 329, 333–5
Axons, 74–5, 96, 100, 129, 132
Axonal end bulbs 75–8

B

Bacon, Sir Francis, 318
Barton, Dr John, 56,
Basal Ganglia, 59, 83, 102–6, 108, 118, 145, 180, 212–3, 237
Beardall, Dr Alan, 54, 65
Becker, Robert, 299–300
Bends
  type one, 9
  cerebro-spinal, 9, 23
Bennett, Terence, 43,
Bennett Reflex Points, 43,
Biocomputer, 54, 65,
Biofeedback, 33,
Blood-brain barrier, 295
Blum, Kenneth, 130, 268,
Body-Mind-Spirit, 35, 48
Bohm, David, 58
Bottom-up processing, 346
Brain damage, 24, 90, 161, 172, 248–50
Brain dominance, 161–3
Brain integration, 174–5, 181, 186, 188, 190–3, 195–7, 200–2, 204–7, 221, 240, 245, 251, 258–9, 262–3, 271, 278, 286, 294, 302–3, 310
Brain nuclei, 97, 102,
Brain stem, 80, 85, 109, 123, 219, 349

Broca's area, 91, 161
Broca, Pierre Paul, 91
Brodmann, Korbinian, 87
Brodmann's areas, 87–91
Burns, Kathy, 3, 12
Byrd, Dr Randolph, 362

C
Callaway, Candice, 57,
Candida, candida overgrowth, 293–7
Candidaiasis, 274, 293–7
  balancing for, 297–8
Cannon, Walter, 111
Castanada, Carlos, 36
Caudate nucleus, 102–4, 179–80
Cell bodies, 74,
Central gyri
  pre 87
  post 87
Central sulcus, 86–7
Central vessel, 50, 210, 223, 226, 228, 298
Cerebellum, 59, 83–4, 102, 106, 108, 146, 1179–80, 212–3, 237
Cerebral cortex, 81, 84–5, 102, 171–2, 211–2, 219
Cerebro-spinal fluid, 166, 275
Chakras, 320–341
  autonomic nerve plexuses 333–5
  colors, 338
  endocrine system, 333–5
  locations, 331, 333
  nadi system, 323, 336
Chapman, Frank, 42
Chapman Reflex Points, 42
Ch'i, 20, 45, 48, 222, 315, 319, 328, 342–3, 359
Chinese medicine, 35, 46
Cingulate gyrus, 111–3
Clairvoyance, 319, 323–4
Cocaine, 130, 268
Collicular commissure, 97–8
Commissural fibres, 96, 117–8, 181–2, 223
Conjugate gaze, 229, 306
Consciousness, 113, 170, 205, 212, 215, 315–30, 340–1, 346–7, 351–7, 363
Conowara, The, 7
Consolidation of memory, 134
Convergence zones, 124, 142, 176, 194
Cook's hookups, 238–40
Corpus callosum, 96–7, 111–2, 117, 172–3, 181–2, 186, 188, 197–8, 220–3, 205, 223, 232, 246–8, 296–7
  shutdown, 208, 251, 256
Corpus striatum, 102
Cortical columns 92–4, 102, 160, 163
Corticospinal tracts, 99, 108, 212
Crickett, Rob, 29, 36
Cross-crawl, 229, 232–4
Crowded teeth, 310–12
Cytowic, Richard, 316

D
D_2 dopamine receptor, 267–9
Dalai Lama, 326
Damasio, Antonio, 113, 194–5, 204
Decompression, 9–10, 12–14, 17
Deductive reasoning, 163–7
Deep-level switching, 208, 222–8, 246, 297
Deformed palate, 309–10
Democritus, 316
Dendrites, 74, 79, 215
Dennison, Dr Paul, 57, 173, 222, 234, 239
Dentate gyrus, 116, 123
Dewe, Dr Bruce, 29–31, 37
Dharma, 343
Diencephalon, 80, 108, 111,
Diet
  amino acids 284–5
  essential fatty acids, 284
  minerals, 279, 282–6
  vitamins, 279, 281, 284–5, 293
Digit Span, 254, 265–6
Dopamine, 128–31, 267–8, 276, 282
Dyslexia, 29, 57, 173, 184, 190, 210, 219, 222, 256

E
Einstein, Albert, 94, 167, 316, 319
Electroencephalogram (EEG), 143–4, 194, 210, 261, 269, 300, 360
Electromagnetic radiation (EMR), 238, 274, 299–306, 327
  fluorescent lights, 303–5
  mobile telephones, 301–3
  neutralisers, 305–6
  televisions and video display units, 302–3
Electromagnetic spectrum, 320–5, 338
Electronystagmograms (ENG), 219–21

Emotional brain, 115
Emotional conditioning, 146
Emotional Stress Defusion, 57–8, 63–7, 221, 240–5
Endocrine system, 333–5
Endorphins, 128–30, 191, 271, 278
Entorhinal cortex, 114, 124, 142,
Entropy, 322, 325–7
Essential fatty acids, 284
Esso (Exxon), 18
Eye muscle balance, 307–8

F
Fight or flight, 150–2
Finger modes, 55
Foetal alcohol syndrome, 171, 296
Food additives, 286–7, 291
Food dyes, 287–91
Fornix, 124
Fourteen muscle balance, 53
Freud, Sigmund, 146
Frontal lobes, 24, 57, 86, 90, 104, 160, 180, 212, 215, 227–8, 241, 263, 279, 295, 360
Frontal occipital holding, 243
Functional Magnetic Resonance Imaging, MRI, 123, 162, 248, 345

G
Gait mechanism, 231
Geniculate nucleus,
  medial, 108
  lateral, 108
Gerber, Dr Richard, 315, 319, 325
Gestalt, 73, 90, 96–7, 163–5, 179, 197, 199, 202, 208, 251
  dominance, 163, 180, 182–4, 256–7
  lead functions, 94, 163, 173–8, 181, 186, 192
Globus pallidus, 102, 104, 212
Goodheart, Dr George, 41–5,
Governing vessel, 50, 226, 228
Grey matter, 85–91, 94–102
Gyrus, 88, 91
  precentral, 87
  postcentral, 87,

H
Habenular commissure, 97
Hannaford, Carla, 239

Hawking, Stephen, 14, 319
Hemispheres, 96–7, 197–8, 202, 228, 232
  left, 94, 97, 161–76, 224, 231
  right 94, 97, 159, 161–76, 180, 224, 231
Hippocampus, 114–8, 123–5, 130, 132, 137, 142, 145, 147–8, 154, 160, 172, 202–3, 275, 356
  left, 97, 117, 203, 250
  right, 117, 203
Hippocampal commissure, 97, 202–4, 259–60
Hippocampal-cortical system, 145–6, 149–50
Hippocampal formation, 113–4, 116, 156, 160
Hippocampal system, 123–5
Hippocrates, 317–8
HM, 116, 123
Homeostasis, 333–6
Hookups, 238–40
Huang-di-Nei-Ching, Inner Classic of the Yellow Emperor, 45, 317
Huxley, Aldous, 317
Hydration, 274–6
Hyperactivity, 219, 266, 276, 278–82, 287–9, 296
Hypothalamic nuclei, 115, 129
  dorsomedial nucleus, 110
  lateral nucleus (hypothalamic area), 110
Hypothalamus, 102, 108–11, 114, 128, 130, 145, 329, 222–5
Hypoxia, 38, 172, 250
Hysterical paralysis, 172

I
Immunoglobin E, Ige, 286
Inductive reasoning, 163–6
Infantile amnesia, 146,
Insertions, 41,
Intention tremour, 213
Ion channel, 76
Interneuron, 75, 100
Interhemispheric fibres, 97–9
Iron, 276, 282–3
Iser, David, 10–12

J
James, Dr Phillip, 14
James William, 363

K

Katz, Michael, 317
Kendall and Kendall, 40
Kinesiology, 29, 32, 55–6
　Academic Kinesiology, 40, 55
　Applied Kinesiology, 43, 53, 173, 222–3
　Applied Physiology, 29, 36, 58
　Biokinesiology, 56
　Brain Gym, 57, 222
　Clinical Kinesiology, 54–5
　Educational Kinesiology, 32, 57, 222, 229, 237–8
　One Brain, 30, 32, 57, 222
　Three-in-One Concepts, 222
　Touch for Health, 53, 222
Kubler-Ross, Elizabeth, 24–8, 250
Kuhn, Thomas 167,

L

Law of five elements 46, 50
Lazy eights
　hand-eye integration, 236
　hearing integration, 237
　visual integration, 234
Lead functions, 94, 169, 173–4, 181, 188, 192
Learning, 122
Learning difficulties, 172–4, 182–5, 190, 195–6, 219, 246, 254–61, 267, 276, 283
LEAP. (Learning Enhancement Advance Program), 253–4, 256, 263, 265–6, 269–70
Leukemia, 300–1
Lentiform nucleus, 102,
Limbic brain, 61, 63, 81–3, 99, 104, 111–20, 226, 241, 247, 279, 356
Limited access Gestalt and Logic, 185–6
Logic, 94, 96–7, 160, 163–77, 197, 202, 251
　dominance, 184–5
　lead functions 163, 173–5, 181, 186, 192
Long-term memory, 114, 116, 119, 124–5, 135–6, 159, 202, 251, 255
Long-term potentiation, 132
Lovett, R.W., 40
LSD, 352
Lymph, 42, 166
Lynch, Gary, 80

M

Macfarlane, Dr Geoff, 10–16
Magnetoelectric energy, 324, 327, 331, 338, 361–62
Mammillary bodies, 111,115
McCrossin, Susan, 38, 248-52, 254–7, 261–5
McLean, Paul, 80,
Meaning assignment, 177, 183
Medial temporal lobes, 111, 123, 127, 142
Meditation, 27, 343, 351–3, 358, 364
Medulla, 80, 219, 349
Memory, 121–3
　auditory, 117, 132, 141, 157, 203, 250
　decay, 145
　declarative, 132, 139, 144, 150
　dual, 148–52
　eidetic, 135, 177, 203
　emotional, 146
　episodic, 139–40, 146
　explicit, 132, 142, 144, 147
　false, 142
　immediate, 132
　implicit, 144, 156, 350
　interference, 135
　loss, 275
　motor, 105
　olfactory, 132, 141, 154–5
　scratchpad, 136, 160
　semantic, 139
　source, 143
　taste, 141
　touch and body sensation, 141
　triggers, 145, 154, 156–8
　visual, 117, 132, 141, 176, 202–3, 255
　working, 90, 136–9, 146, 149, 195, 203
Meridians, 50, 209, 222, 396
Mescalin, 35
Micro-bleeding, 171–2
Miller, Galanter and Pribham, 136
Mind, 342, 345–6, 352, 355–64
Minerals, 282–5
Motor cortex, 99, 103,
Motor homunculus, 90
Motor memory, 84, 105, 146
Motor neuron, 75
Muscle-emotion interface, 61–3
Muscle/Organ/Gland Meridian Complex, 45, 396–7
Muscle testing, 40

Muscle monitoring, 33, 56, 196, 209
Myelin, 95, 100

N
Nadis, 336
Nadi shodan, 224-5
Needham, Jospeh, 48
Neocortex, 81-3, 92
Nerve impulse, 75-79
Neuronal migration, 171, 249
Neurons, 38, 54, 74-80, 94, 171, 193-5, 197, 214, 249, 275
Neurotransmitters, 76-80, 132, 276, 282-3
Neurtophins, 215
Neural nets, 79-80, 100, 172, 215, 217, 296, 347
Newton, Issac, 166, 316
Nitrogen narcosis, 7
Nucleus accumbens, 129, 268

O
Occipital lobes, 86, 90, 108, 263, 360
One trail learning, 159
Optic radiations, 108
Opiates (opiods), brain, 128, 276
Origins, 41
Out-of-body experiences, 315
Over-energy, 46, 209

P
P300 EEG brainwave, 210, 269
Packer, Kerry, 256
Palaomammalian cortex, 81, 241
Parahippocampal gyrus (cortex), 111, 123-124
Parietal lobes, 86, 90
Perirhinal cortex, 111, 123-4
Penfield, Wilder, 87, 139
Periventricular grey matter, 130
Pettersson, Carl, 143
Phantom Limb, 211
Phonetic, 182, 184
Phonological loop, 137
Physis, 318
Pituitary gland, 109, 110, 329, 335
Polaris, The, 10, 12, 18
Polychlorinated biphenyls (PCBs), 345-6
Positron Emission Tomography (PET), 118, 123, 162, 345
Posterior commissure, 97

Prana, 338
Prayer, 362
Prefrontal cortex, 103, 114, 129, 132, 195
Premotor cortex, 90, 103, 105, 108, 282
Pribham, Carl, 58
Primary motor cortex, 88, 90, 212
Primary sensory cortex, 88-9, 92, 99
Projection fibres, 99, 212, 226
Proprioceptor, 213-6
Proust, Marcel, 154
Punishment, 128-31, 159
Putamen, 102, 104, 212

Q
Qualia, 346
Quantum Mechanics, 316, 318

R
Reptilian brain, 80, 361
Retaining mode, 55, 65
Reticular activating system (RAS), 215-9
Reward, 128-31, 159, 278
Reward deficiency syndrome, 268
Ritalin, 267-9, 281, 289

S
Samadhi, 364
Saturation diving, 13
Satya, 28, 35-6
Schacler, Daniel, 143
Sensory Neuron, 74
Septal nuclei, 112
Seratonin, 276, 281-2
Sharon, 25-7
Sibling rivalry, 201
Short-term memory, 115-7, 119, 132-3, 159, 202, 253, 261, 264
Skull Rock, 7, 39
Small brain, 83
Sodium ion channels, 77
Somaesthetic area, 87
Sphenoid bone, 308
Spina Bifida, 171
Spinal cord, 75
Spindrift, 362
Steady State Visually Evoked Potential (SSVEP), 261-3
Stokes, Gordon, 57, 222
Stress avoidance cycle, 189-90
Subcallosal gyrus, 111

Subconscious, 58–60, 102, 105, 107, 114–5, 125, 146–7, 151, 154, 169–70, 174, 181, 100–200, 204–5, 212, 247, 329
Subiculum, 123–4
Subtle bodies, 48, 318, 327–30, 331, 338, 343–45, 349
  astral, 329, 331, 350
  causal, 330, 331
  etheric, 328, 331, 350
  mental, 329, 331, 350
  physical, 327, 331, 350
Substantia nigra, 103, 128–9, 212
Subthalamic nucleus, 103, 212
Success cycle, 271–3
Sugar, 275–81, 294
Sullivan, Johnny, 14, 17
Swami Sivananda, 364
Switching, 222–3
  right/left, 223–5
  top/bottom, 225–7
  front/back, 227–8
Synapse, 76, 79–80
Synovial fluid, 9

T
Tartrazine, 287–9
Telepathy, 319, 340
Temporal lobes, 86–7, 91
Temporomandibular joint (TMJ), 310
Tesla, Nickoli, 299, 305
Thalamus, 106–8, 132, 148, 212
  anterior nucleus, 108, 112
  ventroanterior nucleus, 212
  ventrolateral nucleus, 212
Thalamic-amygdaloid system, 147, 149–50, 152
Thermocline, 8
Thie, Dr John, 52
Thought-form, 329, 345
Tiller, Professor William, 315, 319, 324–5, 330, 361

Tiller-Einstein Model of Negative-Positive Space/Time, 319, 325
Top-down processing, 345
Triune brain, 80–3
Tulving, Endel, 121

U
Under-energy, 46
Utt, Richard, 33–7, 58, 247

V
Vestibular-ocular reflex, 216, 219, 231, 237
Vestibular system, 216, 294
Visual construction, 176
Vitamins, 281–2, 284–5
  B_3, 281–2, 284
  B_6, 276, 281, 284–5
Volume transmisson, 194

W
Wada's test, 162
Water, 274–6
Watson, Dr James, 73
Wechsler Intelligence Scale for Children (WISC), 264
Wernicke, Carl, 92
Wernicke's area, 92, 161–3, 179
White matter, 95–100
Whiteside, Daniel, 57
Will, 21, 330, 343, 359
Wilson's Promontory, 6–7, 10
Working memory, 136–9
  central executive, 137
  phonological loop, 137
  visuospatial scratchpad, 137

Y
Yin and Yang, 48–52, 166, 169, 223
Yoga, 57, 222–4, 318, 364

Z
Zinc, 283, 285, 289

Ordering Information for
A Revolutionary Way of Thinking

Mail check to
Green Angel Press 7121 New Light Trail Chapel Hill, NC 27516

Order online at
www.USkinesiology.com

Bookstores and health care practitioners please inquire about quantity discounts for resale

---

Name_____

Address_____

City_____ State_____ Zip code_____

Phone_____ Email_____

Qty.   Amount

_____ **A Revolutionary Way of Thinking** $29.95 each   _____

NC residents add 7% sales tax - $2.10 per book   _____

Shipping/Handling for U.S. & North America
$4 for the first book, $2.for each additional book to same address   _____

                                                              Total   _____

Green Angel Press